Musculoskeletal Physiotherapy

Musculoskeletal Physiotherapy
Clinical Science and Practice

Edited by

Kathryn M. Refshauge DipPhty, GradDipManipTher (Cumb), MBiomedE (NSW), MAPA, MPAA
Senior Lecturer
School of Physiotherapy
The University of Sydney, Australia

and

Elizabeth M. Gass DipPhty, BAppSc, MAppSc (Cumb), MAPA, MPAA
Senior Lecturer
School of Physiotherapy
The University of Sydney, Australia

With a Foreword by

Professor Lance Twomey
Deputy Vice-Chancellor and Professor of Physiotherapy, Curtin University of Technology, Perth, Australia

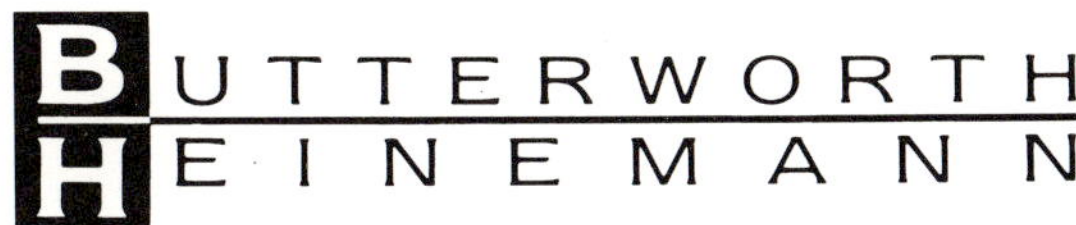

BUTTERWORTH
HEINEMANN

Butterworth-Heinemann
Linacre House, Jordan Hill, Oxford OX2 8DP
A division of Reed Educational and Professional Publishing Ltd

℞ A member of the Reed Elsevier plc group

OXFORD   BOSTON   JOHANNESBURG
MELBOURNE   NEW DELHI   SINGAPORE

First edition 1995
Reprinted 1997

British Library Cataloguing in Publication Data
Musculoskeletal Physiotherapy: Clinical
Science and Practice
  I. Refshauge, Kathryn M. II. Gass,
  Elizabeth M.
  616.7062

ISBN 0 7506 1746 2

Library of Congress Cataloguing in Publication Data
Musculoskeletal physiotherapy: clinical science and practice/
    edited by Kathryn M. Refshauge, Elizabeth M. Gass. - 1st ed.
    p. cm.
    Includes bibliographical references and index.
    ISBN 0 7506 1746 2
    1. Musculoskeletal system - Diseases - Physical therapy.
    2. Physical Therapy - methods. WE 140 1995]
    RC925.5.M89   1995
    616.7'062-dc20
    DNLM/DLC   94-40453
    for Library of Congress   CIP

Composition by Genesis Typesetting, Rochester, Kent
Printed and bound in Great Britain by
Martins the Printers Ltd, Berwick upon Tweed

Contents

Contributors

Grant Bigg-Wither MBChB, FRACR
Consulting Radiologist
Department of Radiology
St Vincent's Hospital
Darlinghurst, Australia

Nikolai Bogduk BSc(Med), MB BS, MD, PhD,
FAFRM, Dip Anat, Hon MPAA
Professor of Anatomy
Faculty of Medicine
The University of Newcastle
Newcastle, Australia

Robert Boland BAppSc, GradDipAppSc
(ManipTher)
Lecturer, School of Physiotherapy
Faculty of Health Sciences
The University of Sydney
Lidcombe, Australia

Marco Campello MA PT
Occupational & Industrial Orthopedic Center,
New York, USA

Janet Carr Dip Phty, MEd, EdD(Columbia)
Associate Professor
School of Physiotherapy
Faculty of Health Sciences
The University of Sydney
Lidicombe, Australia

Philip Conaghan MBBS, FRACP
Consultant Rheumatologist
St Vincent's Clinic
Sydney, Australia

Richard Day MD, FRACP
Professor of Clinical Pharmacology
St Vincent's Hospital and
University of South Wales
Sydney, Australia

Harold M. Frost MD
Orthopaedic Surgeon
Southern Colorado Clinic

Elizabeth M. Gass Dip Phty, BAppSc, MAppSc
Senior Lecturer, School of Physiotherapy
Faculty of Health Sciences
The University of Sydney
Lidcombe, Australia

Michalene Goodsell BAppSc,
GradDipManipTher
Lecturer, School of Physiotherapy
Faculty of Health Sciences
The University of Sydney
Lidcombe, Australia

David W. Gronow MBBS, FFARACS,
FANZCA
Director, Sydney Pain
Management Centre, Newcastle
Pain Management Centre and Royal
Rehabilitation Pain
Management Centre
Sydney, Australia

Lynette Harmond DipPhty, GradDipManipTher
Clinical Physiotherapist
Macquarie Street Physiotherapy
Sydney, Australia

Robert Herbert BAppSc, MAppSc
Lecturer, School of Physiotherapy
Faculty of Health Sciences
The University of Sydney
Lidcombe, Australia

Paul Kelly DipPhty, GradDipManipTher
Manipulative Physiotherapist
St Vincent's Clinic
Sydney, Australia

Dale Larsen BAppSc, MAppSc(Manip Phty)
Lecturer, School of Physiotherapy
Faculty of Health Sciences
The University of Sydney
Lidcombe, Australia

Jane Latimer BAppSc, GradDipAppSc
(ManipTher)
Lecturer, School of Physiotherapy
Faculty of Health Sciences
The University of Sydney
Lidcombe, Australia

Michael Lee BE, BAppSc, MBiomedE
Lecturer, Department of Biomedical Sciences
Faculty of Health Sciences
The University of Sydney
Lidcombe, Australia

Christopher Maher BAppSc, GradDipAppSc
(ExtSpSc), GradDipAppSc (Manip Phty)
Lecturer, School of Physiotherapy
Faculty of Health Sciences
The University of Sydney
Lidcombe, Australia

Susan Mercer BPhty(Hons), MSc
Assistant Professor, Department of Physical
Therapy
Duquesne University
Pittsburgh, USA

Kathryn M. Refshauge Dip Phty,
GradDipManipTher, MBiomedE
Senior Lecturer, School of Physiotherapy
Faculty of Health Sciences
The University of Sydney
Lidcombe, Australia

Roberta Shepherd Dip Phty, MEd, EdD, FACP
Professor, School of Physiotherapy
Faculty of Health Sciences
The University of Sydney
Lidcombe, Australia

Debra Shirley BSc, GradDipPhty,
GradDipManipTher
Lecturer, School of Physiotherapy
Faculty of Health Sciences
The University of Sydney
Lidcombe, Australia

Judith Stenmark BAppSc, MPH
Education Services Manager
Arthritis Foundation of New South Wales
Surry Hills, Australia

Foreword

Musculoskeletal Physiotherapy is a most unusual book. It signals a departure from the traditional prescriptive approach to musculoskeletal physiotherapy toward a more rational science-based methodology, centred around careful, logical examination and clinical decision-making. Indeed, much of this book considers the way in which data is gathered from patients and their surrounds to provide the input necessary for reaching an appropriate clinical judgement. In itself, this process demonstrates the very considerable change in the position to which physiotherapy has moved over the past two to three decades. The classical approach to the physical treatment of musculoskeletal disorders relied on the referring doctor's diagnosis and a rather perfunctory examination, followed by treatment according 'to the book'. The reliance on the clinical judgements of authoritative forebears and their detailed approaches to patient management provided a certain warm security to the physiotherapist, but often provided cold comfort to the captive patient.

In selecting authors to present the material in *Musculoskeletal Physiotherapy*, the editors, Kathryn Refshauge and Elizabeth Gass, have carefully ensured that they follow their guiding theoretical model. Their goal has been to ensure that a close relationship exists between science and practice and that any theoretical base in this area must precede from that premise for it to be included in the manuscript. It is an active book, a book that encourages and celebrates change. As the knowledge base expands and the theoretical models change (as they must), then it is essential that physical treatment adapt appropriately, change (often radically) and that cherished, long-held approaches to treatment may have to be altered or cast-aside. This is not a comfortable situation and physiotherapists whose training is now well into the past, may not always like the new reality which confronts them. However, the various authors in the volume really '. . . have explored the paradigm of contemporary physiotherapy practice', and have re-analysed their examination and treatment procedures appropriately. Enormous change has occurred in the last twenty years, but this is likely to pale into insignificance when compared to the likely changes of the next two decades, as research knowledge and the science base continues to expand exponentially.

The editors pay proper tribute to Geoffrey Maitland in Chapter 1, as the Australian Clinical Physiotherapist who has most profoundly influenced this process of change. Maitland's emphasis on very careful and comprehensive examination leading to the precise application of treatment by movement and followed in turn by the assessment of the effects of that movement on the patient, forms the basis for the modern clinical approach. This is probably as close to the scientific method as is possible within the clinical practice of physical therapy and serves as a model for other special areas of the profession.

The chapter authors and editors of *Musculoskeletal Physiotherapy* have taken great pains to identify the scientific foundation for clinical practice. They have gathered together important research information from both basic and clinical science sources and used it to underpin contemporary physical management and treatment. This is a book which cheerfully faces its own redundancy as circumstances and knowledge expands and changes. It focuses primarily on rationale and less on technique and is I trust, the shape of the world to come. This book must be considered an important contribution to undergraduate physiotherapy education, as well as stimulating reading for all physiotherapists who are interested in exploring the frontiers of their own profession.

Lance Twomey
Deputy Vice Chancellor
Professor of Physiotherapy
Curtin University of Technology
Perth, Australia

Acknowledgements

We are indebted to many people without whom this book would not have been completed. Doubtless, our joy in the book was not shared by them, nevertheless, their enthusiasm and continual guidance was always evident and has been very much appreciated: particularly Chris Schein's typing skills and her endless patience as we changed our minds; Mary Gauci and Di Brennan's assistance with the manuscript; and the whole musculoskeletal teaching team for their enthusiasm in the project, their ideas, the endless editing and their insights. Many other colleagues gave freely of their advice and feedback, in particular Greg Gass, Bulent Turman, Michalene Goodsell and Rob Boland. We particularly would like to acknowledge the input of Ray Howard who designed the graphics and David Robinson who took the photographs, especially demanding tasks. The Staff and students of the School of Physiotherapy, Faculty of Health Sciences, University of Sydney have provided us with the challenging and supportive environment necessary for us to edit and write this book. All contributors were prompt with their manuscripts, and ably met the enormous challenges presented to them. We are grateful to them all for the quality of their contributions and dedication to the project. Finally, our appreciation is extended to all those who helped us with other tasks which had lower priority to us in the excitement of finishing this book, and especially to those who supported us personally through this endeavour.

Chapter 1

The context of musculoskeletal physiotherapy practice

K.M. Refshauge and E.M. Gass

The need for this book

To speak of need is to imply a goal, a means of achieving the goal and a means of measuring deficiency from the goal (Wilkin *et al.*, 1992). A critical goal in musculoskeletal physiotherapy is to possess a sound theoretical basis for a clinical practice which demonstrably achieves relevant and effective outcomes. Achievement of this goal means overcoming deficiencies in both the musculoskeletal physiotherapy theory base and in demonstration of clinical effectiveness. In musculoskeletal physiotherapy the gap between the goal and the measured deficiencies is constantly narrowing.

Many former textbooks on musculoskeletal physiotherapy, while serving the important function of describing practical procedures, were frequently anecdotal, often including incorrect and unsubstantiated information, and describing practical procedures in isolation. In this book current scientific knowledge underlying physiotherapy practice is interpreted and analysed for clinical use, although it is acknowledged that not all clinical practice can currently be fully substantiated.

Information that is well described and easily accessible elsewhere, such as how to perform passive motion procedures for assessment or treatment, will rarely be covered in detail (for examples see Kaltenborn, 1980; Grieve, 1984; Maitland, 1986; Magee, 1987). Rather, this text focuses on an evaluation of examination procedures, the interpretation of tests and evaluation of management strategies. Occasionally procedures are described to enable evaluation and to avoid constant cross-referencing. Knowledge is drawn from related areas to develop a considered interpretation that is both current and clinically applicable. The use of information is illustrated with clinical, examples, this contextual relevance giving the information a realistic perspective.

Examination and treatment of spinal musculoskeletal conditions are discussed, using examples relating to upper and lower quadrants, i.e. the cervical spine and shoulder, the lumbar spine and hip, and the sacroiliac joint and lumbar spine. Although much information is relevant to the peripheral regions, and some illustrations use the periphery for clarification, the periphery will not be dealt with separately.

The musculoskeletal physiotherapy paradigm

The goal of possessing a sound theoretical base for musculoskeletal physiotherapy clinical practice implies a close relationship between science and practice. The extent to which one considers that physiotherapy practice is based on science depends to some degree on one's view of what constitutes 'science'. This book does not explore the relationship between physiotherapy and 'science', but some relevant issues are raised. James Gordon (1987), in a fascinating exposition, explored the way in which science provides a guiding theoretical model, and the tenet that practical needs determine the validity of the theoretical model, using neurological physiotherapy as the example.

A discussion of the developement of 'scientific' thought is relevant here to place in context the development of musculoskeletal physiotherapy. Many philosophers have proferred theories about the development of scientific thought (Kuhn, 1974; Popper, 1974; Chalmers, 1983). One of these is Kuhn and his theory of scientific revolutions. The development of musculoskeletal physiotherapy could be likened to these 'scientific revolutions'.

Kuhn (1974) and others propose that we operate using a theoretical framework and set of assumptions. Kuhn termed this 'scientific' framework a paradigm. He further suggests that in reality scientists direct their work to solving questions determined by, or relevant to, the paradigm. When problems considered important within a discipline can no longer be solved using the current paradigm, a new theoretical framework and set of assumptions is adopted. Kuhn termed this a 'paradigm shift'. There are many examples of paradigm shifts in the historical development of scientific disciplines. A famous example is within the field of astronomy. In medieval times it was assumed that the earth was the centre of the universe, and that all the planets including the sun orbited the earth. In the seventeenth century it became important to solve the problem of the current calendar being inconsistent with the lunar year. Galileo was employed to solve this vexatious problem (Burke, 1985). The results of his work are well-known: the original assumption about the earth being the centre of the universe was no longer tenable. This led to a scientific (and personal for Galileo) crisis or revolution, and ultimately to a paradigm shift. Other examples can be found in the development of Charles Darwin's theories on evolution or Einstein's work on relativity.

A paradigm shift generally results in adopting more appropriate assumptions, although these are not necessarily 'correct' or even 'more correct'. Consequently a paradigm shift also results in a change in the questions that scientists and members of a discipline consider important.

The reason for discussing Kuhn's theories about paradigms and how they shift is that this philosophy provides a particularly apt perspective for interpreting growth of knowledge in physiotherapy. When considering past and future changes in physiotherapy knowledge and practice, it is attractive to believe that we currently operate within a paradigm. This paradigm will most probably 'shift' in the future; however, this book is concerned with our current understanding of science and physiotherapy practice.

The various authors in this book have explored the paradigm of contemporary physiotherapy practice. Current scientific knowledge is interpreted and analysed for use in clinical practice. This, of necessity, involves evaluating prevailing approaches to examination and treatment. This in turn involves attempting to identify assumptions underlying physiotherapy practice. Some assumptions are explicit (such as that a reduction in spinal pain leads to return of normal function), but many are implicit, and therefore very difficult to identify. When identified, these assumptions are evaluated. We make it clear that such a process is not intended to be negative, but is an attempt at identification and analysis of the philosophy underlying physiotherapy practice.

Physiotherapy practice

At any instant, the practice of physiotherapy may appear to be clearly defined and static. This is probably particularly true from the perspective of undergraduate students. The following brief summary of the development of physiotherapy highlights the enormous changes that have actually taken place in physiotherapy practice.

The first descriptions of practice allied to physiotherapy refer to the use of 'therapeutic gymnastics' and 'gymnastic medicine' as preventive and curative treatments in the time of Herodicus (approximately 480 BC), Hippocrates (460–370 BC) and later Galen (AD 129–210). Even in these early times there was controversy about the delineation of roles of physicians and gymnasts in the delivery of these treatments (Berryman, 1987).

The practice of manual therapies did not change substantially until the twentieth century. In 1920 the Chartered Society of Massage and Medical Gymnastics emerged in the UK, amalgamating several small groups which had apparently originated from an initial group formed in 1894, consisting at that time of eight women. The aim of the Chartered Society of Massage and Medical Gymnastics was to bind together those who practised physical treatment in an honourable way (Mennell, 1934). A similar association was formed in the US, the American Womens Physical Therapeutic Association (now the American Physical Therapy Association) which, in 1921, aimed to establish and maintain a professional and scientific standard and disseminate information through medical and professional articles (American Womens Physical Therapeutic Association, 1921).

The First and Second World Wars increased the demand for treatments to deal with stiff joints, weak muscles and associated functional deficits following fractures and gunshot and shrapnel wounds (May, 1954). The poliomyelitis epidemic in the 1950s further increased this demand (May, 1954). Those carrying out physical treatments at this time worked closely under the guidance of medical practitioners. The six-month training course was entirely technical, and predominantly equipped physiotherapists to perform massage and exercise, such as the Swedish Remedial Exercise System (Palmer, 1918; Mennel, 1934). The types of massage and remedial exercises prescribed in the 1920s make interesting readings; however, one wonders whether current practice is actually any more firmly based on theory.

More recently, the writings of many physiotherapists, in particular those of Geoffrey Maitland, profoundly influenced the further development of musculoskeletal physiotherapy practice (Maitland, 1964; Kaltenborn, 1980). Although the emphasis in these first editions was on manipulative treatment, Maitland proposed an extensive system of examination of patients and advocated basing treatment decisions on the patient's signs and symptoms rather than on the diagnosis. The Preface to the First Edition emphasized that all physiotherapy treatments described in the book would require medical referral (Maitland, 1964). In a foreword to a subsequent edition (Brewerton, 1977) the question was posed whether it is sufficient for physiotherapists to apply heat, ice or active exercise when patients have stiff or painful joints, or whether something more specific to restoration of joint movement should be used. The author prophesized that controlled trials would be needed to resolve such a question and noted that, since it might be many years before adequate answers were produced, it was essential to achieve an assessment based on clinical judgement and experience (Brewerton, 1977).

Throughout many editions of the books authored by Maitland (Maitland, 1964, 1968, 1973, 1981, 1986) the emphasis was not only on describing a system of manoeuvres and techniques for assessment and treatment of joints, but also on evaluating results of treatment and prescribing adequate treatment doses. Maitland suggested constant monitoring of changes in the patient's signs and symptoms and introduced the concept of 'irritability' to assist in dose prescription. New concepts of 'comparable joint sign' and 'accessory joint movement' were also described, and suggested as tools to enable more specific examination and treatment of spinal musculoskeletal disorders. Maitland and his peers thus applied a challenge to accepted musculoskeletal physiotherapy practice.

Education of physiotherapy students closely parallels these advances in theoretical frameworks and practical skills. These advances have eventually formed the foundation for our current practice as independent professionals.

Context of current practice: assumptions and theory models

The current environment is again altering the face of physiotherapy. The conditions being treated have changed. Sedentary workers are presenting with back pain in greater numbers than ever before, with few cases of poliomyelitis now presenting for intervention. In addition, the autonomy of the profession means that we need to be accountable; the scarcity of the 'health dollar' and a better informed public also challenge the profession to justify its interventions and prove their efficacy.

In the past most developments in musculoskeletal physiotherapy have been the result of serendipity. This is not inappropriate, because the volume of knowledge from which to derive theoretical models was inconsequential. However, today much more knowledge is available. The availability of knowledge and the search for justification has probably changed the nature of discovery. Today we have the option of developing appropriate treatments from a sound theory base. This raises the issues of whether we should use a treatment because the theory is appropriate, and also whether we should use it because 'it works'. These issues are discussed in Chapter 7 by Bogduk and Mercer. The demand for accountability and justification of physiotherapy practice has applied further pressure to try to discover the mechanism of effect for physiotherapy treatments, many of which have been used for several decades. First, however, it is important to determine whether the treatment does actually 'work'. If indeed the treatment does not achieve stated goals, then it should probably be discarded rather than further examined. The need to explore the mechanism of effect of treatments is of primary importance after we know the value of the treatment. By knowing how treatments achieve their outcomes, we can then improve key aspects of patient management such as who will benefit most from a particular treatment, how to further improve the treatment itself, and whether there is a better method of applying the characteristics of the treatment. By adhering to the principles of inquiry, we can avoid using treatments in a routine way, often described as 'mythical' or 'ritualistic'.

In the current paradigm within which musculoskeletal physiotherapy operates, decisions are made about:

1. diagnosis: particularly about pathological and clinical diagnosis
2. management: particularly about aims of treatment, specific strategies to be used, their dose and how it will be evaluated, and whether aims have been met.

These clinical decisions include making judgements about contraindications and precautions to various treatment options, and about the use of preventive measures. The assumptions underlying such clinical decisions in musculoskeletal physiotherapy are often difficult to identify, probably including assumptions adopted from fields such as physiology, biomechanics, and other disciplines within the health and medical sciences. It may be valuable, however, to attempt to identify some assumptions, to gain a clearer insight into the basis of current musculoskeletal physiotherapy practice.

Some readily identifiable assumptions include:

1. Non-specific mechanical pain is musculoskeletal in origin.
2. Pain and pain behaviour exhibited by the patient are signals that the musculoskeletal system is disordered.
3. Musculoskeletal tissues and organs behave in a predictable way when damaged and, provided that the environment is adequate, will follow a prescribed healing and repair process.
4. Both the patient and the physiotherapist have key roles in achieving goals of treatment. Except in extreme circumstances, a partnership approach is generally assumed to help achieve stated treatment goals.
5. Treatments aimed at affecting the musculoskeletal system will primarily affect the musculoskeletal tissues.
6. Prevention of certain musculoskeletal disorders is possible. This remains an assumption because there is a lack of knowledge of cause and effect of various factors. Some examples of prevention include interventions aimed at altering segmental alignment (or posture) to prevent future pain, or altering the amount of foot pronation to prevent future lower limb or spinal pain. Since there is little evidence about cause and effect of these characteristics, such interventions remain based on assumption.

These assumptions may seem trite or even ridiculous. Paradigms shift, however, when fundamental 'truths' such as these no longer hold. It is extremely difficult to pinpoint implicit assumptions because they are often considered to be known facts; however, identification of common assumptions can provide a basis for challenge and growth. It is useful to recognize that physiotherapists operate in today's paradigm, and that the basis of musculoskeletal physiotherapy may change radically even within a decade if, and as, the paradigm shifts. It is difficult to predict the next major change in a discipline when one is so firmly entrenched in current practice.

The writers and editors of this book have faced the challenge of explicit identification of the scientific basis for musculoskeletal physiotherapy practice. The process of facing this challenge has been stimulating, thought provoking and, at times, uncomfortable and sobering. Physiotherapists are encouraged to read, reflect on and question the material presented in this book, because this material is thought to represent the current foundation of musculoskeletal physiotherapy practice.

References

American Women's Physical Therapeutic Association (1921). Constitution. *Phys. Ther.*, **1**, 5.

Berryman, J.W. (1987). The tradition of the 'six things non-natural': Exercise and medicine from Hippocrates through ante-bellum America. *Exerc. Sport Sci. Rev.*, **17**, 515–59.

Brewerton, D.A. (1977). Foreword. In *Peripheral Manipulation* (2nd edn.) (G.D. Maitland), London: Butterworths.

Burke, J. (1985). *The Day the Universe Changed*. London: British Broadcasting Corporation.

Chalmers, A.F. (1983). *What is This Thing Called Science: An Assessment of the Nature and Status of Science and its Methods* (2nd edn.) St Lucia, Queensland: University of Queensland Press.

Gordon, J. (1987). Assumptions underlying physical therapy intervention: theoretical and historical perspectives. In *Movement Science. Foundations for Physical Therapy in Rehabilitation* (J.H. Carr, R.B. Shepherd, J. Gordon *et al.*, eds), London: Heinemann Physiotherapy.

Grieve, G.P. (1984). *Mobilisation of the Spine*, (4th edn). London: Churchill Livingstone.

Kaltenborn, F.M. (1980). *Mobilization of the Extremity Joints*, (3rd edn.) Oslo: Olaf Norlis Bokhandel.

Kuhn, T.S. (1974). *The Structure of Scientific Revolutions* (2nd edn.), Chicago: University of Chicago Press.

Magee, D.J. (1987). *Orthopedic Physical Assessment*. London: W.B. Saunders Company.

Maitland, G.D. (1964). *Vertebral Manipulation*. London: Butterworths.

Maitland, G.D. (1968). *Vertebral Manipulation*. (2nd edn). London: Butterworths.

Maitland, G.D. (1973) *Vertebral Manipulation* (3rd edn). London: Butterworths.

Maitland, G.D. (1981). *Vertebral Manipulation* (4th edn). London: Butterworths.

Maitland, G.D. (1986). *Vertebral Manipulation* (5th edn). London: Butterworths.

May, F. (1954). The changing face of physical medicine. *Austr. J. Physiother.*, **1**, 6–10.

Mennell, J. (1934). *Physical Treatment by Movement, Manipulation and Massage*. London: Churchill.

Palmer, M.D. (1918). *Lessons on Massage including Swedish Remedial Gymnastics and Bandaging*. London: Ballière, Tindall and Cox.

Popper, K.R. (1974). *Conjectures and Refutations: The Growth of Scientific Knowledge* (5th edn). London: Routledge and Kegan Paul.

Wilkin, D., Hallam, L. and Doggett, M.A. (1992). *Measures of Need and Outcome for Primary Health Care*. Oxford: Oxford University Press.

Chapter 2

Theoretical basis underlying clinical decisions

E.M. Gass and K.M. Refshauge

With the changing role of physiotherapists from one of applying technical skills to one of autonomous professional practice, comes a new requirement; the ability to make independent clinical judgements. The ability to make effective clinical judgements requires a high level of background knowledge. This chapter therefore contains background information considered fundamental to the practice of musculoskeletal physiotherapy. The areas of information included are: acute and chronic pain, physiology and clinical pharmacology, biomechanics, adaptation of various tissues, including bone, muscle and other connective tissue, skill learning following musculoskeletal lesions and the theories concerning clinical reasoning. The extensive and rapid growth of knowledge in each of these areas means that a full review of each is impossible here. We hope that interest will be kindled so that the reader will pursue the reading recommended in each section for a more comprehensive understanding of each area of knowledge. The integration between the presented theory base and clinical practice is explicit in some instances within this chapter or is implicit in material presented in other chapters within this book.

Clinical reasoning in physiotherapy

K.M. Refshauge

Clinical reasoning has, no doubt, been occurring for as long as health professionals have treated patients, but has only recently been identified as a separate and essential skill in good clinical practice (Elstein *et al.*, 1978). Clinical reasoning, sometimes known as decision-making, making clinical judgements or problem-solving (Grant *et al.*, 1988), describes the process of collecting and interpreting information from the patient and formulating predictions about outcomes. The process is heavily influenced by the individual's knowledge base, beliefs or values, and skills associated with clinical practice. Reflecting on new experiences or knowledge allows integration of new information with the existing knowledge base in the context of the person's beliefs.

The clinical reasoning literature is replete with unresolved issues. Many theories have been proposed to describe the way in which clinicians reason, but the process used remains obscure, although it has been argued that different processes may be used in different contexts (Higgs and Jones, 1995). Perhaps reference to research in psychology, especially that on cognition and thinking, could be applied to reasoning with clinical problems. However, the outcomes of introducing explicit study of clinical reasoning into education programs have not been clearly positive (Bowden, 1988). Several reasons have been proposed to account for the lack of positive outcomes, including a disparity between espoused theory and the actual teaching and assessment methods used (Bowden, 1988). The aspects of clinical reasoning most relevant to this book are probably the theories describing clinical reasoning and the influence of knowledge and belief systems on the reasoning process.

Clinical reasoning theory

Reasoning processes, and specifically the clinical reasoning process, have been studied extensively, investigations being predominantly based on either normative theories of decision-making or actual decision behaviour. Normative theories emphasize what clinicians should do. These theories assume that there is an optimal solution to a problem and often use mathematical techniques, such as probability theories, to reach this optimal solution. It is further assumed that, with the addition of new information, clinicians will revise their understanding of the probability of their hypotheses about the patient. A hypothesis, in this context, refers to a supposition made about diagnosis or treatment, for example, that will be modified according to the data subsequently collected. However, it is generally agreed that humans do not reason optimally (Browning, *et al.*, 1988; Grant, 1991).

Other investigations have been directed towards describing actual decision behaviour. These investigations do not assume that there is an optimal decision, nor prescribe an optimal method for reaching a solution to a problem. Rather, this line of inquiry seeks to describe how clinicians reason or use knowledge.

From investigations based on both normative theories and actual decision behaviour, three major models have emerged to explain reasoning in the clinical context:

1. hypothetico-deductive reasoning (Elstein *et al.*, 1978; Jones, 1992),
2. pattern recognition (Scadding, 1967; Barrows and Feltovich, 1987),
3. problem-solving (Bashook, 1976; Paton, 1985).

Other models have been proposed such as the phenomenological model (Mattingly, 1991), backward and forward reasoning models (Ridderikhoff, 1989; Patel and Groen, 1991) and models emphasizing intuition (Benner and Tanner, 1987; Rew and Barrow, 1987). It is most likely that no single model accounts for reasoning in all situations, and that either a more complex model is required or a combination of these proposed models is more representative than a single model.

Hypothetico-deductive reasoning has been investigated in relation to many cognitive tasks, including aspects of clinical reasoning, such as diagnosis. The original hypothetico-deductive reasoning models describe the clinical reasoning process as largely sequential; that clinicians collect information, then form hypotheses about specific aspects of the problem, then confirm or reject these hypotheses. The view that reasoning occurs sequentially (e.g. data acquisition followed by problem identification) underestimates the complexity of the process. Gale and Marsden (1982) provide convincing evidence that clinicians actively evaluate and interpret information during data collection rather than after data collection is complete. In the clinical context, medical practitioners have been most frequently studied, with a consequent high regard for diagnosis (or 'correct' outcome). Although physiotherapists may appear to adopt similar clinical reasoning processes, they probably place greater emphasis on treatment and subsequent evaluation than do these medical models, and therefore the notion of a single 'correct' outcome is inappropriate. Studies designed to describe the use of hypothetico-deductive reasoning in solving abstract tasks also found that people tend to use verification strategies almost exclusively (Gilhooly, 1988). In other words, clinicians tend to engage in a line of questioning or physical testing that would confirm favoured hypotheses about diagnosis and treatment rather than pursue a line of investigation leading to rejection of alternative hypotheses.

The pattern-recognition model suggests that information collected from the patient is compared with existing knowledge and experience until the problem is recognized as a familiar one, with a consequently determined management strategy. This infers that prior to recognizing the pattern, the clinician passively receives information. However, research in psychology demonstrates that humans do not passively receive information; rather they actively structure it and continually interpret it (Gale and Marsden, 1982).

Finally, clinical reasoning skills are often referred to as problem-solving skills. The implication that problem-solving skills are generalizable was taken further by introducing problem-based curricula. Although there are advantages in such curricula, the advantages do not appear to relate to better problem-solving skills (Norman and Schmidt, 1992). Browning *et al.* (1988) tested the correlation between general problem-solving test scores and clinical performance measures, finding no correlation between the two. This preliminary finding for health professionals confirms the findings of studies in other fields (Glass and Holyoak, 1986). Problem-solving is context-specific, requiring rules and knowledge related to the task and context (Glass and Holyoak, 1986).

All the above theories attempt to describe how clinicians currently reason. Another approach might be to find the best way to reason, so that optimal reasoning may be achieved. Investigations into optimal reasoning are found in the literature of mathematics-based sciences and artificial intelligence. Optimal reasoning is therefore usually described in relation to either solving problems with a known best solution (best possible outcome), or in relation to the 'genius' (best possible reasoning process). The former is usually based on mathematical problem-solving techniques, with a known best outcome, which is unlike clinical practice. The latter, exploration of the best possible process, suggests that the 'genius' has a vast knowledge base, often in disparate knowledge areas, makes extensive links between these knowledge areas, and does not accept information at face value (Gilhooly, 1988). These characteristics are probably highly relevant to clinical reasoning and clinical practice.

It is still unclear whether all clinicians reason in the same way. The nature of clinical reasoning does not lend itself to rigorous investigation, since, of necessity, studies are based on either the outcome (e.g. correct diagnosis) or reflection (recalling later what the clinician was thinking at the time the information was given). Therefore perhaps the best we can hope for is a theory or model that seems reasonable and consistent. It is most likely that clinicians use all the models described and possibly other unidentified processes, since no single model would be appropriate in all circumstances. For example, sometimes a key piece of information is immediately recognized as representing a particular condition (pattern recognition), whereas in less familiar cases, a modified hypothetico-deductive reasoning process may be relied upon. Once the general rules for particular classes of clinical problems have been learnt, perhaps problem-solving using learned rules is part of the process.

The role of knowledge in clinical reasoning

Although overlapping substantially, there may be significant differences between scientific, professional and personal knowledge. Knowledge is generally considered to be a person's range of information, which will include knowledge from the scientific discipline and profession to which the person belongs, as well as from experiences of one's own and others. An individual's knowledge base is therefore unique.

To be most useful knowledge needs to be not only broad-based, but also constantly evolving, adequately comprehensive, relevant, accurate, accessible (able to be retrieved for use) and well organized. It appears that a well-organized knowledge base enables the recall of all inter-related information, thus providing a more comprehensive view of a problem. There is increasing evidence that the relevance and depth of knowledge content, the structure of individuals' knowledge bases, and the learners' ability to organize knowledge in a meaningful way are of major importance to clinical reasoning ability (Norman, 1988; Bordage and Lemieux, 1986; Grant and Marsden, 1987; Grant, *et al.*, 1988; Patel and Groen 1991; Jones, 1992).

There is currently no doubt about the role of knowledge in effective clinical reasoning and clinical practice. A compelling question that arises from this understanding is, when striving to improve one's own or another's reasoning process, is it enough to address the knowledge base? The answer to this question may rest in the broader definition of knowledge, i.e. what is considered factual information and what is considered a reasoned deduction about information. Improvement in clinical reasoning probably requires increasing the volume of factual knowledge, as well as making better links between knowledge areas. The process of logical deduction seems to be implicit in making links between items of information. In addition, the impact of each individual's beliefs and values on the interpretation of information should not be overlooked.

A discussion about either the value or the process of increasing the size of an individual's knowledge base is probably unnecessary here. Suffice it to say that being acquainted with disseminated information is important to retain professional currency. However, we now demand our students and practising clinicians to be logical in their thinking and in their use of information. But, what do we mean by logic? Logic is generally defined as the science of reasoning or the chain of reasoning. People do not ordinarily reason using putative (or mathematical/statistical) logic. Rather they tend to rely on their belief systems, and simpler ways of solving problems, providing solutions even in the absence of adequate information (Gilhooly, 1988). In addition, it could be argued that each profession has a 'professional logic', i.e. information is interpreted in a way that is unique to that profession, usually based on empirical evidence, experience and clinical wisdom (for example, pushing on a painful vertebra will reduce pain). The links and interpretations made are not necessarily 'logical' – usually, they could not be deduced from the data alone, as could a problem in geometry from knowledge of deriving theorems from first principles. This is not logic in the pure sense, and must be learnt as the novice joins the profession. To this extent, 'professional logic', or making links, could in fact be considered to be part of 'professional knowledge', and therefore must be learnt from others rather than deduced. When making new links, or evaluating information in a new way, some deduction and logic may be involved. This is often how progress is made in professional practice but probably occurs infrequently.

The other important feature of individuals' reasoning is the system of beliefs and values to which they subscribe, and against which they compare information. If new knowledge or ideas are incongruent with the belief system, individuals may reject the new information. This is consistent with the common tendency to exhibit a confirmatory bias (Elstein *et al.*, 1978; Gilhooly, 1988). Several studies have demonstrated that, in all fields including the health sciences, confirmatory bias is common, that people tend to accept information that supports their beliefs, and reject or ignore information that conflicts with their beliefs. For example, if a physiotherapist strongly believes that segmental alignment is important in the aetiology of back pain, the intervention offered may often include postural correction. There will be a tendency to ignore evidence demonstrating lack of effectiveness of such intervention. In this instance, the physiotherapist may look for other reasons if the intervention fails, e.g. non-compliance with the exercise programme or inadequate dosage of exercise.

Conclusion

The identification of clinical reasoning as a separate skill has been a major influence in causing changes in physiotherapy education. Probably the single most important feature in determining the quality of one's clinical reasoning is the knowledge base, both the type and extent. Obviously, if one has no knowledge, one has nothing with which to reason. The other important feature is the individual's belief system. An inappropriate belief system can impede integration of new and evaluation of old knowledge.

Acute and chronic pain

D. Gronow

The anatomy and physiology of pain perception are areas from which many of us tend to shy away. Our initial teaching in this area was often laborious and not relevant to our subsequent professional practice. Indeed, many early theories of pain perception failed to explain the clinical experience of pain perception.

The *nociceptive system* is a protective or defensive system which enables the body to recognize and defend itself from harmful or potentially harmful stimulus. Pain is commonly defined as an unpleasant sensory and emotional experience associated with actual or potential tissue damage, or described in terms of such damage. Such a definition highlights the two components of pain. The first is the biological function of the body's recognition of a noxious (painful) stimulus. The second is the experience and expression of this stimulus which involves the emotional, cognitive, developmental, behavioural and cultural aspects of pain behaviour. Pain behaviour allows us to show the suffering being experienced which may not be related directly to the level of nociceptive stimulus. The sensation of nociception is always unpleasant, and invokes an emotional experience. The response to this experience is shaped by an individual's ability to communicate this experience and their adaptability to the current environment. In practice, for example, no two patients with a similar injury, such as a Colle's fracture, present with the same pain complaints or behaviour. It is tempting to attribute these differences in pain behaviour to differences in 'pain tolerance' rather than looking for the cause of the suffering. The fundamentals of nociception help us to understand how the signals of noxious stimuli reach the central nervous system to produce a pain response. Nociception can therefore be described as the biological recognition of such a stimulus.

Our understanding of the nociceptive process is progressing rapidly, but is still incomplete. Melzack and Wall (1965), describing the *gate theory of pain*, rekindled the interest of the scientific world in the theory of pain and nociception. The gate theory introduced the idea of modulation of the nociceptive stimulus in the dorsal horn of the spinal cord by the effect of non-noxious stimuli (e.g. touch, proprioception) or descending inhibition reducing the central perception of nociception.

The rapidity of the increase in knowledge in this area and its important clinical application can be illustrated by our growth in understanding of the mechanisms and site of action of morphine. It was not until 1973 that the opiate receptor in the brain was identified (Pert and Sydner, 1973). In 1976 binding sites in the dorsal horn of the spinal cord were described. More recently opiate receptors were found to be formed on peripheral nerves in inflamed tissue suggesting that morphine and other opiates may have a peripheral mechanism of action in some inflammatory pain states. The use of intra-articular morphine in arthroscopy has been shown to reduce joint pain with no systemic effects. This, of course, is contrary to our classical teaching. Each of these basic science discoveries has advanced the understanding of nociception and altered the clinical course of management of various pain states. Considerable research is being undertaken to develop specific pharmacological substances to take advantage of this knowledge. A new group of peripherally acting opioids that do not cross the blood–brain barrier would give a new dimension in the management of certain inflammatory musculoskeletal pain states. Thus the importance of our knowledge and understanding of nociception and pain perception will continue to help in our clinical decision-making.

Nociception can be divided into the peripheral recognition of the stimulus, the modulation of that stimulus in the spinal cord, in particular the dorsal horn, and the central interaction allowing localization of the stimulus and the behavioural and learnt responses. Over the last two decades much of the work has been directed at understanding the dorsal horn responses to nociception, initially in acute pain and in understanding the changes in some chronic pain states, particularly following peripheral nerve injury. More recently studied are the peripheral receptor responses and the changes that may occur in acute and chronic pain. A brief outline of the nociceptive experience will hopefully entice the reader to gain further knowledge in this area.

Peripheral nerves are divided into those carrying non-noxious and noxious information. The non-noxious nerves, typically those that respond to sensation such as touch, vibration, heat and proprioception, are classified as responding to mechanical and thermal stimulation. Noxious nerves respond to strong stimulation by heat (thermal), mechanical (such as pinprick) and chemical stimuli, e.g. inflammation. These nerves normally have a high threshold to stimulation with pathways to the dorsal horn via the small diameter unmyelinated C fibres and the small diameter myelinated A-Delta fibres. The distribution of the termination of these nerves in deep tissue is still under debate. In the joint, free nerve endings of the small diameter fibres have been demonstrated in the fibrous capsule, adipose tissue, ligaments, menisci and periosteum but their presence is disputed in the synovial and cartilage tissue.

In the pathological state following tissue damage or nerve injury *hyperalgesia* (an increased response to noxious stimuli), *allodynia* (where non-noxious stimulus is felt to be painful) or *persistent pain* (prolongation of the response to brief stimulation) may develop. During the early stages of tissue damage when acute inflammation is still present, peripheral neural mechanisms contribute to the development of on-going pain. After healing has occurred, however, spinal mechanisms are increasingly involved in the persistence of pain.

Sensitization of both non-noxious and noxious afferents occur in the inflamed joint. This sensitization lowers the threshold to noxious stimuli, also causing non-noxious afferents to respond as if to a noxious response. Thus the normal range of movement or loading to an inflamed joint will be perceived as being painful. In addition there will be an increased barrage into the dorsal horn causing further changes.

Further, it has been postulated that there are a group of mechano-insensitive afferents or 'silent nociceptors' which become functional in the inflamed joint.

Protracted afferent input, particularly with stimulation through the C-fibre receptors and afferents, will cause sensitization of other peripheral afferents which will enhance the peripheral response to any stimuli. In turn this ongoing input will alter the dorsal horn responsiveness to produce a state of secondary hyperalgesia (i.e. increased responsiveness to the same level of noxious input) and hyperaesthesia. This area of responsiveness can be in a much wider area than the original stimulus or injury and is often non-dermatomal. Such a state partly accounts for prolongation of the post-injury response to pain and may explain the maintenance of some pain states.

The prostaglandins (PGE_1, PGE_2 and PGI_2), bradykinin, serotonin, leukotrienes, substance P and histamine are known to sensitize the peripheral afferents, altering their threshold to stimulation and their intracellular processing and, as mentioned above, can cause the production of new receptors that are responsive to application of opiate (and therefore possibly of others?).

Prolonged or repetitive noxious stimuli of C-fibres leads to sensitization of neurons in the dorsal horn, leading to the phenomenon of 'wind-up'. Wind-up is characterized by these dorsal horn cells developing reduced thresholds, prolonged after-discharges and increased spontaneous activity with expansion of peripheral fields. At least two receptors in the dorsal horn are implicated in this process. These are neurokinin$_1$ (NK_1) activated by substance P and the *N*-methyl-D-aspartate (NMDA) which is activated by the amino acid neurotransmitters glutamate and aspartate. Substance P and glutamate can coexist in primary peripheral afferents, being released on noxious stimulation. Activation of the NMDA receptor allows Ca^{2+} ions to enter the neuron, increasing intracellular Ca^{2+} and precipitating a series of events. Through mechanisms such as the formation of nitric oxide (NO) and changes in gene expression, the responsiveness of the neuron will be further altered. These changes in Ca^{2+} and NO alter synaptic transmission and may account for the development of chronic pain states of hyperalgesia, allodynia and wind-up. If therapeutic approaches could be developed that would interfere with this process, then such pain states may be reversed.

The implication is that, even by reducing peripheral nociceptive input which occurs naturally with tissue healing, the magnitude of the painful response may not reduce. This can have important clinical considerations in the management of acute pain states. Importantly, reduction of this spinal effect improves the recovery time. Providing adequate analgesia at the time of the acute injury response has been shown to reduce the wind-up effect in the dorsal horn and lead to quicker return of normal function. Providing adequate analgesia at the time of physiotherapy is an important consideration in clinical practice.

Many mechanisms operate to reduce the excitatory responsiveness of the dorsal horn and spinal systems. These inhibitory systems have a complex interaction. One inhibitory system acts via the opiate receptors and explains the ability for both endogenous and exogenous opioids to reduce dorsal horn activity and the perception of pain. In addition, descending pathways from the brain may reduce or inhibit spinal cord activity via action of noradrenaline, serotonin and enkephalin, thus improving the spinal effect of analgesia. The central control mechanisms synapsing on to the dorsal horn are influenced via these inhibitory systems by such states as relaxation and agitation, providing possible application in clinical practice.

The ascending pathways to the higher levels within the central nervous system are even more complex. Classically, these pathways ascend in the spinothalamic tract. However, other reported pathways have been noted to contain or have the ability to contain nociceptive input. Although their clinical relevance is not yet known, we are aware, that after cordotomy or tractotomy of the spinothalamic tract, one can still develop pain states that are very resistant to treatment. The thalamus is an important major relay site for nociceptive information, but not necessarily all nociceptive information is relayed through the thalamus. Fibres will then project to some extent to the cortex and to the limbic system where the emotional, memory and learning component of pain perception is caused. The role of the cortex in the perception of pain is unclear. Although pain must be perceived as a result of activity in the corticoneurons, focal stimulation of the cortex rarely results in pain, and lesions of the cortex of the brain rarely affect pain perception. The frontal cortex may have a role in the affective motivational aspects of pain, although this is not the only area where this occurs. Interestingly frontal lobotomy was first used to treat phantom limb pain in amputees after the First World War. Further work will enhance understanding of the role of the cortex. Positron emission tomography is now being used to localize the region of cortex activity during noxious stimulation.

It is hoped that this section has produced an awareness in the reader of the importance of the basic sciences of pain, nociception and pain perception in the understanding and treatment of the patient in pain. References to other texts are recommended to further the understanding of this area of science and to provide a basis for thoughtful informed physiotherapy practice and research.

Physiology and clinical pharmacology: inflammation, pain and anti-inflammatory drugs and analgesics

P. G. Conaghan and R. O. Day

Inflammation

In clinical practice the signs of inflammation are heat, redness, swelling, pain and loss of function. Inflammation represents the response of living tissues to injury. Acute inflammation involves:

1. Increased blood supply in the region of injury. Inflammatory mediators or the traumatizing agent itself act on smooth muscle in the vessel walls to cause vasodilation. Sometimes there are stimuli for new vessel formation.
2. An increase in local capillary permeability. This process involves active contraction of the capillary lining cells or endothelium leading to gaps between cells, again in response to chemical mediators.
3. Exudation of vascular fluid. This inflammatory exudate follows the increased capillary permeability. It contains many plasma proteins and antibodies.
4. Migration of inflammatory cells out of the blood vessels into the surrounding tissue. This involves adhesion of cells in the bloodstream (leucocytes such as neutrophil granulocytes, lymphocytes and monocytes) to the vascular endothelium and the subsequent 'squeezing' of the leucocytes through the intercellular junctions of the endothelium. Adhesion requires specific molecules on the surfaces of involved cells. Some of these adhesion molecules are constitutively expressed and others are only expressed in response to inflammatory mediators; certain cell types can then be selectively recruited. Migration also involves chemotaxis, which is the directional movement of cells in response to inflammatory mediators.
5. Molecular mediators of inflammation. Many chemicals are released by cells and many plasma proteins are activated in inflammation. Examples of these mediators are histamine, which is released by mast cells, prostaglandins, which are formed from phospholipids in cell membranes, and bradykinin, formed by activation of a precursor molecule in plasma.

Acute inflammation may be followed by tissue death or necrosis, scarring or fibrosis, or chronic inflammation. The best example of chronic inflammation in musculoskeletal medicine is rheumatoid arthritis and because all classes of anti-inflammatory drugs are used to treat this condition, it is appropriate to discuss its underlying features.

Rheumatoid arthritis

Rheumatoid arthritis is a chronic inflammatory arthritis that presents usually as a symmetrical destructive polyarthritis. It affects about 1% of the adult population, with females being more frequently affected than males. The aetiology of this condition is still unknown, although genetic and environmental factors play a role.

The normal joint has a thin lining layer or synovium overlying a thick fibrous joint capsule and cartilagenous articular bony surfaces. This synovium consists of cells termed synoviocytes overlying a matrix of extracellular proteins. The initial changes on light microscopy of the synovium in rheumatoid arthritis include thickening of the lining layer due to accumulation of cells and fluid. This thickened lining can be seen macroscopically and is called the pannus. Early in the disease white cells migrate into the joint lining from the blood vessels. The predominant leucocytes invading the synovium are lymphocytes, whereas the predominant leucocytes in the synovial fluid are neutrophil granulocytes. As well as infiltration of cells, there is proliferation of synoviocytes and local replication of lymphocytes and phagocytic cells or macrophages.

All the cells involved, especially the lymphocytes and macrophages, produce a group of soluble molecules called cytokines, which act as intercellular messengers over short distances. The most important of the cytokines involved are interleukin 1, tumour necrosis factor α, interferon-γ, platelet-derived growth factor and interleukin 6. These molecules act as chemoattractants for more inflammatory cells and stimulate other cells such as fibroblasts to produce collagen and glycosaminoglycans, i.e. the proteins that make up the substance or matrix of the synovium. This increase in extracellular protein together with the cytokine effects leads to increased fluid retention within the inflamed synovium.

The initial inflammatory mediators activate an enzyme, phospholipase A_2, in cell membranes which consequently releases arachidonic acid. Arachidonic acid is then converted into prostaglandins by an enzyme called cyclo-oxygenase and then into leukotrienes via the lipoxygenase pathway. Prostaglandins and leukotrienes play an important role in amplifying the inflammatory response.

The thickened synovium or pannus grows slowly across the articular surface. As well as producing proteins that lay down material, fibroblasts and other cells produce a range of molecules which are important in local tissue destruction. Cytokines such as interleukin 1 are important in stimulating cells to produce these enzymes, which include collagenase and stromelysin which are important in breaking down collagen. Reactive oxygen molecules (called reactive oxygen species) are produced and play an important pro-inflammatory role. As disease progresses, the invading pannus causes destruction of cartilage and adjacent bone. These bony changes may be seen on radiographs and are called erosions. Soft tissues surrounding the inflamed synovium such as ligaments may also be involved in the inflammatory process and destroyed. Many ligament and tendon ruptures are associated with ongoing inflamma-

tion, resulting in many of the common deformities seen in rheumatoid arthritis.

The above is a necessarily brief description of the complex interaction between cells, cytokines and structural proteins.

Clinical pharmacology

Before discussing any therapeutic agent, it is appropriate to consider not only how it works, its effects and side effects (termed the pharmacodynamics) but how it reaches its site of action and is metabolized by the body (the pharmacokinetics of the drug). Pharmacokinetics looks at drug absorption, distribution throughout different body compartments, metabolism and eventual excretion. Only a few key concepts of pharmacokinetics will be discussed.

The half-life ($t_{1/2}$) of a drug refers to the time required for the amount in the body to fall to 50%, and it is important when calculating dosage schedules. It is dependent on two other important parameters, drug clearance (C) and the volume of distribution (V). The terms are related by the following formula:

$$t_{1/2} = 0.7V/C$$

The volume of distribution gives an index of drug binding to tissues and plasma proteins and gives an indication of the initial or loading dose. It is important to remember that it is the free or unbound concentration of a drug that is active or available to bind to appropriate receptors. Drug clearance determines daily dosage and largely relates to hepatic metabolism and renal excretion of drugs. Some drugs undergo extensive metabolism on their first passage through the liver: this is referred to as a first-pass effect.

Anti-inflammatory drugs

The anti-inflammatory drugs are usually classified into categories of steroidal and non-steroidal medications. The drugs will be discussed below under the categories:

1. glucocorticosteroids,
2. non-steroidal anti-inflammatory drugs (NSAIDs),
3. disease-modifying antirheumatic drugs (DMARDs).

Rheumatoid arthritis patients will often use an NSAID and a DMARD, often with additional glucocorticosteroid.

Glucocorticosteroids

Glucocorticosteroids are produced naturally in the body by the cortex of the adrenal gland. The adrenal gland responds to hormones released by the pituitary gland which in its turn is responsive to hormonal commands from the hypothalamus in the brain. The hypothalamus secretes corticotrophin-releasing hormone which acts on the anterior pituitary gland to cause production of adrenocorticotrophic hormone (ACTH). ACTH, which is released with a diurnal rhythm, then acts on the adrenal cortex resulting in glucocorticoid production. Cortisol (or hydrocortisone) is the main glucocorticoid produced in humans.

A number of glucocorticosteroids are available for use in Australia, including cortisone, prednisolone, methylprednisolone, triamcinolone, betamethasone and dexamethasone. Some are only available for intramuscular or intravenous use. These glucocorticoids have different degrees of effect, for example on a milligram for milligram basis prednisolone is four times more potent than hydrocortisone.

Glucocorticosteroids are powerful immune-suppressant and anti-inflammatory drugs and have a large role in the treatment of inflammation based conditions. Their modulation of immune and inflammatory conditions is an extension of the natural action of cortisol which is physiologically released at times of stress and illness. Many mechanisms of glucocorticoid action have been described and it is known that these corticosteroids bind to receptors in the cell cytoplasm and that the receptor–steroid complex enters the cell nucleus, modifying DNA transcription. In inflammatory states, exogenous glucocorticoids can inhibit the function and even decrease the circulating numbers of various leucocytes, especially lymphocytes and macrophages. They can reduce prostaglandin and leukotriene production and antagonize the effect of some pro-inflammatory cytokines.

Steroid therapy is usually given orally or intra-articularly. Intra-articular therapy is commonly used in inflammatory arthritis where a small number of joints are inflamed and not being controlled by systemic therapy. These injections may need to be repeated depending on the duration of response of an individual joint. Intra-articular steroid can also be used in other musculoskeletal problems, for example in inflammation secondary to rotator cuff tendon damage in the shoulder, or in lateral epicondylitis or tennis elbow. Glucocorticosteroids may damage cartilage and therefore the number of injections into a given joint is usually limited to three or four per year. Intravenous corticosteroids may be used when a very rapid effect is required in severe or life-threatening inflammatory conditions. Intramuscular steroids are occasionally used in intermittent doses as an alternative to continuous daily oral therapy.

Glucocorticoids have many adverse effects and these are listed in Table 2.1. The most important long-term adverse effects include weight gain, osteoporosis with concomitant increased risk of fracture, and increased susceptibility to infection. It is obvious from this list of complications that a decision must be made when starting a patient on long-term oral steroids that there is a significant inflammatory component to the disease. Every effort is made to try to reduce the oral steroid dose to the minimum that has the required anti-inflammatory effect. The dose required of anti-inflammatory steroid varies with conditions. A common maintenance anti-inflammatory dose in rheumatoid arthritis would be in the range of 5–10 mg per day.

Table 2.1   Adverse effects of glucocorticosteroid therapy

Musculoskeletal	Osteoporosis Myopathy Avascular necrosis of femoral head
Immunological	Increased susceptibility to infection
Endocrine	Truncal obesity, 'moon-like' facies Hyperglycaemia or frank diabetes Acne Hirsutism Salt and water retention
Dermatological	Thinning of skin Increased fragility of skin
Cardiovascular	Hypertension Exacerbation of congestive cardiac failure
Gastrointestinal	Peptic ulceration Reduced rate of ulcer healing Pancreatitis
Neurological	Cataracts Psychosis Change in mood (especially with high doses)

Long-term oral glucocorticoid therapy leads to suppression of the body's own hypothalamic–pituitary–adrenal axis. Consequently any attempt to reduce the dose of prednisolone is carried out slowly, often in a stepwise manner, or else the risk of hypocortisolaemia occurs.

Non-steroidal anti-inflammatory drugs (NSAIDs)

NSAIDs are drugs that work quickly to help reduce the symptoms and signs of inflammation such as pain, stiffness and swelling. Although anti-inflammatory, they do not modify the long-term course of a disease process, hence the differentiation with disease-modifying drugs. It should be noted, however, that there is some overlap between these categories. Common NSAIDs are classified according to their chemical derivation (Table 2.2). As well as being used as anti-inflammatory drugs, they can be used as analgesics, antipyretic agents and antithrombotic agents. They can be given orally, rectally and topically.

NSAIDs seem to work by preventing the formation of prostanoid derivatives by inhibiting cyclo-oxygenase. Many other mechanisms have however, been suggested for their mode of action because their anti-inflammatory actions are seen at drug concentrations greater than those required to inhibit cyclo-oxygenase. NSAIDs also interfere with the lipoxygenase pathway and the consequent formation of leukotrienes. There is evidence that they affect neutrophil leucocyte function, interfering with both the chemotactic response of the cell and the generation of reactive oxygen species by the cell membrane.

NSAIDs are generally mildly acidic and concentrate at sites of lowered pH, such as the sites of inflammation, and also in gastric and renal tissue. The latter findings are of note because of the side effects of these drugs (Table 2.3). In terms of pharmacokinetics the drugs are all very well absorbed in the gastrointestinal tract and are highly plasma-protein bound with only a very small amount of the drug being available for equilibration in tissues. NSAIDs undergo only little first-pass effect.

All NSAIDs appear to be of equivalent efficacy but have different pharmacokinetic properties. They can be divided into those having short and long half-lives (see Table 2.2). In general, the more potent anti-inflammatory NSAIDs are seen to have higher side effect profiles, but this may only reflect their increased relative dosage. NSAIDs are required in smaller dose than aspirin to have equivalent anti-inflammatory potency.

Adverse effects of NSAIDs

The common adverse effects of NSAIDs are listed in Table 2.3. Of these side effects the gastrointestinal ones are the most commonly encountered. Although the risk of peptic ulceration or complication of ulcers is small for an individual, the frequency of encountering problems increases with age, such that people over 65 years old have much higher risk of gastrointestinal problems. The causes of toxicity are again thought to be due to inhibition of prostaglandin formation. In the kidney

Table 2.2   Common non-steroidal anti-inflammatory drugs (NSAIDs)

Class	Drug	Usual daily dose (mg/day)
2-Arylacetic acids	Indomethacin*	50–150
	Diclofenac*	75–150
	Sulindac	200–400
2-Arylpropionic acids	Ibuprofen*	1200–3200
	Ketoprofen*	100–400
	Naproxen	375–1500
	Tiaprofenic acid*	200–600
Oxicams	Piroxicam	10–20
	Tenoxicam	10–20
Salicylates	Acetylsalicylic acid*	1200–5200
	Diflunisal	500–1000

* These NSAIDs have short half-lives (< 6 h). The others have half-lives > 10 h.

Table 2.3   Adverse effects of NSAIDs

Gastrointestinal	Dyspepsia
	Peptic ulceration
	Gastritis
	Hepatitis
Renal	Reversible renal impairment
	Interstitial nephritis
Neurological	Confusion, especially in elderly
	Headaches
Endocrine	Fluid retention
Cardiovascular	Exacerbation of congestive cardiac failure
Haematological	Interference with platelet function

where prostaglandins play an important role in regulating intrarenal blood flow and glomerular filtration, lack of prostaglandins secondary to NSAIDs can precipitate acute renal failure and hyperkalaemia amongst other problems. Patients with pre-existing renal impairment are especially at risk of adverse effects.

There are also important clinical pharmacodynamic interactions with NSAIDs. NSAIDs can antagonize antihypertensive medications, including drugs that work via vasodilation and diuretic mechanisms. Hyperkalaemia may occur in conjunction with certain diuretics and antihypertensives. The concomitant use of warfarin, and perhaps alcohol, increases the risk of NSAID-induced gastrointestinal bleeding.

Disease-modifying antirheumatic drugs (DMARDs)

As the name implies, these drugs are used in the treatment of rheumatoid arthritis and are seen to modify the course of the disease. A particular DMARD (or combination) is started early in the disease in an attempt to prevent permanent joint damage. These drugs are listed in Table 2.4. These drugs are also known as the slow acting antirheumatic drugs (SAARDs) referring to their slow onset of action, often 4–6 weeks. For most of these agents the exact mechanism by which they have their effect is unknown. The DMARDs are also used in inflammatory arthritides such as psoriatic arthritis and ankylosing spondylitis although not all agents are effective in these other conditions.

Table 2.4   Disease-modifying antirheumatic drugs (DMARDs)

Class	Drug
Antimalarials	Hydroxychloroquine
Cytotoxics and immunosuppressives	Methotrexate Azathioprine Chlorambucil Cyclophosphamide Cyclosporin
Gold complexes	Auranofin Sodium aurothioglucose Sodium aurothiomalate
Others	D-Penicillamine Sulphasalazine

Methotrexate

Methotrexate is a folate antagonist which was initially used in treating malignant disease. As with the other DMARDs its mode of action is unclear. It acts as a folate antagonist by inhibiting the enzyme dihydrofolate reductase which reduces the amount of intracellular folate. This folate is required for synthesis of purine, important in cell replication. However, as well as being an antiproliferative agent, methotrexate is immunosuppressive and it is not clear which of these actions accounts for its activity as a disease suppressant. Although there are few data to compare directly the efficacy of the DMARDs, methotrexate is the quickest acting with onset of efficacy at about 3–5 weeks. Methotrexate is moderately well absorbed orally and can be given intramuscularly. It has an elimination half-life of 5–6 h. About 50% is excreted renally and therefore the drug can be toxically retained in the presence of chronic renal impairment.

Methotrexate is usually given in doses of 5–15 mg as a single weekly oral or intramuscular dose. Because it works against rapidly dividing cells the side effects involve the gastrointestinal tract and the bone marrow. Nausea and mouth ulcers occur in about 10% of people. Abnormal liver function tests may occur and this warrants regular blood testing. One of the serious complications of methotrexate therapy is hepatic fibrosis which may rarely lead to cirrhosis: this is related in some patients to previous liver damage or ongoing alcohol use. Effects on the bone marrow can reduce cell counts and frequent full blood counts are also part of monitoring. Pneumonitis may rarely occur with severe hypoxia.

Gold

Gold can be used for rheumatoid arthritis in an oral or intramuscular form. The intramuscular form is more commonly used and has a very good response rate but higher side-effect profile.

Intramuscular gold is normally given as a 10 mg test dose and then quickly increased up to a maintenance dose of 20–50 mg per week. This is continued up to a total dose of 1 g or until clinical improvement is seen, at which stage the dosage interval may be increased.

Side effects of gold include skin rashes, which may or may not necessitate discontinuation of therapy, mouth ulcers, and sometimes bone marrow depression with low white cell and platelet counts. Gold can also affect the kidneys causing proteinuria and even glomerulonephritis, so as well as regular blood screening, routine urine analysis is performed before each injection.

Oral gold or auranofin is given as a dose of 3 mg twice a day but does not seem to be as effective as the intramuscular form. It has a milder side-effect profile with diarrhoea being the most frequent problem and renal side effects much less common.

Sulphasalazine

Sulphasalazine is a combination of sulphapyridine which is an antibacterial agent and 5-aminosalicylic acid which has anti-inflammatory properties. This drug is most commonly used for treatment of inflammatory bowel disease and it was subsequently found to be an effective disease-modifying agent. It is normally given in doses up to 1 g twice a day, and again like other DMARDs may require weeks before onset of action. The common side effects of sulphasalazine include nausea and dyspepsia, along with rash. Very occasionally low white blood cell counts are seen and therefore regular blood monitoring is again required. Headache is another occasional side effect.

Penicillamine

Penicillamine is another commonly used disease-modifying antirheumatic drug. Again its action is unclear and it is normally used in an oral dose of 500–750 mg daily. Penicillamine's side effects include nausea, rash, thrombocytopenia, mouth ulcers and proteinuria. It is also associated with a number of unusual immunological diseases such as drug-induced systemic lupus erythematosus. Again, as with gold, many of the side effects are reversed when therapy is ceased.

Hydroxychloroquine

Hydroxychloroquine is related to chloroquine which was first used as an antimalarial drug. It is probably the mildest acting of the disease-modifying antirheumatic drugs, but similarly it has a very good side-effect profile. It is normally given in a dose of 200–400 mg per day orally. The major but rare potential side effect of hydroxychloroquine is damage to the retina; six monthly thorough eye examinations are required since patient symptoms are a poor guide to ongoing damage.

Other immunosuppressive agents

The agents listed above are the commonest currently used for treatment of rheumatoid arthritis and other inflammatory arthritides. Other agents are used that are true immunosuppressive agents. Azathioprine is commonly used as a steroid-sparing agent, i.e. to lower the dose of prednisolone required, and cyclophosphamide and cyclosporin A are also used for resistant inflammatory arthritis.

Pain

Pain is a complex phenomenon and although many pain pathways have been described, the actions of many of the components of these pathways are not clearly defined. Pain travels from both peripheral and central pathways within the nervous system. Peripheral pain or noxious stimuli receptors are called nociceptors and they transmit their signals centrally via small myelinated nerve fibres called A-Delta fibres or unmyelinated C fibres. These afferent fibres synapse in the dorsal horn of the spinal cord. The ascending pathways within the spinal cord have inputs from other spinal pathways which modify their signals. The supraspinal terminations of these pathways are complex and various parts of the brain including the thalamus are important in pain reception and perception.

The body also contains its own systems for modifying and modulating pain. In particular, opioid receptors are found on nerve cell membranes. The body produces its own opioids which are called enkephalins, endorphins and dynorphins. The endogenous opioids are present in only small amounts and although the locations of their receptors and neural pathways have been determined, their exact roles are not clear. Pain has therefore been classified as neurogenic- or nociceptive-mediated pain, or central if generated by central nervous system (CNS)-mediated damage.

It is useful to think of pharmacological therapy for pain according to the type of pain involved. There are many analgesic agents available. In nociceptive-type pain, paracetamol, aspirin, NSAIDs and opioids are all used. For neurogenic pain opioids are also used but other drugs such as dothiepin and other antidepressants or carbamazepine, an anticonvulsant, can be used. Members of the benzodiazepine family, e.g. diazepam can be used as muscle relaxants although they are of limited efficacy.

Aspirin and the NSAIDs are excellent analgesics as well as anti-inflammatory agents and their pharmacology has already been discussed. Paracetamol and the opioids will be discussed below.

Paracetamol

Paracetamol, also known as acetaminophen, is a very weak anti-inflammatory agent but is probably equal to aspirin in analgesic properties. Although it is also thought to work by inhibiting prostaglandin synthesis, its site of action seems to be more in the CNS than at peripheral sites of inflammation. It is well absorbed orally and reaches maximum blood concentrations between 15 min and 2 h after dosing. It is extensively metabolized by the liver and therefore it can accumulate in chronic liver disease. Paracetamol does not have the same degree of adverse effects as the more potent anti-inflammatory agents, and its most serious side effect is acute hepatic necrosis in overdose situations. The presence of alcohol enhances this overdose-induced hepatic toxicity. Paracetamol is usually recommended in doses of less than 4 g per day because of possible hepatic toxicity in long-term studies.

Opioids

As the name suggests these drugs are derived from the opium poppy. These agents are not frequently used in acute musculoskeletal pain and only a few are discussed but other short- and long-acting oral agents are available. They all work by acting on endogenous opioid receptors, though not all are active at each subtype of receptor.

Morphine

Morphine is derived from opium and is a very potent analgesic and euphoria-producing agent. Although oral preparations are available and are used extensively in palliative care, the drug undergoes sustantial first-pass effect after oral dosing and so the parenteral route of administration is commonly used. It has a half-life of 2.5–3 h and for an otherwise fit 70 kg adult would be given intramuscularly in a dose of 5–15 mg at 3–4-hourly intervals

Morphine has substantial side effects and the drug should be individualized with these in mind. It acts centrally to produce nausea and vomiting and depresses respiratory drive. It reduces gastrointestinal motility leading to constipation and acts as a vasodilator to reduce blood pressure. Physical dependence can occur with regular use.

Pethidine

Unlike morphine, pethidine is a synthetic narcotic but it works in a similar way. Again it is well absorbed orally with a short half-life but undergoes extensive first-pass metabolism and so is used parenterally. A dose of 50–150 mg intramuscularly every 3–4 h is used in a 70 kg adult. The side effects are very similar to those of morphine. However, norpethidine, which is a breakdown product of pethidine metabolism, can cause convulsions and other CNS adverse effects. This metabolite accumulates in renal impairment so care must be exercised in patients with this problem and in the elderly. Pethidine is not recommended for use in chronic situations.

Codeine

Codeine is another opium derivative although less potent than morphine. It is available in tablets on its own or in combination with paracetamol or aspirin. It is not as extensively metabolized on first pass through the liver as morphine or pethidine and so it is often given in oral preparations. It is metabolized in part to morphine and this probably explains its analgesic efficacy. The daily dose will depend on whether it is used alone or in combination. The major side effect at common dosage is constipation.

Biomechanics of joint movements

M. Lee

The discipline of biomechanics can provide a useful perspective on a number of aspects of the musculoskeletal system. In this section we will consider some of the principles of biomechanics related to movement of the joints of the body. Studying joint movements can tell us a great deal about the way the musculoskeletal system is working. If a child has a disordered movement control system, then joint movements may be *jerky*, or may be abnormally *fast* or *slow*. A person with a group of muscles showing abnormal mechanical behaviour may have one of more joints that show a smaller or larger *amount of movement* than normal. Pathological changes to the structural elements of an intervertebral joint may produce alterations in the *pattern of joint movement*. In this section I will concentrate on aspects of joint movement that might give clues about abnormalities of the system that produces the movement. In doing so I will restrict the discussion to the data that can readily be obtained by clinicians. Many aspects of joint dynamics, such as the details of forces and torques acting across joints, would make the study of joint movement more complete, but are not commonly available to clinicians.

Descriptions of joint movement

How do we describe joint movement? There are a number of aspects that need to be included if we are to identify those elements of joint movement that are likely to be signs of a disorder of the musculoskeletal system. The major elements involved are the *amount* and *pattern* of movement.

During movement of a limb, it appears as though the limb segments rotate around the joints. The most complete method for describing joint movements begins with this basic observation. The first parameter to be defined when describing a joint movement is the *axis*, about which the joint rotation occurs. In the case of human joints that behave as 'hinge' joints, such as the elbow, we can define the *pattern* of joint movement by simply defining the location of the joint axis. The *amount* of movement can be measured as the angle of rotation about the axis. This axis of movement is sometimes known as the *helical axis of motion* (Woltring *et al.*, 1985). In practice very few joints, if any, have an axis that remains completely fixed in space throughout the entire range of movement. Therefore to precisely define the pattern of movement at a joint we need to locate the axis of the movement at each instant during the movement.

Sometimes a joint moves in such a way that, as well as the main rotation about the axis, there are also very small amounts of movement *along* the axis. For example, during knee flexion, for which the axis lies in a medial–lateral orientation, there may be slight medial or lateral movements of the tibia during the range of movement. Although the amount of this type of movement would be expected to be small, a complete description of joint movement requires that we incorporate this translation as one of the parameters describing the joint movement.

We can now see that there are three parameters required for full definition of the movement at a joint:

1. location of the axis of movement, including information about how this location changes during the movement;
2. amount of rotation – the angle through which the joint rotation occurs about the axis during the movement,
3. amount of translation – the displacement (if any) that occurs along the axis during the movement.

Knowledge of the normal pattern and amount of movement allows us to detect abnormalities of movement. If we knew that the axis was normally fixed in a particular direction throughout the movement, then any movement that involved a differently oriented axis, or in which the axis moved during the range of movement, could be regarded as having an abnormal pattern.

Inevitably we are not able to obtain complete information about movement of a joint and an approximate description of joint motion is given. The first aspect of approximation occurs in the way we describe the changes in axis position throughout a movement. Usually we do not know the location of the axis at every instant. In fact, we do not know the axis location at *any* instant. Each axis location is usually derived by knowing the location of the body segments on either side of the joint on two occasions (*A* and *B*) in time, where these two occasions are separated by a finite angle. A procedure is then applied to calculate the location of the axis about which rotation seems to have occurred between the two positions. This axis is known as the *finite axis of rotation* between *A* and *B* (Woltring *et al.*, 1985). The degree to which this finite axis approximates the locations of the instantaneous axes as the joint moves between *A* and *B* depends on how close *A* and *B* are together. In some cases *A* may correspond to full flexion and *B* may correspond to full extension. In such a situation, the finite axis between *A* and *B* tells us nothing about the variation of axis location during the movement and may tell us very little about the pattern of movement at all.

The second aspect of approximation in describing joint motion occurs in the way we describe the axis. Imagine that we located a knee flexion axis and found it to lie in a horizontal medial–lateral direction. If we view this axis from the front, the axis will be a horizontal line. Where the axis passes through a mid-sagittal plane, the axis will appear as a point in that plane. Any such point on the axis of rotation is known as a *centre of rotation* for the movement. Provided the axis is perpendicular to the plane, the location of the centre of rotation in a plane can accurately represent the axis. However, if the axis travels obliquely, then it cannot be fully represented by one point in the mid-sagittal plane. To be an accurate representation of the axis of motion, we need to know the orientation of the axis as it passes through the centre of rotation. We must also note whether there is any translation along the axis during rotation if we are to fully define the pattern of movement. In addition, as with the axis of rotation, we need to know this information at as many occasions as possible during a complete movement.

rotation method remains a valid way of describing non-planar movements, it is difficult to use because of the need to employ a three-dimensional method to show the positions and orientations of the axes.

To deal with the complexity of three-dimensional movement a simpler method of joint movement description is often used. In particular, much of the detail of the pattern of movement is usually omitted. The method used involves considering the joint motion as comprising rotations in each of the three cardinal planes (sagittal, frontal and horizontal) and three components of translation (antero–posterior, medial–lateral, cephalo–caudal). For physiological movements, where rotation is the desired motion, one of the rotations is designated as the *main movement*. All other movements, including rotation in other planes and translations in any direction, are called *coupled movements*. For example, if we attempt to produce right lateral flexion at a normal C4–C5 joint, right axial rotation will occur as well as the desired right lateral flexion. In this case the *main movement* is right lateral flexion, and the right axial rotation is a *coupled movement*. Note that this approach to describing joint movement gives a simplified, but quantitative method of describing the pattern and amount of motion. For example, Goel *et al.* (1985) measured the main and coupled motions to assess the effect of discectomy on the kinematics of the whole lumbar spine. They applied torques in each of the cardinal planes and measured the resulting main and coupled rotations and the three coupled translations. For a 3 N.m right lateral flexion load applied to an intact specimen, the main rotation was 12 degrees with a coupled lateral translation to the side of movement of 8 mm. The other coupled rotations and translations were found to be an order of magnitude smaller: less than 1 mm or degree. These data give us useful information about the normal pattern and extent of lumbar lateral flexion.

Coupled movements

The axis-of-rotation method, whether used in its complete form or simplified to centre of rotation, is most useful for describing movements that occur in a *single plane*. If a movement is fully three-dimensional, then the axis moves into orientations that are oblique to those corresponding to previous parts of the movement. Although the axis-of-

Passive joint movements

Passive joint movements are often divided into two categories (Maitland, 1986). Passive *physiological* movements involve the same sorts of movement patterns as active movements, but are performed by the therapist while the patient is passive. These movements can be described using the methods given above for active movements. Passive *acces-*

sory movements occur when the therapist moves the joint in a way that is not normally done by the patient's muscles. A body segment is *translated* by the therapist during accessory movements, rather than rotated, so the axis-of-rotation concept is not relevant.

In the case of passive accessory movements, the therapist may be especially interested in the movements occurring at the joint surfaces in relation to the surface movements that take place during physiological movements. An anatomist, MacConaill, has developed a complicated system of classification and description of joint types and movements which emphasizes the anatomical aspects of joints (MacConaill, 1964). We will just consider one small aspect of MacConaill's ideas.

MacConaill focused very much on the shape of joint surfaces. He declared that there were only two different joint surface shapes: ovoid (egg-shaped; convex in all directions or concave in all directions) and sellar (saddle-shaped; convex in one direction and concave in another direction). Most joints comprise two ovoid surfaces, one concave and one convex. MacConaill divided the movements between the joint surfaces into three categories: spin, roll and slide. When spin occurs there is essentially no movement through space of the body segments. Rotation occurs about the segment axis while the axis remains in a fixed position. Both roll and slide produce translation of a body segment. When roll occurs there is rotation of the segment about an axis that is located at the point of contact between the joint surfaces. Slide involves translation of the body segment without rotation.

In a typical joint, roll and slide occur together. If roll occurs alone then the point of contact between the surfaces moves (such as when a ball rolls on a table). The combination of roll and slide allows the point of contact to remain approximately stationary. The roll alone may tend to move the point of contact in one direction, but if this is combined with a slide in the opposite direction the point of contact can remain in one place. This combination of movements is desirable if the amount of cartilage-covered area of one joint surface is small such as in the case of the glenoid fossa that forms one surface of the glenohumeral joint. Passive accessory movements produced by the therapist involve slide movements between the joint surfaces without the concomitant roll. Therefore joint movements produced in this manner may not normally occur during physiological motion.

Passive joint dynamics

Up to this point we have only examined kinematic issues. Here we will briefly discuss the passive resistance to movement, considering separately the cases of passive physiological and passive accessory movement. For *physiological* movements, the torque-angle curve is usually similar to that shown in Figure 2.1 (Berme *et al.*, 1985). Depending on the joint and the direction of movement, the low stiffness region AB may be of variable length. Generally there will be a substantial low stiffness region because joints are designed to allow physiological movements to occur freely within a certain range. At the highly mobile glenohumeral joint the low stiffness zone AB is relatively large for most movements while at the ankle joint this zone is much smaller.

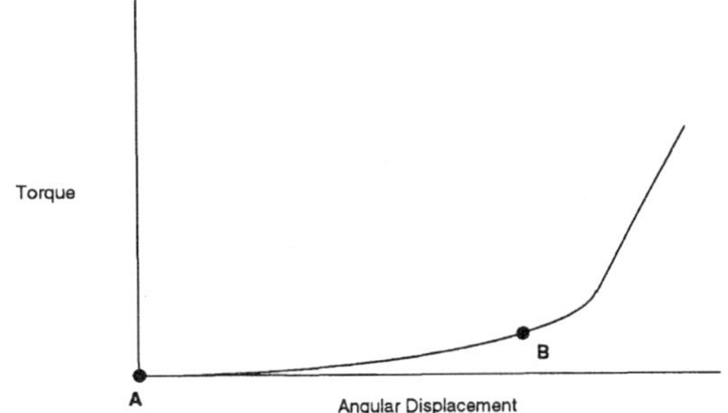

Figure 2.1 Resistance of typical physiological movement

For *accessory* movements the resistance varies in a different way. For these movements it appears that there is only minimal low stiffness phase which is probably caused by compression of compliant soft tissue overlying the bone. Although very few data are available, it seems likely that in accessory movements there is resistance to the entire movement, probably increasing linearly with the amount of translation.

For both physiological and accessory movements there is very little information available about which structures are responsible for the tissue resistance measured (or perceived) at the skin surface. It is often assumed that muscles provide most of the resistance to physiological movements, and accessory movements are resisted mostly by ligaments and joint capsule. There is some evidence, largely based on animal studies, to support the dominant role of muscles in resisting passive physiological movements (Akeson *et al.*,

1974). There is very little evidence to implicate any particular tissues in the resistance to passive accessory movements. In the case of the accessory movements in the spine, the therapist is not necessarily able to produce pure translation of the vertebra to which she or he applies a force, nor is she or he able to stabilize adjacent vertebrae so that movement only occurs at one or two intervertebral joints. Indeed, research indicates that when a force is applied to, for example, an L3 vertebra, then appreciable vertebral movements occur as far away as T8 (Lee and Svensson, 1993). In this situation there will be contributions to the movement resistance from a very large number of structures. Therefore the clinical meaning of the behaviour of resistance will be very difficult to determine.

Instability

There is one issue related to passive joint dynamics that is worthy of special consideration here – instability. The major issue to consider in relation to instability is one of definition. The term instability is used in two different ways in the clinical literature related to joint movements and these two uses involve quite different meanings. As a result there is considerable confusion about the concept of instability. The confusion can be resolved by defining two separate concepts: *mechanical (true) instability* and *clinical instability.*

The key to understanding *mechanical instability* lies in consideration of the changes in potential energy of a joint system. Therefore, before we consider instability further we need to understand how the potential energy of a joint system can be changed. In relation to a joint there is one major form of potential energy, elastic potential energy. The amount of elastic potential energy possessed by a body depends on the amount of elastic deformation. In the case of a joint, the elastic deformation is the stretch of the spring-like soft tissues around the joint. For a linearly elastic tissue, the potential energy stored when it is deformed is equal to $\frac{1}{2}kx^2$, where k is the stiffness and x is the amount of elastic deformation. Where a bone is restrained (at a joint) by a number of soft tissues, such as ligaments and muscles, the total potential energy is the potential energy stored in all of those restraining structures. In general, a system will tend to come to rest in a position in which the total stored potential energy is least.

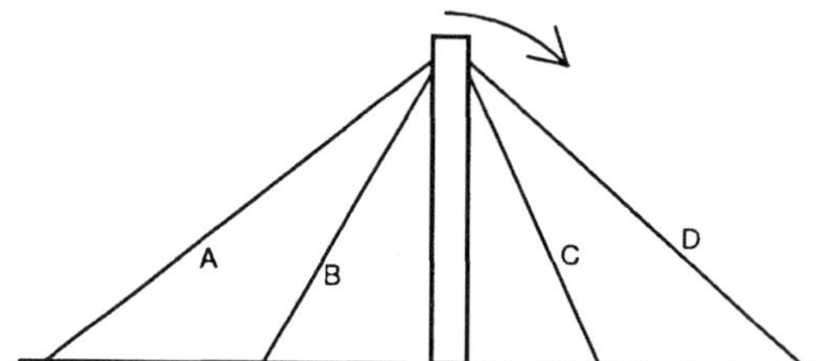

Figure 2.2 Example of a stable system

Mechanical instability can now be defined as the situation where small joint movements result in a decrease in total stored potential energy. Where there is instability, small initial movements will result in further movement, until a position of stability is reached and the potential energy is at a minimum. Conversely, in the case where stability exists, small initial movements result in an increase in stored potential energy and the joint tends to return to its original position. Consider the example shown in Figure 2.2. A post is restrained by four elastic cables A, B, C and D. If the post is displaced in the direction of the arrow, then restraints A and B will become stretched and will store potential energy. Therefore, according to our definition, the post is stable. If the post is released, it will tend to return to the original vertical position.

In a joint, some of the restraining structures (such as A and B) may be deficient as the result of trauma, disease or other factors and there is no strong tendency for the joint to return to its original position after a small perturbation. Consider the case shown in Figure 2.3 which is a better representation of a peripheral joint. There are two objects (equivalent to bones) held together by restraints, with at least one of the objects having an irregularly shaped surface on which the other object can spin, slide or roll. Imagine for the moment that object 1 can move and object 2 is fixed. There are a number of restraining tissues (A, B, C, D, E) that are tending to hold the joint in position. In addition, the shape of the surface of one of the objects tends to produce a normal equilibrium position. However, if some of the restraints are weak or missing (such as A and B)

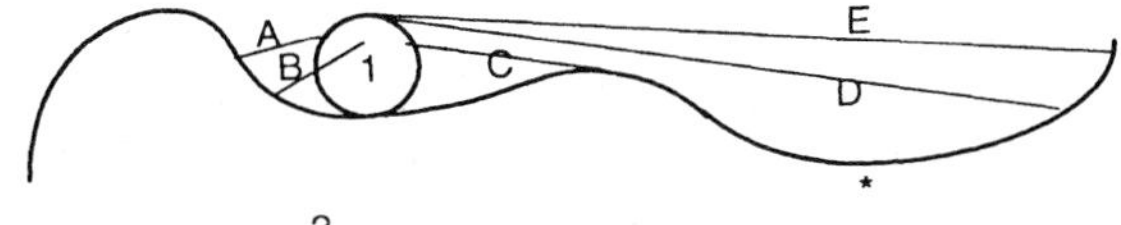

Figure 2.3 Simple representation of a peripheral joint

then we may find that we can move object 1 to the right through a small distance and it will not return to its original position. If we plot the change in potential energy against the amount of movement to the right (Figure 2.4 – the arrow shows the initial position) we see that there is an initial small increase in potential energy but then with further movement the potential energy decreases.

Figure 2.4 tells us that if we move object 1 beyond the peak in potential energy then it will keep moving by itself until it reaches a point where the potential energy is at a minimum, in the position marked *. The corresponding physical position is shown on Figure 2.3. The peak of energy corresponds to the point at which the joint becomes unstable. If restraints A and B were normal, then the initial position would be much more stable. There would be much more energy required to move the joint beyond the peak of potential energy into a position of instability.

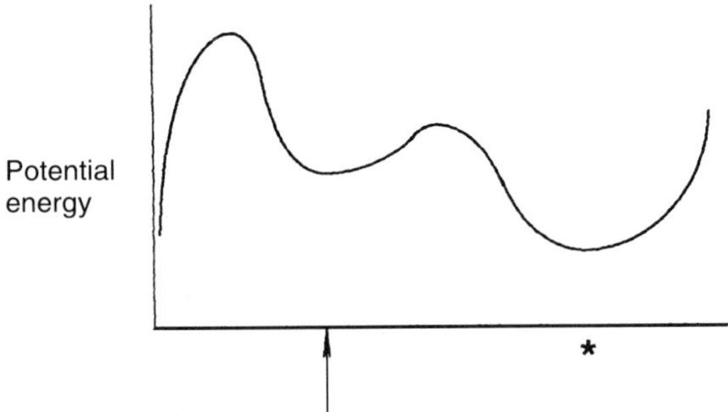

Figure 2.4 Change in potential energy with movement from initial position (marked with arrow)

It is well known that some peripheral joints show an instability not unlike that which has just been described. For example, in some individuals the glenohumeral joint can be unstable, with dislocation resulting if the humerus is moved too far in a particular way. In Figure 2.3 an accessory movement was shown to produce instability. Instability can also occur in physiological movements. In a physiological movement muscles provide much of the resistance that tends to restore the joint to the initial position. It is possible that a sudden change in activation of a muscle, when an external torque is being applied, may allow a joint to quickly move away from the neutral position with minimal resistance. This phenomenon could rightly be also called instability.

Clinical instability is a much simpler concept, but does not really involve instability at all! A more correct name would be *pathological hypermobility*. This term is most often applied to the spine. In this context the term instability usually means excessive movement at an intervertebral joint which is likely to compromise the spinal cord. A person who has damage to the structures that restrain intervertebral movement (caused by disease or trauma) can show an amount of intervertebral movement that can endanger the spinal cord so that surgical 'stabilization' is required. The judgement as to whether instability exists is often made on the basis of the amount of coupled intervertebral antero-posterior translation that is exhibited during movement through the full flexion – extension range. Cases of *clinical instability* may not show the decreasing potential energy that is the characteristic of *true* instability.

Bone: recent concepts important to musculoskeletal physiotherapy

H.M. Frost

Introduction

This section summarizes recent developments in bone research that finally seem ready for physical therapists, coaches, trainers and other health professionals to apply to clinical practice. Definition of key terms is provided in Table 2.5. Values for some important parameters are also provided. The following facts should be noted:

1. Our daily mechanical usage (MU) provides the loads that cause strains and stress in bones (Martin and Burr, 1989; Burr and Martin, 1992). Strains are deformations (Table 2.5); stress is the internal force in bone that resists them. Increased vigor of MU means larger forces on bones, not more frequent ones.

2. The largest bone loads and strains come from muscles, not bodyweight. On a soccer player's

Table 2.5   Definitions of key terms used for bone involvement in musculoskeletal physiotherapy

---

Fracture strain: the strain at which normal lamellar bone usually fractures (its ultimate strength). Equal to about 25 000 microstrain (a little more in children and less in adults), it corresponds to a compression or tension stress of about 16 000 lbf/in^2 or 130 MPa.

MESm*: the minimum effective strain range that controls remodelling. A strain threshold range at and above which remodelling begins to conserve bone, but below which it removes bone (in humans, centred near 50–100 microstrain?).†

MESr*: the minimum effective strain range that controls remodelling. A strain threshold range at and above which remodelling begins to conserve bone, but below which it removes bone (in humans, centred near 50–100 microstrain?).†

Microdamage threshold: the strain range at and above which more new microdamage arises than its repair mechanism can handle, so it begins to accumulate (for bone, centred near 3000 microstrain).

Microstrain: a measure of deformation, which can be in tension, compression, shear, bending or/and torque; 25 000 microstrain in compression equals a 2.5% shortening of a bone, e.g. from 100% to 97.5% of its original length; 1500 microstrain in compression (or tension) equals 0.15% shortening (or stretching) of a bone, e.g. from 100% to 99.85% (or 100.15%) of its original length. Whereas strain can be measured directly in tissues, stress must be inferred from other measurements.

MU: mechanical usage of the skeleton, with far more emphasis on the size of the resulting bone loads or forces than on their number and frequency.

---

* These MES ranges correspond to the natural criteria that determine if too little or too much bone exists for its usual MU. If they differ in different people, that could make some people unusually resistant to injury and others unusually susceptible to it.

† Studies of *in vivo* bone strains revealed these thresholds and suggested their approximate values with respect to the fracture strain of bone. As their systematic study began quite recently, the above values may need revision in the future.

femur those loads can briefly exceed five times bodyweight (Frost, 1986; Martin and Burr, 1989; Burr and Martin, 1992).

3. Bone fractures at about 25 000 microstrain (Martin and Burr, 1989; Burr and Martin, 1992).

4. Two biological mechanisms, modelling and remodelling, help to control a bone's architecture, mass and strength, and to fit it to its MU, minimize its fatigue damage and keep strains below its fracture strain (Figure 2.5).

5. Each mechanism responds to stimuli in its own way but both use osteoclasts and osteoblasts to do it (Frost, 1986; Jee, 1989; Martin and Burr, 1989; Burr and Martin, 1992).

6. Modelling can add to and strengthen bone and remodelling can remove it when a mechanical need for it ceases, but neither can do the other's work.

Microdamage

Repeated load–deload cycles (as in running) cause microscopic damage or *microdamage* in bone (Frost, 1986; Martin and Burr, 1989; Parfitt, 1990; Schnitzler, 1993). This damage increases with the size and number of the loads and can weaken bone enough to let normal MU cause stress fractures and spontaneous fractures. Excessive microdamage always causes such fractures (Frost, 1986; Burr and Martin, 1992).

Bone has a *microdamage threshold* well below its fracture strain and can repair lesser but not larger amounts. At 2000 microstrain it can take over 40 years of normal activities to fracture a bone in fatigue, but less than 2 months at 4000 microstrain. Doubling the size of the strains in that 2000–4000 microstrain region increases microdamage hundreds of times (Pattin and Carter, 1991; Frost, 1993). The remodelling mechanism (see below) normally repairs microdamage by removing and replacing damaged bone with new bone (Frost, 1986; Burr, 1993).

Creating too much microdamage, depressing its repair, or both can cause stress fractures and spontaneous fractures. Small amounts of microdamage seldom cause pain but enough microdamage to threaten a fracture usually causes bone pain during MU. This can happen in particular conditions, such as osteoporosis, at particular sites, such as around artificial joints and teeth, and can affect particularly active groups such as aggressive athletes and military trainees (Frost, 1986).

Modelling: strengthening and adding bone

Strains in or above an MESm range (see Table 2.5) can make modelling drifts (henceforth called 'modelling') begin to strengthen bone by adding more to it and/or changing its shape and size (Figure 2.5) (Frost, 1990a; Jee *et al.*, 1991). These changes usually reduce further strains towards the

Remodelling and conserving or removing bone

Over approximately 4 months a typical remodelling basic multicellular unit (BMU) replaces a small packet of older bone with new bone (Frost, 1986; Martin and Burr, 1989; Heaney, 1993), for example, the secondary osteon (Figure 2.5). By changing how much bone completed BMUs resorb and make, remodelling can conserve or remove bone but does not normally add to it (Frost, 1990b). Here 'remodelling' means by BMUs. Remodelling normally repairs microdamage, an important if belatedly accepted function (Frost, 1986; Burr, 1993; Heaney, 1993; Parfitt, 1993). Remodelling usually *removes* bone where strains stay below an MESr strain range, as in disuse (Table 2.5), but *conserves* it where strains exceed that range (Frost, 1990b; Burr and Martin, 1992).

In summary, global remodelling can remove or conserve but does not normally add to and strengthen bone. It also repairs microdamage. The MESr distinguishes mechanically needed from unneeded bone during normal MU.

There are a number of questions which should be asked by physiotherapists working in the musculoskeletal area.

1. Which *mechanisms* determine bone mass and strength? In children longitudinal bone growth adds new trabecular bone and length to cortical bone. Then modelling can thicken and strengthen both, while remodelling can conserve or remove them. Adults lack longitudinal growth and effective cortical bone modelling, so remodelling mostly controls conservation of the bone mass and strength they accumulated during growth (Frost, 1986, 1993; Jee, 1989). Hence this is a reason to encourage children to accumulate good bone banks (see next).
2. What *controls* those mechanisms? MU exerts the most important control over them.
   (a) For bone mass and strength. In children increased MU tends to increase the above additions and to reduce losses from remodelling, so bone mass and strength increase. Disuse reduces such gains and increases the losses, so bone mass and strength decrease. In adults who lack longitudinal growth and efficient modelling of cortical bone, the remodelling responses to MU control most conservation and losses of bone (Frost, 1986, 1992; Burr and Martin, 1992).

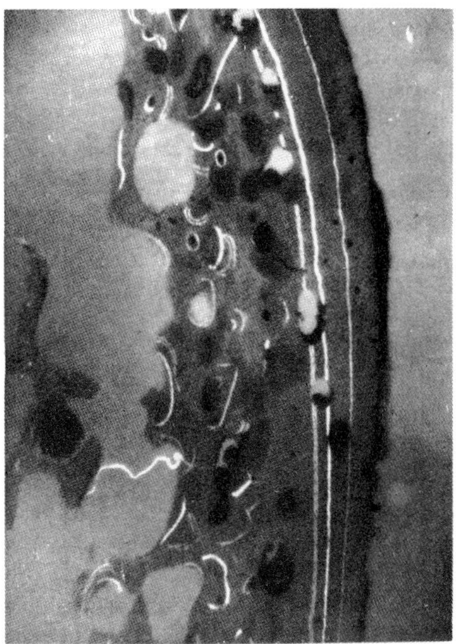

Figure 2.5 Modelling and remodelling. Undecalcified cross-section of the cutaneous cortex, sixth rib, of an adolescent girl, removed at cardiac surgery. Blue-light fluorescence microscopy, magnification about 5×. Periosteal surface on the right, marrow cavity on the left. The bright bands are bone labels of tetracycline taken for infections three times in the past. The long, vertical white bands on the right label periosteal lamellar bone formation drifts, which were faster near the top than the bottom of the Figure. The short white arcs to the left of the drifts are secondary osteons labelled during their formation. Newer osteons partly replaced many of them and remodelling basic multicellular units (BMUs) produced all of them. This whole cortex was drifting towards the reader's right. A stray cotton fibre fluoresces in the marrow cavity towards the bottom (reprinted by permission: Frost, H.M. (1963) *Introduction to Biomechanics.* Springfield: Charles C. Thomas)

bottom of this MESm range, an arrangement that makes bones very strong. Since the MESm normally lies below the microdamage threshold of bone (Table 2.5), modelling keeps strains below that threshold also (Jee *et al.*, 1991; Frost, 1992).

In summary, global modelling can add to and strengthen bone but does not normally remove and weaken it. During normal MU, the MESm indicates whether and where a bone needs strengthening.

Throughout life the largest loads and strains have far more influence on bone mass and strength than small ones. This gives weight lifters stronger bones than marathon runners (Frost, 1986).

MU effects dominate non-mechanical ones long thought to be more important, but which can help or hinder the MU ones (Frost, 1986; Jee and Frost, 1992). Examples of non-mechanical influences include: Vitamin D, calcium and protein in the diet; the adrenal cortical, growth, parathyroid and sex hormones; homoeostatic needs; genetics, some drugs.

(b) For microdamage. Some hormones, drugs and diseases can depress microdamage repair in bone, and in fibrous tissues (Frost, 1986; Schnitzler, 1993), causing stress fractures, tendon and ligament ruptures and aseptic necroses of the hip, knee and humeral head (Frost, 1986). Although agents that improve microdamage repair should exist, future research must find and prove them.

3. What are the explanations for some of the problems encountered in sports medicine? True bone pain in athletes, special forces trainees or patients with other problems usually reflects increased microdamage, which may cause local inflammation also. Greatly reducing the vigor of the MU that caused this pain usually lets microdamage repair catch up to the need, but that can take many months (Frost, 1992).

4. How long does it take for adaptation to occur? Throughout life a BMU needs at least 4 months to repair a bit of microdamage. In children, modelling needs similar time to react effectively to increased vigor of MU (Frost, 1986; Frost 1990a, b). Many factors (ageing, disease, genetic influences, drugs) can prolong those times but *so far nothing has been found to shorten them*, including drugs, hormones and, sorry to say, all treatment methods in use in physical therapy and rehabilitation medicine, and by athletic coaches and trainers. Although agents that could shorten them should exist, future research must find and prove them also.

5. How can adaptation be maximized? Firstly the vigor of the MU that caused the microdamage should be greatly decreased. This should be done for the months bone needs to adapt to the need. The vigor of new strenuous activity should be increased slowly towards maximum, over 6–12 months (Frost, 1986) Physiotherapists should also know that aggressive training can sometimes increase muscle strength faster than bone, tendon and ligament can adapt to it. This regimen has obvious applications to the postoperative management of bone and ligament repair and reconstruction.

6. How can one distinguish microdamage in fibrous tissues? Distinguishing true bone pain from the pain caused by excessive microdamage in ligament, tendon and fascia (Charley horse, fascitis, shin splints, tendinitis) requires diagnostic acumen and experience and, even with this, is not always possible. Excessive fibrous tissue microdamage usually results from any regimen based upon the timeframe for adaptation of bone outlined in the answer to question 4.

7. How does research guide us with healing problems? *Small* strains, in the MESm region, of a healing fracture or spinal fusion probably improve their healing (Frost, 1989). Achieving this outcome can pose problems, however, because very small loads cause such small strains in healing tissues, and apply trivial loads to them, but they may accrue more from this phenomenon than from the gross joint and limb motion itself.

8. Are there other roles for bone remodelling? In the past many assumed that the major function of remodelling lay in controlling the blood calcium and acid–base status (homoeostasis). However, this is not so (Jee and Frost, 1992), although some clinicians do not yet understand this. The role of remodelling in microdamage repair and control of bone conservation and loss for mechanical requirements usually dominates its homoeostatic function (Martin and Burr, 1989; Jee *et al.*, 1991; Jee and Frost, 1992; Burr, 1993; Parfitt, 1993).

Adaptations of muscle and connective tissue

R. Herbert

Muscles and connective tissues perform fundamentally important roles. Firstly, and most obviously, muscles *actively* generate forces which move body segments. Muscle forces interact with gravitational forces and forces associated with the acceleration of body segments to produce controlled movement. If muscles become unable to generate tension, normal motor performance may be impaired. Normal motor performance also requires that muscles be able to appropriately gradate the tension which they produce, and sustain the production of tension for the duration of the task.

Both muscles and connective tissues also perform an equally important *passive* role. They function to constrain the movement of joints so that other body tissues are not injured, and so that the muscles are able to act effectively to move body segments. This is no more evident than in the spine, because the spinal column is an inherently unstable structure. During the performance of almost any task in which the trunk is upright, the paraspinal muscles and ligaments act to constrain intervertebral motion, preventing subluxation of adjacent vertebrae (Crisco and Panjabi, 1990). Muscles need not always actively contract to perform this role, as it is possible that some muscles generate functionally significant amounts of passive tension with the amounts of stretch they experience during task performance. Of course muscles and connective tissue must not overly constrain joint motion – the spine cannot function effectively as rigid column. Clearly muscles and connective tissues must prevent potentially damaging movement at joints, but they must also permit sufficient movement for task performance.

The mechanical properties of muscle and connective tissues can undergo functionally significant changes as a result of trauma, pathology of non-traumatic origins, or as an adaptation to altered patterns of use.

Trauma alters the mechanical properties of muscle or connective tissue when, for example, a joint is forced through a greater than usual degree of stretch (for reviews see Woo and Buckwalter (1988)). Under these conditions muscles, tendons or ligaments can tear. With a complete tear, tissues become unable to produce forces which act on the skeletal system. Muscles may also experience contusion injuries in which muscle fibres are damaged by a direct blow. Contusion injuries can impair the ability of muscle to actively generate tension, and they can initiate pathological changes in muscle which alter the muscle's passive properties as well.

Trauma may also act to damage the nervous system. Damage to upper motor neurons (for example, head injury or cervical or thoracic spinal cord injury) or lower motor neurons (for example, lumbar spinal nerve injury or peripheral nerve lesions) may result in weakness (Guttman, 1976; Vinken *et al.*, 1990; Sunderland, 1978).

Pathologies of non-traumatic origin include neuropathies (such as Guillain Barré), myopathies (such as the muscular dystrophies) and connective tissue diseases (such as rheumatoid arthritis). For overviews see Walton (1974, 1985), Hughes (1977), Mastaglia and Walton (1982), Dyck *et al.* (1984) and Millikan *et al.* (1987).

Adaptations to altered patterns of use

Many of the pathologies mentioned above cause restriction of joint movement and disuse of muscles. For example, a person with a recent rotator cuff tear may be capable of full arm elevation, but may choose not to elevate the arm because movement of the shoulder causes severe pain. In effect the person's shoulder joint complex is immobilized by pain. As another example, following fracture of the humeral shaft the joints of the shoulder complex may be intentionally immobilized, because this facilitates fracture healing. The consequence, again, is that muscles and connective tissues are deprived of movement and stretch, and muscles experience disuse. In general, pathologies may act both directly to alter the mechanical properties of muscle and connective tissues (e.g. a tendon avulsion may prevent muscles from generating force) and indirectly to initiate deleterious tissue adaptations (in this example by initiating muscle atrophy and muscle shortening). Sometimes the indirect effects, adaptations of tissues to altered patterns of use, are referred to as 'complications' of the original pathology, which tends to obscure the fact that they may ultimately have a greater impact on function than the primary pathology.

Muscles and connective tissues are remarkable for the degree to which they can adapt their mechanical properties to the mechanical environment. Muscles respond to immobilization at short lengths by becoming shorter, less extensible and less able to produce or sustain force. The peri-articular connective tissues (specifically, ligaments and joint capsule) respond to immobilization in a less consistent way; some connective tissues become inextensible, whereas others become more extensible.

Adaptations of the mechanical properties of muscle and connective tissues cause disability in two ways. Firstly, they can directly affect the ability to perform motor tasks. Prolonged immobilization and disuse can initiate adaptations which can impede the performance of everyday tasks, such as standing up and walking. For example, a person who experiences prolonged immobilization after a femoral shaft fracture may be unable, following the period of immobilization, to ascend stairs independently because of immobilization-induced muscle weakness and joint stiffness. At the other extreme, subtle musculoskeletal adaptations, such as 'tightness' in key muscle groups, can impair optimal performance in elite sports-people. The prevention and treatment of adaptations of muscle and connective tissues that impede the performance of motor tasks is a core part of the practice of musculoskeletal physiotherapy.

It is also thought that adaptations of muscle and connective tissues can produce disability in a more indirect way, by causing excessive stress on the body and thereby painful tissue damage. For example, it is widely held that short structures lateral to the patella can cause patellar misalignment and retropatellar pain (McConnell, 1993), and that muscle tightness or weakness that flattens the normal lumbar lordosis can stress intervertebral discs, causing low back pain (McKenzie, 1981). The idea that adaptation of muscles and connective tissues can be a cause of many sorts of musculoskeletal pain underlies the concern of many physiotherapists with 'posture' or the alignment of body parts (see Gould and Davies (1985), Donatelli and Wooden (1989) and Kendall *et al.* (1993) for more examples). Implicitly, abnormal posture and the resulting abnormal stresses are thought to be the result of maladaptation of muscles or connective tissues (and sometimes also, of inappropriate activation of muscles). The concept is intuitively appealing because it means that some

sorts of musculoskeletal pain can be understood in terms of problems that are amenable to treatment; they therefore need not be seen as being of unknown cause, the treatment of which is guided by the behaviour of symptoms alone. At present, the working hypotheses of the mechanical causes of various sorts of pain are driven by clinical observations and to a lesser degree by biomechanical and orthopaedic research, but they mostly lack tight empirical support. It is hoped that, over the next few decades, the relationship between 'poorly functioning' muscles and connective tissues and the development of musculoskeletal pain will become better understood.

Many clinical syndromes are associated with immobilization and disuse. Sometimes, with these syndromes, it is not clear whether the signs with which the person presents primarily reflect the basic pathology, or whether they result from adaptation to the patient's altered patterns of movement. One example is the loss of mobility commonly seen after injury and surgical repair to the flexor tendons of the fingers. Until recently it was thought that the tendon 'adhesions' which form on the surface of the healing tendon and which restrict joint movement were a necessary part of the tendon repair process. More recently it has been demonstrated that fewer adhesions are produced when the fingers and wrist are immobilized for the shortest possible duration, suggesting that the adhesions are as much a consequence of immobilization as of the injury itself (Gelberman *et al.*, 1983; Gelberman and Manske, 1987; Gelberman and Woo, 1989).

Much has been written on the causes of musculoskeletal pathology. However, while an enormous range of musculoskeletal pathologies cause disability, they are largely beyond the influence of conservative physical treatment – physiotherapists cannot repair torn muscles or influence the progress of muscle pathology in Duchenne muscular dystrophy. Conservative physical treatment can, however, profoundly influence the adaptations of muscle and connective tissues to altered patterns of use. By manipulating the mechanical environment of the tissues (for example, by giving stretches or prescribing exercise) physiotherapists can prevent or reverse disabling adaptations.

The remainder of this section describes some of the immobilization and training-induced changes in mechanical properties of muscle and connective tissues which may adversely or positively affect the function of the musculoskeletal system.

Disuse weakness and training

When muscles are immobilized in casts, or by traction, bed-rest or pain, they become deprived of the tension which they normally experience, i.e. they experience disuse. In response, disused muscles lose the ability to generate tension, and the person becomes weak [for reviews see St-Pierre and Gardiner (1987) and Herbert (1993a)]. The time course of the development of this process is highly variable, especially in the heterogeneous population of patients with whom physiotherapists usually deal, but mean strength losses of 30–60% with 5 weeks of bed-rest or cast immobilization are typical (Herbert, 1993a). Chronic low-level disuse, such as may occur in response to arthritic disease, may induce equally significant strength losses. This degree of weakness is likely to impair motor function in many people, particularly those whose strength before the period of immobilization only marginally exceeded their requirements for normal function.

Disuse is often accompanied by clinically observable wasting of tissues. The circumference of disused limbs decreases, in the most extreme cases to apparently little more than the circumference of the underlying bones. Measures of limb circumference do not, however, provide a good measure of muscle atrophy (or, more specifically, of the decrease in muscle cross-sectional area, which is the most important determinant of muscle force-generating capacity) because tissues other than muscle also atrophy, and because there may be large differences in the amount of atrophy in different muscle groups crossing one joint (Davies and Sargeant, 1975; Ingemmann-Hansen and Halkjaer-Kristensen, 1980; Young *et al.*, 1982). For experimental purposes, reasonably reliable measures of muscle or muscle fibre cross-sectional area can be obtained by muscle biopsy, ultrasonography, computed tomography (CT) scans or nuclear magnetic resonance (NMR) imaging. Even with these techniques, valid measures are difficult to obtain, not least because of the complex architecture of most major human muscle groups (Fukunaga *et al.*, 1992). The best available data suggest that the magnitude of the atrophy varies from muscle to muscle, and it probably also depends on the degree of disuse that the muscle experiences, the muscle's biochemical characteristics, and the length at which the muscle was immobilized [for reviews see St Pierre and Gardiner, (1987) and Herbert (1993a)]. It might be expected that decreases in muscle cross-sectional area would occur in proportion to the degree of muscle weakness, because in normal (non-immobilized) muscles tetanic tension is approximately proportional to muscle cross-sectional area. However, when decreases in muscle cross-sectional area have been measured, they have usually been found to be much less than the decrease in strength (McDougall *et al.*, 1980; Le Blanc *et al.*, 1988; Wigerstad-Lossing *et al.*, 1988; Rutherford *et al.*, 1990).

There are several explanations of why strength may decline much more than the data for muscle or fibre cross-sectional area would predict. Perhaps the most compelling is that, with disuse, people become less able to activate motor units at sufficiently high frequencies to obtain near-tetanic muscle contractions. Some electromyographical studies provide support for this hypothesis (e.g. Duchateau and Hainaut, 1987, 1990), although electromyographical studies may be biased by changes in tissue impedance and muscle fibre dimensions that accompany immobilization. A few animal studies suggest that immobilization (particularly in a shortened position) may decrease the specific tension of muscle, so that the amount of tension produced per unit of muscle cross-sectional area becomes less (e.g. Edgerton *et al.*, 1975; Witzmann *et al.*, 1982a). There is also a more mundane explanation. It could be that the methods used to measure muscle cross-sectional area grossly underestimate the atrophy that occurs because they are incapable of accounting for complex muscle architectures.

Disuse adaptations of muscle cross-sectional area and muscle strength appear to be largely reversible, at least in some circumstances. One study found that even without structured exercise the weight and tension-generating ability of rat hindlimb muscles returned to near-normal values within 28 days of termination of a 6-week period of immobilization (Witzmann *et al.*, 1982b). This suggests that demands put upon the neuromuscular system in the performance or attempted performance of everyday motor tasks provide a powerful stimulus for favourable adaptations to occur. Nevertheless some clinical reports suggest that some people still have less than normal strength several years after knee injury and reconstruction (e.g. Rutherford *et al.*, 1990). It is widely believed, although not yet clearly demonstrated, that structured exercise provided by therapists can hasten recovery after a period of disuse, and, where complete recovery would not have occurred, exercise can produce a better recovery of strength.

The effect of exercise on able-bodied subjects is less ambiguous. There is no doubt that well-designed training programmes can cause large and rapid increases in strength. Over the past few decades an enormous volume of research has been directed towards explicating the mechanisms by which these strength increases are mediated. Despite a major research effort, however, the mechanisms remain obscure.

One mechanism which certainly does mediate training-induced increases in muscle strength is muscle hypertrophy. Measures of fibre and muscle cross-sectional areas made before and after training using muscle biopsies or ultrasound, CT scan or NMR imaging procedures demonstrate hypertrophy with training (Narici *et al.*, 1989). Typically, measurable muscle hypertrophy is not manifested until several weeks after the start of training (see McDonagh and Davies (1984) for review).

In addition, it has been suggested that training may bring about an increased ability to activate muscle, and that this could increase voluntary force production. Evidence for this comes from studies that have measured changes in electromyography (EMG), motor neuron excitability or muscle fibre membrane excitability. Also, the observations that training responses are largely specific to the type of contractions employed in training, manifest contralaterally, and may be induced by imagined contractions all support the view that increases in strength are neurally mediated (Sale, 1987, 1992; Enoka, 1988; Yue and Cole 1992). In contrast, measures of muscle activation suggest that, at least during isometric contraction of isolated muscle groups, most subjects can activate their muscles almost fully before training (Jones and Rutherford, 1987; Gandevia and McKenzie, 1988), which might suggest that the training effect is **not** mediated neurally, and perhaps that it is mediated instead by an increase in muscle-specific tension.

A common problem is that none of the proposed mechanisms seem capable of explaining the magnitude of strength increases observed in the early stages of a training programme. This may be because of technical problems, many of the measurements of muscle cross-sectional area and activation employed in research to date have been fraught with such problems. Perhaps with the better muscle imaging procedures (Fukunaga *et al.*, 1992; Narici *et al.*, 1992) and better measures of activation now available (Hales and Gandevia, 1988) these issues may soon be resolved.

At a more behavioural level, the literature provides some useful guidelines for the prescription of exercise aimed at increasing muscle strength [for reviews see Atha (1981) McDonagh and Davies (1984) and Herbert (1993a)]. Most importantly, studies on able-bodied subjects clearly indicate that, if training is to be effective, it must employ high intensity contractions (McDonagh and Davies, 1984). As a rule of thumb, the most rapid increases in strength can be obtained when subjects train with weights no lighter than the weight they can just lift 10 times without resting (Berger, 1962). Fewer data are available for the prescription of isometric exercise, but it appears that optimal isometric training programmes should also employ high but submaximal intensity contractions (Szeto *et al.*, 1989). There is some evidence that both isometric and dynamic training programmes will be most effective if training is structured so that it induces fatigue (Davies and Young, 1983; Rooney *et al.*, 1994). This can be done by ensuring that subjects continue lifting training weights without rest until they can perform no further lifts (Rooney *et al.*, 1994), or, for isometric exercise, by sustaining contractions (Davies and Young, 1983) and perhaps by employing brief rests between contractions.

The response to training is often said to be training specific, i.e. the increases in strength are most evident with the type of contractions employed in training [for reviews see Sale (1987, 1992); and Herbert (1993a)]. The implications of this phenomenon for training are discussed by Carr and Shepherd in the final section of this chapter.

A concern amongst clinicians has been that intense exercise may damage the muscles of people with neuromuscular disorders such as Duchenne muscular dystrophy or poliomyelitis (Bennett and Knowlton, 1958; Johnson and Braddom, 1971). Fear of inducing 'overwork weakness', as it is sometimes called, has made many therapists reluctant to provide intensive exercise programmes for people with neuromuscular disorders. However, evidence for the existence of overwork weakness is not strong (Vignos, 1983). In fact, both moderate and high-intensity training programmes have been shown to induce rapid strength increases in some patients (McCartney *et al.*, 1988; Milner-Brown and Miller, 1988). The current consensus appears to be that suitably intense exercise can safely be prescribed for people with mild or moderate weakness, provided that the exercise is introduced gradually and is carefully supervised. In carefully selected patients, exercise may prolong functional independence.

Adaptive muscle shortening

Clinicians have known for a long time that, under some conditions, an increase in the resistance of resting muscles to stretch may limit the amount of movement at joints. This phenomenon, perhaps one of the most functionally significant adaptations of muscle, has been called many things, including 'contracture', 'muscle shortening' and 'muscle tightness'. I will use the term 'adaptive shortening' of muscles when referring to this phenomenon.

Only in the past few decades have significant insights been gained into the nature of adaptive muscle shortening. Most of these have come from studies in which animals have been immobilized in casts [for reviews see Gossman *et al.* (1982), O'Dwyer *et al.* (1989), Herbert (1988, 1993b)]. Other models of muscle shortening (including congenital spasticity, the injection of tetanus toxin and bone shortening procedures) have demonstrated changes in muscle that are broadly similar to those induced by cast immobilization, but it is not yet clear how well these models represent the problems of adaptive muscle shortening seen by physiotherapists in clinical practice.

When an animal limb is immobilized so that some muscles are held in their most shortened position, the length of the muscle–tendon units decreases and the muscles become stiffer (Herbert and Balnave, 1993). Some of these changes can be attributed to changes in muscle tissue. Specifically, fibres of adaptively shortened muscles are usually found to have fewer sarcomeres in series and a greater proportion of their volume is comprised of connective tissue (Tabary *et al.*, 1972; Williams and Goldspink, 1978; Józsa *et al.*, 1990; but see Heslinga and Huijing, 1993). Changes in muscle morphology such as these may be responsible for decreasing the length and increasing the stiffness of muscle tissue, and they affect the contractile properties of the muscle too. The effect of sarcomere loss is to cause fibres to develop their greatest active tensions at shorter lengths and over a shorter range of lengths (Williams and Goldspink, 1978; Witzmann *et al.*, 1982a). Sarcomere number increases in fibres of muscles immobilized in a lengthened position, and this means that the length at which these muscles are best able to develop tension becomes greater than normal (Williams and Goldspink, 1978).

Changes in the tendinous portion of muscle have been much less extensively investigated than the changes in muscle fibres. One of the first studies of adaptation of tendon length found significant length and compliance changes in the part of the tendon that blends with the muscle belly (the 'tendinous aponeurosis' or 'tendon plate'; Heslinga and Huijing, 1993) of immobilized rat gastrocnemius. In the immobilized rabbit soleus muscle, nearly two-thirds of the decrease in length of the muscle–tendon unit occurs in the tendon (Crosbie and Herbert, unpublished data). Perhaps this is not surprising, because in normal rabbit soleus muscle, as with many important human muscles, the tendon constitutes the greater part of the length of the muscle–tendon unit.

One of the most important findings to come from studies on length adaptation in muscles is that the length of the muscle and tendon adapt to the position at which the muscle is habitually held: if the muscle is immobilized in a shortened position, it becomes short, but if it is immobilized in a lengthened position, it does not. Muscle shortening is, therefore, a response to deprivation of stretch, rather than to deprivation of movement. By implication, treatment aimed at preventing or treating adaptive muscle shortening should involve ensuring muscles receive adequate stretch. Little is known about what constitutes an adequate stretch to maintain the length of muscles, but animal studies suggest that relatively short durations of stretch (30 min every day in mouse soleus muscle) is sufficient to maintain the length of muscles immobilized in a shortened position (Williams, 1990). The available human studies are less prescriptive. Perhaps the best trial to date, a clinical trial on non-ambulatory nursing home residents with knee flexion 'contractures' (which may have been the result of adaptive muscle shortening or adaptations of other soft tissues) has shown that low-load prolonged stretch is more effective at increasing joint range of motion than briefer high load stretches (Light *et al.*, 1984).

Insufficient connective tissue extensibility

Connective tissues have sometimes been thought of as relatively incapable of adapting their mechanical properties. However, the connective tissues that surround joints can undergo functionally significant changes within the periods of immobilization that are commonly seen clinically.

Studies on immobilized rabbit joints indicate that, when taken together, the connective tissues that surround the knee (i.e. all the tissues that cross the knee except muscle–tendon units and skin) become stiff in the flexion–extension direction with prolonged immobilization [for review see Akeson *et al.* (1980)]. But immobilization also causes some ligaments to become less stiff [Noyes, 1977; see Woo (1986) for a brief review]. Together these findings translate in clinical terms to a loss of range of motion at the joint and an increase in joint laxity. These changes have been found to be at least partly reversible in animal studies (Akeson *et al.*, 1977), although animal studies may not provide good models of chronic immobilization following injury which is often seen clinically. There are many clinical cases where people develop intractably stiff joints, or permanently lax (and sometimes, therefore, unstable) joints.

After injury, musculoskeletal tissues undergo repair. These repair processes are imperfect, at least in that a generic connective tissue (scar) is used to replace specialized connective tissues (scar tissue is the 'Spak-filla' or 'boggo' of the musculoskeletal system). Scar tissue performs a 'quick-fix' role by rapidly providing structural integrity for injured tissues, but it is often mechanically inferior to the original tissues [for a review see Hardy (1989)]. In particular, in binding together damaged parts of one tissue, scar may adhere injured tissues to other tissues (for example, muscle may adhere to skin or bone, and tendons may adhere to tendon sheaths) preventing the motion between tissues which must occur with normal joint movement. A consequence can be the loss of a normal range of joint movement.

Long after injury and immobilization, muscle, tendon and ligament remain mechanically inferior to uninjured tissues – they tear at lower forces, and they are capable of absorbing less energy before tearing [for review see Järvinen and Lehto (1993)]. However, injured muscles, tendons and ligaments undergo smaller losses of strength when the period of immobilization is minimized. This indicates that at least part of the decrease in tensile strength can be attributed to the effects of immobilization following injury. While some degree of immobilization is usually necessary to prevent further damage to injured tissues in the period immediately after injury, these findings suggest that the duration of immobilization should be kept as short as possible without risking further injury.

Skill learning after musculoskeletal lesions

J. Carr and R. Shepherd

A theoretical framework for skill learning in rehabilitation

The process of clinical reasoning in physiotherapy practice requires an understanding of the problems with which the disabled person presents and the processes involved in recovery including the regaining of skill. Information is relevant, therefore, if it relates to the underlying pathological and adaptive mechanisms and the effects of these mechanisms on normal functioning.

Since movement is the only means by which we can interact with the environment, any breakdown of normal motor control, whether through disease, injury or disuse of the musculoskeletal system, will affect the individual's ability to produce goal-directed movements and interact with the environment. Clinical reasoning also involves, therefore, an understanding of the importance of context and task in the organization of skilled movement, as well as of the naturally occurring morphological, musculoskeletal and biomechanical constraints. The individual with movement dysfunction is faced not only with having to cope with the demands normally imposed by the environment but also with the changing demands imposed by the damaged and/or recovering musculoskeletal system.

In rehabilitation, the physiotherapist is concerned not only with the physical treatment of symptoms (such as pain, joint stiffness or muscle weakness) but also with the restoration of health, physical fitness and optimal functional motor performance. This section is concerned with the theoretical basis of that part of clinical reasoning that has to do with the planning and implementation of what could be called restorative motor training; that is, training to regain skilled performance in those actions relevant to the individual recovering from a lesion of the musculoskeletal system.

Physiotherapy intervention is based on theoretical assumptions regarding how movement is controlled and organized, what happens when the neuromusculoskeletal system is damaged and how recovery takes place. The last two decades have seen a substantial increase in the number of investigations into human movement, the results of which require a change in our underlying assumptions and, therefore, a change in practice. Recent scientific investigations have provided new information related to such aspects of movement as: its neural control and dyscontrol; skill learning; the biomechanical characteristics of functional motor tasks and the changes in these when motor control is impaired; the effects of environmental factors on movement control; muscle adaptability; and the muscle length and velocity-specific effects of exercise. Part of the process of clinical reasoning involves deriving implications from relevant scientific research, whether in the physiological, behavioural or health sciences. Such research enables the development of a theoretical framework for rehabilitation and the generation of hypotheses that can be tested in the clinic.

A brief historical perspective

Rehabilitation in large part is a learning process in which individuals must regain the ability to perform previously well-learned skills, for example, reaching for an object, standing up from a seated position, walking, or serving in tennis. Some individuals must master new skills, for example, walking with crutches or a prosthesis, or moving by means of a wheelchair. Physiotherapists intervene in the learning process to facilitate the regaining of mastery in the performance of actions. Learning is an abstract concept and difficult to define. Generally motor learning is viewed as a set of processes involving practice and exercise leading to a relatively stable change in motor behaviour (Schmidt, 1988). It involves the acquisition of the ability to perform an action effectively in a flexible manner in different environmental contexts.

In the early 1970s, Gentile (1972) published a seminal article which examined learning as a function of the interaction of the individual and the environment in the pursuit of goal attainment. The focus of Gentile's article was the understanding of movement as it becomes organized and differentiated in varying environmental contexts. This was shortly followed by other influential papers by, for example, Schmidt (1975), Martenuik (1976) and Stelmach (1978) who viewed movement as the product of a centrally represented and generalized motor programme. This period marked the beginning of an intense focus within the field of motor learning on understanding movement itself and on investigating issues of motor control. [For reviews of theories of skill learning and related experimental studies see Newell (1981), Johnson (1984), Gentile (1987) and Schmidt (1988)].

Over the last two or three decades the study of movement has been influenced in particular by the ecological perspectives of Gibson (1966) in the study of perceptual processes, and by the perspective of the Russian physiologist, Bernstein (1967). Out of this work has developed a dynamic systems approach in which the structure of movement is seen as emergent, dynamic and responsive to both internal and external mechanisms.

In the Gibsonian view, vision is not only considered as an exteroceptive sense but also as a proprioceptive sense, providing subjects with information about their own movements and playing an essential role in the regulation of action (Gibson, 1986). In order to investigate this theory, Lee and Aronson (1974) and Lee and Lishman (1975) had subjects stand on a stable floor surrounded by a movable chamber made of three walls and a ceiling. The question of interest was how subjects would respond when the surrounding chamber was moved. Normal adults swayed in relation to the movement of the room, i.e. when the wall in front of the subjects approached them, subjects swayed backward and when the wall receded, the subjects swayed forward. In some instances, small children over-corrected and fell over when the wall approached them. It appeared that subjects in both experiments were responding to visual inputs even when other inputs (e.g. proprioception) would have provided contradictory (and, in this case, accurate) information.

Bernstein (1967) was instrumental in pointing out the need to understand the biomechanical or dynamic characteristics of linked segments, what he called the problem of coordinating and controlling a complex system of biokinetic links. He noted the need for movement organization to be in some way simplified. Such simplifications may involve constructing functional linkages or synergies (Gelfand *et al.*, 1971; Turvey *et al.*, 1982), or forming a simplified 'virtual' limb as suggested for reaching to grasp (Greene, 1982; Arbib *et al.*, 1986).

Bernstein (1967) recognized that the study of movement could not simply focus on the muscle forces produced by the individual but must also include inertial and reactive forces. It is important in rehabilitation to be aware that, during active movement, the dynamic coupling that exists between body segments can bring about movement at joints that are distant from the site of active movement. That is to say, joint torques may result from mechanical linkage effects as well as from muscle contraction.

Following on from Bernstein, either directly or indirectly, much of the recent human movement research has concentrated on increasing the understanding of intersegmental dynamics. Investigations of actions such as the vertical jump have contributed to an understanding of the dynamic effects of the sequencing of segmental rotation (Gregoire *et al.*, 1984; Bobbert and van Ingen Schenau, 1988). Hypotheses have been generated regarding the function of biarticular compared with monoarticular muscles (Jacobs and van Ingen Schenau, 1992).

As a consequence of this theoretical and research effort, it is generally accepted that movements of the body take place as the result of cooperative activity between muscle action and segmental movement. This activity is dynamic and flexible, enabling the individual to be effective in different environmental contexts, and to modify the action according to changing task and other demands.

Movement rehabilitation as a science has been relatively slow to take up the opportunities offered by recent research into human movement and the acquisition of skill. However, we have proposed for some years now that rehabilitation should be based on this research and have illustrated how research findings and theoretical perspectives can be utilized in clinical practice (e.g. Carr and Shepherd 1987a,b, 1989; Shepherd and Carr, 1994). It is interesting that this perspective is increasingly being seen as critical to the rehabilitation of individuals after brain damage (e.g. Anderson and Lough, 1986; Winstein and Knecht, 1990; Mulder, 1991; Malouin *et al.*, 1992). This perspective is also, however, a useful one for the physiotherapist working with individuals with lesions of the musculoskeletal system.

Wherever the lesion, whether it directly or indirectly affects the musculoskeletal system, the individual must manage to control a multisegmental linkage in order to accomplish the goals of everyday life. A lesion of the motor effector apparatus, because of the complex musculoskeletal linkages and interactive forces produced during movement, must affect neural control and the performance of everyday actions.

Adaptive motor behaviour

Recovery involves physiological changes that take place as the lesioned system repairs itself, after, for example, a muscle tear, ligament injury or surgical lesion. Recovery also involves regaining the ability to function effectively in recreation, daily living tasks, sport or workplace activity.

During the acute period, the individual functions adaptively. This may be enforced by bed-rest, splinting or pain. Such adaptive motor behaviour may persist after the symptoms have gone, particularly if the length of immobilization or disability is long; for example, after joint replacement surgery, an individual is very likely to persist with motor patterns developed during the period of pain and stiffness that developed over a considerable time before the surgery.

Immediately after a lesion of the musculoskeletal system, the individual's attempts at action reflect the emergence of adaptive motor behaviour. For example, such an adaptation may include a change in the pattern of swing phase of walking when a splint constrains the knee. This constraint demands altered biomechanics at the unconstrained joints (ankle, hip, upper body joints) if function is to be maintained. Detailed biomechanical analyses of adaptations to gait occurring as a result of functional limitations imposed by surgery and prosthetic devices have been reported, for example, by Winter *et al.* (1991). Adaptive movement seems to emerge out of what can be used of the lesioned system. To put it another way, the individual moves in the most effective way possible given the effects of the lesion (e.g. pain, stiffness), the biomechanical possibilities inherent in the musculoskeletal linkage, and the requirements of the task. The adaptations reflect, therefore, the flexibility available in the system.

Skill learning in rehabilitation: restoration of optimal functional motor performance

The major aim of physiotherapy, beyond the stage where treatment of specific symptoms may be the principal issue, is the restoration of optimal motor performance. It cannot be assumed that improvement in the presenting symptoms (e.g. pain, stiffness) will necessarily generalize into improved performance of functional activities. A study of subjects 6 weeks after hip replacement surgery (Westwood, 1993) showed, for example, that, although all the subjects had been discharged from rehabilitation, they continued to stand up from a seat using their arms to assist in propelling the body mass vertically. The subjects who were given specific training in sit-to-stand over a period of 6 weeks were able to stand up without using their arms, whereas an untrained control group were still using their arms when measured at the end of the 6 weeks. Another study (Jevsevar *et al.*, 1993) has shown that 15 subjects considered to be fully rehabilitated after knee arthroplasty had performance deficits during walking, stair ascent and descent and sit-to-stand that included decreased peak knee moments of force and decreased knee angular velocities.

In planning a training programme, the physiotherapist utilizes the results of research into motor learning or how people acquire skill in action. Training is planned to optimize motor performance to enable the individual to return to everyday life, the athlete to return to sport, the worker to the workplace, without repeating the injury. Annett (1971) has defined skill as any activity that has become better organized through practice. Skilled action is defined in terms of consistency in attaining a goal with some economy of effort through movement patterns shaped by dimensions of the performer and configured to fit the environment (Gentile, 1987). Several factors have been shown to be important in the acquisition of skill, for example, task-specific training, feedback, practice, and modification of the task or environment.

Task-specificity in training

One of the most interesting areas of research in recent times which is pertinent to rehabilitation has developed out of investigations of the task- and context-specific effects of training. This information has required a considerable shift in rehabilitation strategies used in clinical practice.

Many studies (e.g. Sale and MacDougall, 1981) report that the major changes accompanying strength training are seen in the training exercise itself. Conventional leg-extension exercises to strengthen quadriceps, for example, have been shown to increase the weight lifted (by 200%) whereas the isometric strength of the muscle increased very little (by 11%) (Rutherford and Jones, 1986).

Typically the major changes in load lifted occur early in the training period (Rutherford and Jones, 1986), suggesting that, since isometric strength does not increase much during this period, the early changes may be due to the individual becoming more skilled at the weight-lifting rather than increasing intrinsic muscle strength. In other words, the earliest changes may be due to learning, suggesting that neural factors may play the primary role in the early stages of training (Hakkinen and Komi, 1983). In an early study, Rasch and Morehouse (1957) came to a similar conclusion when they reported that subjects who performed resisted elbow flexion exercises in standing increased the strength of these muscles in standing but not in supine. From work on the specificity of postural adjustments (e.g. Nashner, 1976; Cordo and Nashner, 1982), it becomes apparent that, in performing the strengthening exercise in standing, the subjects in Rasch and Morehouse's study were learning a pattern of muscle activation specific to weight-resisted elbow flexion in standing.

Although particular muscles, for example the lower limb extensors, may need to be strong enough to generate the necessary power for such varied actions as stair climbing, sit-to-stand and cycling, the context in which the muscles must generate force varies from action to action. This means that the pattern of muscle activation differs according to task and context. As Rutherford (1988) points out, particular neural connections that become established as a result of the lower leg extensor training may not be the connections necessary for other actions. It appears that the neural adaptation that occurs as a result of training is itself specific (Sale, 1988).

The effects of exercise have been found to be *velocity-specific* (e.g. Lesmes *et al.*, 1978; Caiozzo *et al.*, 1981; Wooden *et al.*, 1992), perhaps because of velocity-specific adaptations within the muscle (by altering force–velocity characteristics of the muscle) and/or the neural system (by altering the motoneuron recruitment pattern) (Rutherford, 1988). A recent study (Ellenbecker *et al.*, 1988) reported that, although significant strength improvements in shoulder rotator muscles occurred through both concentric and isokinetic (fixed-speed, variable resistance) training, tennis serving speed increased only in the concentrically trained group of subjects.

Exercise effects have also been reported to be muscle *length-specific* (e.g. Kitai and Sale, 1989), with isometric training being followed by an increase in strength at the joint angle at which the exercise is practised (Sale and MacDougall, 1981; Lindh, 1979). There is some evidence from electromyography that there is a greater increase in motor unit activation at the joint angles trained (Thepaut-Mathieu *et al.*, 1985).

Considerable research interest centred on the differential effects of *concentric* versus *eccentric* training. Komi and Buskirk (1972) reported that eccentric exercise was followed by a greater increase in strength than concentric exercise. A characteristic of human muscle action in functional activities is its use in stretch–shortening cycles (e.g. Asmussen and Bonde-Petersen 1974; Bosco *et al.*, 1982; Komi, 1986). It is has been shown, principally in studies of the vertical jump, that eccentric muscle contraction immediately before the major concentric force generation can augment the amount of force delivered by the prime mover muscles.

Although non-specific exercise is unlikely to carry over into improved performance of specific actions, there is some evidence of a positive transfer to similar tasks (e.g. Robinson, 1927; Oxendine, 1984). In a recent study consistent with this hypothesis, Gottlieb and colleagues (1988) had their subjects perform a simple two-segment elbow flexion exercise in the frontal plane as fast as possible. Subjects flexed their elbows repetitively over a range of 54 degrees. When they were tested moving over ranges of 36, 54 and 72 degrees, although the maximum improvement occurred at the distance practised, subjects also improved their movement speed at all three distances.

The implication for rehabilitation from these studies of normal subjects is that practice of an action is necessary for there to be improvement in the performance of that action. This hypothesis is supported by a few rehabilitation or quasi-rehabilitation studies reported within the last few years. In one study of able-bodied young men (Godges *et al.*, 1993), passive hip flexor stretching and training of an isolated movement (a trunk flexion exercise) did not improve the 'economy' of walking or running as inferred from the measurement of open-circuit spirometry with subjects running on a treadmill. That is, although passive hip flexor stretching improved hip extension range of motion and trunk flexor exercises improved trunk flexor muscle performance, these isolated improvements did not affect functional activities. As the authors suggest, 'coaching' of subjects may be required so that they can integrate the localized improvements in strength and flexibility into a more efficient pattern of, in this case, walking. Baker and colleagues (1991) showed that walking training (using a treadmill) after total hip replacement (THR) was associated with a decrease in double support time and a normalization of stance/swing ratio for the affected leg. In another study of subjects after THR (Henderson *et al.*, 1992), a 6-month programme of walking and weight-bearing activities was followed by a significant increase in walking speed.

Attention

Action comprises not only motor factors but also cognitive/perceptual factors. The obvious conceptual links between knowing and doing (Newell, 1981), i.e. cognition and action, are increasingly being recognized in the movement and neurosciences. However, the emphasis in rehabilitation remains largely on the motor system and perceptual–cognitive aspects of function tend to be ignored (Mulder, 1991). This is despite an increasing body of theoretical clinical literature in which the need to recognize and incorporate the action–cognition link in rehabilitation is advocated (Carr and Shepherd, 1987a, b; Mulder, 1991).

In everyday life, virtually every movement we make is linked to an intention. As we move we are selecting, from all the information that is available (both internally derived sensations and those coming from the environment), the most essential to the task at hand. That is, we select what it is we must pay attention to (Wise and Desimone, 1988) and ignore the rest. It is unlikely, therefore, that skill in action will be (re)gained unless that action is practised under the appropriate environmental conditions. We are learning not only the appropriate motor pattern but also learning to select the most appropriate information in order to match the intention or the goal to the action and the environment (Higgins, 1972). One of the important functions of the therapist (as coach) is setting up the conditions of practice to facilitate this process.

Information: instruction, demonstration and feedback

Information about performance that is available to the learner, either before, during or after the performance, is an important factor in optimizing skill acquisition (Newell, 1981) and is, therefore, of practical importance for both therapist and patient in rehabilitation.

The most commonly used methods for conveying information about the goal and appropriate action sequences are verbal instructions and demonstrations (e.g. Newell, 1981; Johnson, 1984; Gentile, 1987). Information may focus on kinematic description, for example, angular displacements, paths of body parts and timing of action sequences, which requires an understanding by the therapist of linked segment dynamics and the biomechanical necessities of the action to be learned.

Instructions are given in such a way as to present a clear goal and to reduce uncertainty. There is evidence that individuals perform better when an action is presented as a concrete task as opposed to an abstract task. These two types of task differ in the degree to which the required action is directed toward controlling physical interaction with the environment as opposed to producing movement for its own sake.

For example, Leont'ev and Zaporzhets (1960) had patients with restricted range of motion of the elbow or shoulder as a result of injury to raise their forearm or whole arm (depending on the site of injury) in four actions that varied from abstract to concrete. The actions were to raise the arm: (1) as far as possible with eyes shut; (2) as far as possible with eyes open; (3) to a specific point on a ruled screen; and (4) to grasp an object. The results indicated that the amplitude of movement increased progressively from task 1 to task 4, i.e. as the task became more concrete. Similar results have been reported recently in children with cerebral palsy who obtained a greater range of forearm supination when the task involved supinating the forearm to beat a drum than when they were instructed to perform the more abstract task of supination for its own sake (van der Weel *et al.*, 1991).

The goal of the action and the movements to be executed can be demonstrated either live or on videotape. Empirical work on the effectiveness of demonstration, however, has been sporadic and the results equivocal. One of the reasons for equivocal results is that the videotaped demonstration is sometimes distant from actual practice in both time and place. Gonella and colleagues (1981), however, demonstrated that self-instruction using an audiovisual medium was effective in enabling normal subjects to learn the new skill of crutch walking. The hypothesis that subjects could learn the cognitive aspects of the motor task in one viewing of the film was supported and transfer of learning to the physical performance of the task was found to occur.

Feedback can be positive or negative, subjective or objective and it may motivate the learner as well as provide information. Knowledge of results (KR) is information related to achievement of the goal of the action and it is known to be one of the most potent variables in learning (Annett and Kay, 1957; Newell, 1976). A second type of feedback, commonly referred to as knowledge of performance (KP), provides information about how the movement was performed. Both KP and KR can be augmented by the therapist verbally, through demonstration and through the use of electronic devices (e.g. videotape, EMG, forceplate system). Feedback should provide clues to the learner about how to improve the next attempt.

Practice

Practice can be considered as a continuum of procedures from overt practice at one extreme to covert or mental practice at the other (Johnson, 1984). As a general rule, skill in performance increases as a direct result of the amount of practice. It has been shown, for example, that repetition of a task can improve performance, although thousands of repetitions may be necessary (Crossman, 1959; Beggs and Howarth, 1972; Kottke, 1980; Canning, 1987). Repetitive practice is known to be important for learning to occur, as the repetitions enable the system to coordinate the muscular synergies which move the segmental linkage in the desired manner to accomplish the goal of action. However, in rehabilitation, repetitive practice of an action may also be necessary to increase the strength of the muscle contractions to that necessary to accomplish the goal.

One issue of research focus which has considerable importance for rehabilitation is the whole versus part method of practice. As a general rule, it seems that the action should be practised in its entirety, particularly when one part of the action is to a large part dependent upon the performance of a preceding part. For example, several studies of sit-to-stand (Schenkman *et al.*, 1990; Pai and Rogers, 1991; Shepherd and Gentile, 1994) have pointed to the importance of trunk flexion in setting up the conditions for ascent into standing. The implications from these studies is that the vertical movement of the body mass is facilitated by the initial upper body flexion.

Performing the whole action seems important for giving the individual the idea of the action to be achieved. However, when the individual in rehabilitation is having difficulty in activating muscles and generating and timing force, it may be necessary to practise eliciting activity in a particular group of muscles, or to practise one part of the action in order to strengthen a muscle group critical to the performance of the action. Part practice should, however, be followed by an attempt at performing the entire action (Johnson, 1984). Furthermore, variable practice, i.e. practice on a range of related tasks, has been found to lead to better performance than consistent practice of the one task (e.g. Newell, 1981; Johnson, 1984; Schmidt, 1988).

In order to facilitate optimal practice conditions and increase performance of a particular action, the environment or task may need to be varied by the therapist. This could involve, for example: (1) the use of an external support such as taping (e.g. McConnell, 1993) to facilitate a muscle or group of muscles to contract and generate force at the appropriate length for a specific action; (2) practising standing up from a higher than average chair to decrease the muscle force requirements while still ensuring that the individual is strengthening leg extensor muscles in the appropriate context; (3) ensuring that crutch walking is practised not only in the protected environment of the physiotherapy area but also in a busy corridor where people and objects in the environment are moving; and (4) having patients with an injury to one hand practise bimanual tasks in order to facilitate cooperative control between hands and object and particularly to enhance timing.

Summary

The primary purpose of this section is to stress the importance of skill learning in musculoskeletal rehabilitation. This concept differs from the traditional medical model of rehabilitation in which it is expected that the effects of 'treatment' will generalize into improved functional performance. This concept is theoretically applicable to the rehabilitation of any individual with a musculoskeletal lesion which interferes with essential or desired actions. In some cases, an individual may need to practise a sporting activity in order to regain skill; in others, the most pressing need may be to specifically strengthen lower limb extensor muscles to optimize stair climbing and descent; a novel task such as walking with crutches may need to be learned; or the manner in which a task must be performed in the workplace may need to be modified to ensure that the individual's back injury is not repeated. What seems certain at the present time is that the process of rehabilitation should include practice of specific actions and that such 'exercise' is likely to be remedial in itself.

References and further reading

Clinical reasoning in physiotherapy

Barrows, H.S. and Feltovich, P.J. (1987). The clinical reasoning process. *Med. Educ.*, **21**, 86–91.

Bashook, P.G. (1976). A conceptual framework for measuring clinical problem-solving. *J. Med. Educ.*, **51**, 109–14.

Benner, P. and Tanner, C. (1987). Clinical judgement: How expert nurses use intuition. *Am. J. Nurs.*, January, 23–31.

Bordage, G. and Lemieux, M. (1986). Some cognitive characteristics of medical students with and without diagnostic reasoning difficulties. In *Proceedings of the 25th Annual Conference of Research in Medical Education of the American Association of Medical Colleges, New Orleans, Louisiana*, pp. 185–90.

Bowden, J. (1988). Achieving change in teaching practices. In *Improving Learning: New Perspectives*, (P. Ramsden, ed.), pp. 255–67, London: Kogan Page Ltd.

Browning, C., Thomas, S. and Oates, J. (1988). Clinical decision making and clinical performance. In *Proceedings of the 2nd International Health Sciences Education Conference, Sydney*.

Elstein, A.S., Shulman, L.S. and Sprafka, S.A. (1978). *Medical Problem Solving: An Analysis of Clinical Reasoning.* Cambridge, Massachusetts: Harvard University Press.

Gale, J. and Marsden, P. (1982). Clinical problem solving: the beginning of the process. *Med. Educ.*, **16**, 22–6.

Gilhooly, K.J. (1988). *Thinking: Directed, Undirected and Creative.* (2nd edn). London: Academic Press.

Glass, A.L. and Holyoak, K.J. (1986). *Cognition* (2nd edn). New York: Random House.

Grant, J. and Marsden, P. (1987). The structure of memorized knowledge in students and clinicians: an explanation for diagnostic expertise. *Med. Educ.*, **21**, 92–8.

Grant, R. (1991). Obsolence or lifelong education: choices and challenges. In *Proceedings of the World Confederation for*

Physical Therapy 11th International Congress, London

Grant, R., Jones, M. and Maitland, G.D. (1988). Clinical decision making in upper quadrant dysfunction. In *Clinics in Physical Therapy – Physical Therapy of the Cervical and Thoracic Spine* (R. Grant, ed.), pp. 51–79, New York: Churchill Livingstone.

Higgs, J. and Jones, M.A. (1995). *Clinical Reasoning in the Health Professions*. London: Butterworth-Heinemann.

Jones, M.A. (1992). Clinical reasoning in manual therapy. *Phys. Ther.*, **72**, 875–84.

Mattingly, C. (1991). The narrative nature of clinical reasoning. *Am. J. Occup. Ther.*, **45**, 998–1005.

Norman, G.R. (1988). Problem-solving skills, solving problems and problem-based learning. *Med. Educ.*, **22**, 279–86.

Norman, G.R. and Schmidt, H.G. (1992). The psychological basis of problem-based learning: a review of the evidence. *Acad. Med.*, **67**, 557–65.

Patel, V.L. and Groen, G.J. (1991). The general and specific nature of medical expertise: a critical look. In *Toward a General Theory of Expertise: Prospects and Limits* (A. Ericsson and J. Smith, eds), New York: Cambridge University Press.

Paton, O.D. (1985). Clinical reasoning process in physical therapy. *Phys. Ther.*, **65**, 924–8.

Rew, L. and Barrow, E. (1987). Intuition: a neglected hallmark of nursing knowledge. *Adv. Nurs. Sci.*, **10**, 49–62.

Ridderikhoff, J. (1989). *Methods in Medicine: A Descriptive Study of Physicians' Behaviour*. Dordrecht: Kluwer Academic Publishers.

Scadding, J.G. (1967). Diagnosis: the clinician and the computer. *Lancet*, **i**, 877–82.

Acute and chronic pain

Dubner, R. and Hargreaves, K.M. (1989). The neurobiology of pain and its modulation. *Clin. J. Pain*, **5 (Suppl. 2)**, S1–S6.

Hargreaves, K.M. and Joris, J.L. (1993). The peripheral analgesic effects of opioids. *Am. Pain Soc. J.*, **2**, 51–9.

Meller, S.T. and Gebhart, G.F. (1993). Nitric oxide (NO) and nociceptive processing in the spinal cord. *Pain*, **52**, 127–36.

Melzack, R. and Wall, P.D. (1965). Pain mechanism: a new theory. *Science*, **150**, 971.

Pert, C.B. and Sydner, S.H. (1973). Opiate receptor: demonstrated in nervous tissue. *Science*, **179**, 1011.

Schaible, H.G. and Grubb, B.D. (1993). Afferent and spinal mechanisms of joint pain. *Pain*, **55**, 5–15.

Physiology and clinical pharmacology: inflammation, pain and anti-inflammatory drugs and analgesics

Inflammation and basic pathology

Cotran R.S., Kumar, V. and Robbins S.L. (eds) (1989). *Robbins Pathologic Basis of Disease* (4th edn). Philadelphia: W.B. Saunders.

Rheumatology

Klippel, J.H. and Dieppe P.A. (eds) (1994). *Rheumatology*. London: Mosby.

Immunology

Roitt, I.M. (1991). *Essential Immunology*, (7th edn). Oxford: Blackwell Scientific Publications.

Pharmacology

Goodman-Gilman, A., Rall, T.W., Nies, A.W. and Taylor, P. (1990). *Goodman and Gilman's The Pharmacological Basis of Therapeutics*. New York: McGraw-Hill.

Anti-inflammatory drugs

Williams, K.M., Day, R.O. and Breit, S.N. (1993). Biochemical actions and clinical pharmacology of anti-inflammatory drugs. *Adv. Drug Res.*, **24**, 121–98.

Pain

Victorian Medical Postgraduate Foundation (1992). *Analgesic Guidelines*, (2nd edn).

Biomechanics of joint movements

Akeson, W.H., Woo, S.L.Y., Amiel, D. and Matthews, J.V. (1974). Biomechanical and biochemical changes in the periarticular connective tissue during contracture development in the immobilised rabbit knee. *Connect. Tissue Res.*, **2**, 315–23.

Berme, N., Engin, A.E. and de Silva, K.M.C. (1985). *Biomechanics of Normal and Pathological Human Articulating Joints*. Dordrecht: Martinus Nijhoff.

Goel, V.K., Goyal, S., Clark, C., Nishiyama, K. and Nye, T. (1985). Kinematics of the whole lumbar spine: effect of discectomy. *Spine*, **10**, 543–54.

Lee, M. and Svensson, N.L. (1993). Effect of frequency on response of the spine to lumbar posteroanterior forces. *J. Manipulative Physiol. Ther.*, **16**, 439–46.

MacConaill, M.A. (1964). Joint movements. *Physiotherapy*, **50**, 359–67.

Maitland, G.D. (1986). *Vertebral Manipulation*, London: Butterworth-Heinemann.

Woltring, H.J., Huiskes, R., de Lange, A. and Veldpaus, F.E. (1985). Finite centroid and helical axis estimation from noisy landmark measurements in the study of human joint kinematics. *J. Biomech.*, **18**, 378–89.

Descriptions of joint movement

Lee, M. and Moseley, A. (1994). *Dynamics of the Human Body* (3rd edn). Sydney: Zygal.

Passive joint movements

MacConaill, M.A. and Basmajian, J.V. (1969). *Muscles and Movements*. Baltimore: Williams and Wilkins.

Williams, P.L., Warwick, R., Dyson, M. and Bannister, L.H. (1989). *Gray's Anatomy* (37th edn). Edinburgh: Churchill Livingstone.

Passive joint dynamics

Herbert, R. (1993). Preventing and treating stiff joints. In *Key Issues in Musculoskeletal Physiotherapy* (J. Crosbie and J. McConnell, eds.), Sydney: Butterworth-Heinemann.

Instability

Lee, M. (1991). *Introduction to the Analysis of Human Movement* (2nd edn). Sydney: Zygal.

Pope, M.H. and Panjabi, M.M. (1985). Biomechanical definitions of spinal instability. *Spine*, **10**, 55–6.

White, A.A. and Panjabi, M.M. (1990). *Clinical Biomechanics of the Spine*, (2nd edn). Sydney: J.B. Lippincott.

Bone: recent concepts important to musculoskeletal physiotherapy

Biewener, A.A. (1993). Safety factors in bone strength. *Calcif. Tissue Int.*, **53**, (Suppl.), 68–74.

Burr, D.B. (1993). Remodelling and the repair of fatigue damage. *Calcif. Tissue Int.*, **53**, (Suppl.), 75–81.

Burr, D.B. and Martin, R.B. (1992). Mechanisms of bone adaptation to the mechanical environment. *Triangle (Ciba-Geigy)*, **31**, 59–76.

Frost, H.M. (1986). *Intermediary Organisation of the Skeleton*, vols I and II. Boca Raton: CRC Press.

Frost, H.M. (1989). The biology of fracture healing. *Clin. Orthop. Relat. Res.*, Part I: **248**: 283–93; Part II: **248**: 294–309.

Frost, H.M. (1990a). Structural adaptations to mechanical usage (SATMU): 1. Redefining Wolff's Law: The bone modeling problem. *Anat. Rec.*, **226**, 403–13.

Frost, H.M. (1990b). Structural adaptations to mechanical usage (SATMU): 2. Redefining Wolff's Law: The bone remodeling problem. *Anat. Rec.*, **226**, 414–22.

Frost, H.M. (1992). Perspectives: bone's mechanical usage windows. *Bone Miner.*, **19**, 257–71.

Frost, H.M. (1993). Suggested fundamental concepts in skeletal physiology. *Calcif. Tissue Int.*, **52**, 1–4.

Heaney, R.P. (1993). Is there a role for bone quality in fragility fractures? *Calcif. Tissue Int.*, **53** (Suppl.), 3–6.

Jee, W.S.S. (1989). The skeletal tissues. In *Cell and Tissue Biology. A Textbook of Histology* (L. Weiss, ed.), pp 211–59, Baltimore: Urban and Schwartzenberg.

Jee, W.S.S. and Frost, H.M. (1992). Skeletal adaptations during growth. *Triangle (Ciba-Geigy)*, **31**, 77–88.

Jee, W.S.S., Li, X.J. and Ke, H.Z. (1991). The skeletal adaptation to mechanical usage in the rat. *Cells Matter Suppl.*, **1**, 131–42.

Martin, R.B. and Burr, D.B. (1989). *Structure, Function and Adaptation of Compact Bone*. New York: Raven Press.

Parfitt, A.M. (1990). Bone-forming cells in clinical conditions. In *Bone, Vol. I: The Osteoblast and Osteocyte* (B.K. Hall, ed.), pp. 351–429, West Caldwell, NJ: Telford Press.

Parfitt, A.M. (1993). Bone age mineral density, and fatigue damage. *Calcif. Tissue Int.*, **53**, (Suppl.), 82–6.

Pattin, C.A. and Carter, D.R. (1991). *Bone Mechanical Energy Dissipation during Cyclic Loading* (Transactions of the Orthopaedic Research Society, 37th Annual Meeting), p. 129.

Schnitzler, C.M. (1993). Bone quality: a determinant for certain risk factors for bone fragility. *Calcif. Tissue Int.*, **53** (Suppl.), 27–31.

Adaptations of muscle and connective tissue

Akeson, W.H., Amiel, D. and Woo, S.L.Y. (1980). Immobility effects on synovial joints. The pathomechanics of joint contracture. *Biorheology*, **17**, 95–110.

Akeson, W.H., Woo, S.L.Y., Amiel, D. and Doty, D.H. (1977). Rapid recovery from contracture in rabbit hindlimb. *Clin. Orthop. Relat. Res.*, **122**, 359–65.

Atha, J. (1981). Strengthening muscles. *Exerc. Sports Sci. Rev.*, **9**, 1–74.

Bennett, R.L. and Knowlton, G.C. (1958). Overwork weakness in partially denervated skeletal muscle. *Clin. Orthop.*, **12**, 22–9.

Berger, R. (1962). Effect of varied weight training programs on strength. *Res. Q. Exerc. Sport*, **33**, 168–81.

Crisco, J.J. and Panjabi, M. (1990). Postural biomechanical stability and gross muscle architecture in the spine. In *Multiple Muscle Systems* (J.M. Winters and S.L.Y Woo, eds), New York: Springer Verlag.

Davies, C.T.M. and Sargeant, A.J. (1975). Effects of exercise therapy on total and component tissue leg volumes of patients undergoing rehabilitation of lower limb injury. *Ann. Hum. Biol.*, **2**, 327–37.

Davies, C.T.M. and Young, K. (1983). The effects of training at 30 and 100% maximal isometric force (MVC) on the contractile properties of the triceps surae in man. *J. Physiol.*, **336**, (Abstr.), 22–3P.

Donatelli, R. and Wooden, M.J. (1989). *Orthopaedic Physical Therapy*. New York: Churchill Livingstone.

Duchateau, J. and Hainaut, K. (1987). Electrical and mechanical changes in immobilised human muscle. *J. Appl. Physiol.*, **62**, 2168–73.

Duchateau, J. and Hainaut, K. (1990). Effects of immobilisation on contractile properties, recruitment and firing rates of human motor units. *J. Physiol.*, **422**, 55–65.

Dyck, P.J., Thomas, P.K., Lambert, E.H. and Bunge, R. (1984). *Peripheral Neuropathy (Volume II).* Philadelphia: W.B. Saunders.

Edgerton, V.R., Barnard, R.J., Peter, J.B. *et al.*, (1975). Properties of immobilised hindlimb muscles of the *Galago senegalensis. Exp. Neurol.*, **46**, 115–31.

Enoka, R.M. (1988). Muscle strength and its development: new perspectives. *Sports Med.*, **6**, 146–68.

Fukunaga, T., Roy, R.R., Shellock, F.G. *et al.* (1992). Physiological cross-sectional area of human leg muscles based on magnetic resonance imaging. *J. Orthop. Res.*, **10**, 926–34.

Gandevia, S.C. and McKenzie, D.K. (1988). Activation of human muscles at short muscle lengths during maximal static efforts. *J. Physiol.*, **407**, 599–613.

Gelberman, R.H. and Manske, P.R. (1987). Effects of early motion on the tendon healing process: experimental studies. In *Tendon Surgery in the Hand* (J.M. Hunter, L.H. Schneider and E.J. Mackin, eds) St Louis: C.V. Mosby.

Gelberman, R.H., Vandenberg, J.S., Lundborg, G.N. and Akeson, W.H. (1983). Flexor tendon healing and restoration of the gliding surface. *J. Bone Joint Surg.*, **65-A**, 70–80.

Gelberman, R.H. and Woo, S.L.Y. (1989). The physiological basis for application of controlled stress in the rehabilitation of flexor tendon injuries. *J. Hand Ther.*, April–June, 66–70.

Gossman, M.R., Sahrmann, S.A. and Rose, S.J. (1982). Review of length-associated changes in muscle: experimental evidence and clinical implications. *Phys. Ther.*, **62**, 1799–808.

Gould, J.A. and Davies, G.J. (1985). *Orthopaedic and Sports Physical Therapy.* St Louis: C.V. Mosby.

Guttman, L. (1976). *Spinal Cord Injuries: Comprehensive Management and Research.* (2nd edn). Oxford: Blackwell.

Hales, J.P. and Gandevia, S.C. (1988). Assessment of maximal voluntary contraction with twitch interpolation: an instrument to measure twitch responses. *J. Neurosci. Methods*, **25**, 97–102.

Hardy, M.A. (1989). The biology of scar formation. *Phys. Ther.*, **69**, 1014–24.

Herbert, R. (1988). The passive mechanical properties of muscle and their adaptations to altered patterns of use. *Austr. J. Physiother.*, **34**, 141–9.

Herbert, R. (1993a). Human strength adaptations – implications for therapy. In *Key Issues in Musculoskeletal Physiotherapy* (J. Crosbie and J. McConnell, eds), pp. 142–71, Oxford: Butterworth-Heinemann.

Herbert, R. (1993b). Preventing and treating stiff joints. In *Key Issues in Musculoskeletal Physiotherapy* (J. Crosbie and J. McConnell, eds), pp. 114–41, Oxford: Butterworth-Heinemann.

Herbert, R.D. and Balnave, R.J. (1993). The effect of position of immobilisation on rabbit soleus muscle resting length and stiffness. *J. Orthop. Res.*, **11**, 358–66.

Heslinga, J.W. and Huijing, P.A. (1993). Muscle length–force characteristics in relation to muscle architecture: a bilateral study of gastrocnemius medialis muscles of unilaterally immobilized rats. *Eur. J. Appl. Physiol.*, **66**, 289–98.

Hughes, G.R.V. (1977). *Connective Tissue Disease.* Oxford: Blackwell.

Ingemann-Hansen, T. and Halkjaer-Kristennsen, J. (1980). Computerised tomography determination of human thigh components. *Scand. J. Rehabil. Med.*, **12**, 27–31.

Järvinen, M.K. and Lehto, M.U.K. (1993). The effects of early mobilisation and immobilisation on the healing process following muscle injuries. *Sports Med.*, **15**, 78–89.

Johnson, E.W. and Braddom, R. (1971). Overwork weakness in facioscapulohumeral muscular dystrophy. *Arch. Phys. Med. Rehabil.*, **52**, 333–6.

Jones, D.A. and Rutherford, O.M. (1987). Human muscle strength training: the effects of three different regimes and the nature of the resultant changes. *J. Physiol.*, **391**, 1–11.

Józsa, L., Kannus, P., Thöring, J. *et al.* (1990). The effect of tenotomy and immobilisation on intramuscular connective tissue. *J. Bone Joint Surg.*, **72-B**, 293–7.

Kendall, F.P., McCreary, E.K. and Provance, P.G. (1993). *Muscles: Testing and Function* (4th edn). Baltimore: Williams and Wilkins.

LeBlanc, A., Gogia, P. and Schneider, V. (1988). Calf muscle area and strength changes after five weeks of horizontal bed rest. *Am. J. Sports Med.*, **16**, 624–9.

Light, K.E., Nuzick, S., Personius, W. and Barstrom, A. (1984). Low-load prolonged stretch vs. high-load brief stretch in treating knee contractures. *Phys. Ther.*, **64**, 330–3.

Mastaglia, F.L. and Walton, J. (1982). *Skeletal Muscle Pathology.* Edinburgh: Churchill Livingstone.

McCartney, N., Moroz, D., Garner, S.H. and McComas, A.J. (1988). The effects of strength training in patients with selected neuromuscular disorders. *Med. Sci. Sports Exerc.*, **20**, 362–8.

McConnell, J. (1993). Promoting effective segmental alignment. In *Key Issues in Musculoskeletal Physiotherapy* (J. Crosbie and J. McConnell, eds.), pp. 172–94, Oxford: Butterworth-Heinemann.

McDonagh, M.J.N. and Davies, C.T.M. (1984). Adaptive response to mammalian skeletal muscle to exercise with high loads. *Eur. J. Appl. Physiol.*, **52**, 139–55.

McDougall, J.D., Elder, G.C.B., Sale, D.G. *et al.* (1980). Effects of strength training and immobilisation on human muscle fibres. *Eur. J. Appl. Physiol.*, **43**, 25–34.

McKenzie, R.A. (1981). *The Lumbar Spine: Mechanical Diagnosis and Therapy.* Lower Hutt: Spinal Publications.

Millikan, C.H., McDowell, F. and Easton, J.D. (1987). *Stroke.* Philadelphia: Lea and Febiger.

Milner-Brown, H.S. and Miller, R.G. (1988). Muscle strengthening through high-resistance weight training in patients with neuromuscular disorders. *Arch. Phys. Med. Rehabil.*, **69**, 14–19.

Narici, M.V., Landoni, L. and Minetti, A.E. (1992). Assessment of human knee extensor muscle stress from in vivo physiological cross-sectional area and strength measurements. *Eur. J. Appl. Physiol.*, **65**, 438–44.

Narici, M.V., Roi, G.S., Landoni, L. *et al.* (1989). Changes in force, cross-sectional area and neural activation during strength training and detraining of human quadriceps. *Eur. J. Appl. Physiol.*, **59**, 310–19.

Noyes, F.R. (1977). Functional properties of knee ligaments and alterations induced by immobilisation. *Clin. Orthop. Relat. Res.*, **123**, 210–42.

O'Dwyer, N.J., Nielson, P.D. and Nash, J. (1989). Mechanisms of muscle growth related to muscle contracture in cerebral palsy. *Dev. Med. Child Neurol.*, **31**, 543–7.

Rooney, K., Herbert, R. and Balnave, R. (1994). Fatigue contributes to the strength training stimulus. *Med. Sci. Sports Exerc.*, **26**, 1160–4.

Rutherford, O.M., Jones, D.A. and Round, J.M. (1990). Long-lasting unilateral muscle wasting and weakness following injury and immobilisation. *Scand. J. Rehabil. Med.*, **22**, 33–7.

Sale, D.G. (1987). Influence of exercise and training on motor unit activation. *Exerc. Sport Sci. Rev.*, **15**, 95–151.

Sale, D.G. (1992). Neural adaptation to strength training. In *Strength and Power in Sport* (P.V. Komi, ed.), Oxford: Blackwell.

St-Pierre, D., and Gardiner, P.F. (1987). The effect of immobilisation and exercise on muscle function: a review. *Physiother. Can.*, **39**, 24–36.

Sunderland, S. (1978). *Nerve and Nerve Injuries* (2nd edn), London: Churchill Livingstone.

Szeto, G., Strauss, G.R., De Domenico, G. and Lai, H.S. (1989). The effect of training intensity on voluntary isometric strength improvement. *Aust. J. Physiother.*, **35**, 210–18.

Tabary, J.C., Tabary, C., Tardieu, C. *et al.* (1972). Physiological and structural changes in the cat's soleus muscle due to immobilisation at different lengths by plaster casts. *J. Physiol.*, **224**, 231–44.

Vignos, P.J. (1983). Physical models of rehabilitation in neuromuscular disease. *Muscle Nerve*, **6**, 323–38.

Vinken, P.J., Bruyn, G.W., Klawans, H.L. and Braakman, R. (1990). *Head Injury*. Amsterdam: Elsevier.

Walton, J. (1985). *Brain's Diseases of the Nervous System* (9th edn). Oxford: Oxford University Press.

Walton, J.N. (1974). *Disorders of Voluntary Muscle* (3rd edn). Edinburgh: Churchill Livingstone.

Wigerstad-Lossing I., Grimby G., Jonsson T. *et al.* (1988). Effects of electrical muscle stimulation combined with voluntary muscle contractions after knee surgery. *Med. Sci. Sports Exerc.*, **20**, 93–8.

Williams, P.E. (1990). Use of intermittent stretch in the prevention of serial sarcomere loss in immobilised muscle. *Ann. Rheum. Dis.*, **49**, 316–17.

Williams, P.E. and Goldspink, G. (1978). Changes in sarcomere length and physiological properties in immobilised muscle. *J. Anat.*, **127**, 459–68.

Williams, P.E. and Goldspink, G. (1984). Connective tissue changes in immobilized muscle. *J. Anat.*, **138**, 343–50.

Witzmann, F.A., Kim, D.H. and Fitts, R.H. (1982a). Hindlimb immobilisation: length–tension and contractile properties of skeletal muscle. *J. Appl. Physiol.*, **53**, 335–45.

Witzmann, F.A., Kim, D.H. and Fitts, R.H. (1982b). Recovery time course in contractile function of fast and slow skeletal muscle after hindlimb immobilisation. *J. Appl. Physiol.*, **53**, 677–82.

Woo, S.L.Y. and Buckwalter, J.A. (1988). *Injury and Repair of the Musculoskeletal System*. Illinois: American Academy of Orthopaedic Surgeons.

Woo, S.L.Y. (1986). Biomechanics of tendons and ligaments. In *Frontiers in Biomechanics* (G.W. Schmid-Schönbein, S.L.Y. Woo and B.W. Zweifach, eds), New York: Springer-Verlag.

Young, A., Hughes, I., Round, J.M. and Edwards, R.H.T. (1982). The effect of knee injury on the number of muscle fibres in the human quadriceps. *Clin. Sci.*, **62**, 227–34.

Yue, G. and Cole, K.J. (1992). Strength increases from the motor program: comparison of training with maximal voluntary and imagined muscle contractions. *J. Neurophysiol.*, **67**, 1114–23.

Skill learning after musculoskeletal lesions

Anderson, M. and Lough, S. (1986). A psychological framework for neurorehabilitation. *Physiother. Theory Pract.*, **2**, 74–82.

Annett, J. (1971) Acquisition of skill. *Br. Med. Bull.*, **27**, 266–71.

Annett, J. and Kay, H. (1957). Knowledge of results and skilled performance. *Occup. Psychol.*, **31**, 69–79.

Arbib, M.A., Iberall, T. and Lyons, D. (1986). Coordinated control programs for movements of the hand. In *Hand Function and the Neocortex* (A.W. Goodwin and I. Darian-Smith, eds), pp. 111–29, Berlin: Springer-Verlag.

Asmussen, E. and Bonde-Petersen, F. (1974). Storage of elastic energy in skeletal muscles in man. *Acta Physiol. Scand.*, **91**, 385–92.

Baker, P.D., Evans, D.M. and Lee, C. (1991). Treadmill gait retraining following fractured neck of femur. *Arch. Phys. Med. Rehabil.*, **72**, 649–52.

Beggs, W.D.A. and Howarth, C.I. (1972). The movement of the hand towards a target. *Q. J. Exp. Psychol.*, **24**, 448–53.

Bernstein, N.A. (1967). *The Co-ordination and Regulation of Movement*. Oxford: Pergamon Press.

Bobbert, M.F. and van Ingen Schenau, G.J. (1988). Coordination in vertical jumping. *J. Biomech.*, **21**, 249–62.

Bosco, C., Viitasalo, J.T., Komi, P.V. and Luhtanen, P. (1982). Combined effect of elastic energy and myoelectrical potentiation during stretch-shortening cycle exercise. *Acta Physiol. Scand.*, **114**, 557–65.

Caiozzo, V.J., Perrine, J.J. and Edgerton, V.R. (1981). Training-induced alterations of the in vivo force–velocity relationship of human muscle. *J. Appl. Physiol.*, **51**, 750–4.

Canning, C. (1987). Training standing up following stroke – a clinical trial. In *Proceedings of the Tenth International Congress of the World Confederation for Physical Therapy (Sydney)*, pp. 915–19.

Carr, J.H. and Shepherd, R.B. (1987a). *A Motor Relearning Programme for Stroke* (2nd edn). London: Butterworth-Heinemann.

Carr, J.H. and Shepherd, R.B. (1987b). A motor learning model for rehabilitation. In *Movement Science: Foundations for Physical Therapy in Rehabilitation* (J.H. Carr and R.B. Shepherd, eds), Rockville: Aspen Publishers.

Carr, J.H. and Shepherd, R.B. (1989). A motor learning model for stroke rehabilitation. *Physiotherapy*, **75**, 372–80.

Cordo, P.J. and Nashner, L.M. (1982). Properties of postural adjustments associated with rapid arm movements. *J. Neu-*

rophysiol., **47**, 287–302.

Crossman, E.R.F.W. (1959). A theory of the acquisition of speed-skill. *Ergonomics*, **2**, 153–66.

Ellenbecker, T.S., Davies, G.J. and Rowinski, M.J. (1988). Concentric versus eccentric isokinetic strengthening of the rotator cuff: objective data versus functional test. *Am. J. Sports Med.*, **16**, 64–9.

Gelfand, I.M., Gurfinkel, V.S., Tsetlin, M.L. and Shik, M.L. (1971). Some problems in the analysis of movements. In *Models of the Structural–Functional Organisation of Certain Biological Systems* (I.M. Gelfland, V.S. Gurfinkel, S.V. Fomin and M.L. Tsetlin, eds), Cambridge: MIT Press.

Gentile, A.M. (1972). A working model of skill acquisition with applications to teaching. *Quest*, **17**, 3–23.

Gentile, A.M. (1987). Skill acquisition: action, movement, and neuromotor processes. In *Movement Science: Foundation for Physical Therapy in Rehabilitation* (J.H. Carr and R.B. Shepherd, eds), pp. 93–154, Rockville: Aspen.

Gibson, J.J. (1966). *The Senses Considered as Perceptual Systems.* Boston: Houghton Mifflin.

Gibson, J.J. (1986). *The Ecological Approach to Visual Perception.* Hillsdale: Lawrence Erlbaum.

Godges, J.J., MacRae, P.G. and Engelke, K.A. (1993). Effects of exercise on hip range of motion, trunk muscle performance, and gait economy. *Phys. Ther.*, **73**, 468–77.

Gonnella, C., Hale, G., Ionta, M. and Perry, J.C. (1981). Self-instruction in a perceptual motor skill. *Phys. Ther.*, **61**, 177–84.

Gottlieb, G.L., Corcos, D.M., Jaric, S. and Agarwal, G.C. (1988). Practice improves even the simplest movements. *Exp. Brain Res.*, **73**, 436–40.

Greene, P.H. (1982). Why is it easy to control your arms? *J. Mot. Behav.*, **14**, 260–86.

Gregoire, L., Veeger, H.E., Huijing, P.A. and van Ingen Schenau, G.J. (1984). Role of mono-and biarticular muscles in explosive movements. *Int. J. Sports Med.*, **5**, 301–5.

Hakkinen, K. and Komi, P.V. (1983). Electromyographic changes during strength training and detraining. *Med. Sci. Sports Exer.*, **15**, 455–60.

Henderson, S.A., Finlay, O.E., Murphy, N. *et al.* (1992). Benefits of an exercise class for elderly women following hip surgery. *Ulster Med. J.*, **61**, 144–59.

Higgins, J.R. (1972). Movements to match environmental demands. *Res. Q.*, **43**, 312–36.

Jacobs, R. and van Ingen Schenau, G.J. (1992). Control of an external force in leg extensions in humans. *J. Physiol.*, **457**, 611–26.

Jevsevar, D.S., Riley, P.O., Hodge, W.A. and Krebs, D.E. (1993). Knee kinematics and kinetics during locomotor activities of daily living in subjects with knee arthroplasty and in healthy control subjects. *Phys. Ther.*, **73**, 229–39.

Johnson, P. (1984). The acquisition of skill. In *The Psychology of Human Movement* (M.M. Smyth and A.M. Wing, eds), pp. 215–40, London: Academic Press.

Kitai, T.A. and Sale, D.G. (1989). Specificity of joint angle in isometric training. *Eur. J. Appl. Physiol.*, **58**, 744–8.

Komi, P.V. (1986) The stretch-shortening cycle and human power output. In *Human Muscle Power* (N.L. Jones, N. McCartney and A.J. McComas, eds), pp. 27–39, Champaign,

Illinois: Human Kinetics Publisher.

Komi, P.V. and Buskirk, E. (1972). Effect of eccentric and concentric muscle conditioning on tension and electrical activity of human muscle. *Ergonomics*, **154**, 417–34.

Kottke, F.K. (1980) From reflex to skill: the training of coordination. *Arch. Phys. Med. Rehabil.*, **61**, 551–61.

Lee, D.N. and Aronson, E. (1974). Visual proprioceptive control of standing in infants. *Percept. Physchophys.*, **15**, 529–32.

Lee, D.N. and Lishman, J.R. (1975). Visual proprioceptive control of stance. *J. Hum. Movement Stud.*, **1**, 87–95.

Leont'ev, A.N. and Zaporozhets, A.V. (1960). *Rehabilitation of Hand Function.* London: Pergamon.

Lesmes, G.R., Costill, D.L., Coyle, E.F. and Fink, W.J. (1978). Muscle strength and power changes during maximal isokinetic training. *Med. Sci. Sport*, **10**, 266–9.

Lindh, M. (1979). Increase of muscle strength from isometric quadriceps exercises at different knee angles. *Scand. J. Rehabil. Med.*, **11**, 33–6.

Malouin, F., Potvin, M., Prevost, J. *et al.* (1992). Use of an intensive task-oriented gait training program in a series of patients with acute cerebrovascular accidents. *Phys. Ther.*, **72**, 781–93.

Marteniuk, R.G. (1976) *Information Processing in Motor Skills.* New York: Holt, Rinehart and Winston.

McConnell, J. (1993). Promoting effective segmental alignment. In *Key Issues in Musculoskeletal Physiotherapy* (J. Crosbie and J. McConnell, eds), pp. 172–94, Oxford: Butterworth-Heinemann.

Mulder, T. (1991). A process-oriented model of human motor behavior: toward a theory-based rehabilitation approach. *Phys. Ther.*, **71**, 157–64.

Nashner, L.M. (1976). Adapting reflexes controlling the human posture. *Exp. Brain Res.*, **26**, 59–72.

Newell, K.M. (1976). Knowledge of results and motor learning. *Exerc. Sport Sci. Rev.*, **4**, 195–227.

Newell, K.M. (1981). Skill learning. In *Human Skills* (D. Holding, ed.), pp. 203–26. New York: John Wiley.

Oxendine, A. (1984) *Psychology of Motor Learning* (2nd edn). Englewood Cliffs: Prentice-Hall.

Pai, Y. and Rogers, M.W. (1991). Segmental contribution to total body momentum in sit-to-stand. *Med. Sci. Sports Exerc.*, **23**, 225–30.

Rasch, P.J. and Morehouse, C.E. (1957). Effect of static and dynamic exercises on muscular strength and hypertrophy. *J. Appl. Physiol.*, **11**, 29–34.

Robinson, E.S. (1927). The 'similarity' factor in retroaction. *Am. J. Psychol.*, **39**, 297–312.

Rutherford, O.M. (1988). Muscular coordination and strength training implications for injury rehabilitation. *Sports Med.*, **5**, 196–202.

Rutherford, O.M. and Jones, D.A. (1986). The role of learning and coordination in strength training. *Eur. J. Appl. Physiol.*, **55**, 100–5.

Sale, D.G. (1988). Neural adaptation to resistance training. *Med. Sci. Sports Exerc.*, **20**, 135–45.

Sale, D. and MacDougall, D. (1981). Specificity in strength training: a review for the coach and athlete. *Can. J. Appl. Sports Sci.*, **6**, 87–92.

Schenkman, M., Berger, R.A., Riley, P.O. *et al.* (1990). Whole-body movements during rising from sitting to standing. *Phys. Ther.*, **70**, 638–48.

Schmidt, R.A. (1975). A schema theory of discrete motor learning. *Psychol. Rev.*, **82**, 225–60.

Schmidt, R.A. (1988). *Motor Control and Learning: A Behavioral Emphasis* (2nd edn). Champaign: Human Kinetics.

Shepherd, R.B. and Gentile, A.M. (1994). Sit-to-stand: Functional relationships between upper body and lower limb segments. *Hum. Mov. Sci.*, **13**, 817–84.

Shepherd, R.B. and Carr, J.H. (1994). Reflections on physiotherapy and the emerging science of movement rehabilitation. *Aust. J. Physiother.*, 40th Jubilee Issue, 39–47.

Stelmach, G.E. (1978). *Information Processing in Motor Control and Learning.* New York: Academic Press.

Thepaut-Mathieu, C., Van Hoecke, J. and Maton, B. (1985). Length specificity of strength and myoneural activation improvements following isometric training. In *Biomechanics X-A* (B. Johnson, ed.), pp. 513–17, Champaign: Human Kinetics.

Turvey, M.T., Fitch, H.L. and Tuller, B. (1982). The Bernstein perspective: 1. The problems of degrees of freedom and context-conditioned variability. In *Human Motor Behavior: An Introduction* (J.A.S. Kelso, ed.) Hillsdale: Lawrence Erlbaum.

van der Weel, F.R., van der Meer, A.L.H. and Lee, D.N. (1991). Effect of task on movement control in cerebral palsy: implications for assessment and therapy. *Dev. Med. Child Neurol.*, **33**, 419–26.

Westwood, P. (1993). An investigation into the effect of task-specific training on the biomechanics of standing up in patients following total hip replacement. MAppSc Thesis, School of Physiotherapy, University of Sydney, Australia.

Winstein, C.J. and Knecht, H.G. (1990). Movement science and its relevance to physical therapy. *Phys. Ther.*, **70**, 759–62.

Winter, D.A., McFadyen, B.J. and Dickey, J.P. (1991). Adaptability of the CNS in human walking. In *Adaptability of Human Gait* (A.E. Patla, ed.), Amsterdam: Elsevier Science Publishers B.V.

Wise, S.P. and Desimone, R. (1988). Behavioral neurophysiology: insights into seeing and grasping. *Science*, **242**, 736–40.

Wooden, M.J., Greenfield, B., Johanson, M. *et al.* (1992). Effects of strength training on throwing velocity and shoulder muscle performance in teenage baseball players. *J. Sports Physiother.*, **15**, 223–8.

Chapter 3

Diagnostic imaging in musculoskeletal physiotherapy

G. Bigg-Wither and P. Kelly

Introduction

Successful physiotherapy management of musculoskeletal disorders depends on a thorough physical examination. In many musculoskeletal conditions a detailed history and physical examination may suffice, but in other cases the neglect of radiological investigations may lead to inappropriate or harmful treatment. To make best use of the results of these investigations, physiotherapists need to be aware of the principles and practices of radiology.

There are few instances in musculoskeletal disorders where radiological findings solely determine diagnosis and management, but there are many cases where appreciation of these findings will have a large impact on clinical decisions regarding treatment and prognosis. In some countries (e.g. Australia and some states and provinces of North America) physiotherapists act as primary contact practitioners and may order X-rays. The subject of radiological investigation in the practice of physiotherapy has received little attention to date. Because of recent technological developments in the diagnosis of musculoskeletal problems this topic now deserves more attention from the profession.

Imaging is an extension of the history and physical examination and plays a key role in helping to arrive at an accurate diagnosis by confirming a clinical impression, excluding unsuspected pathology and providing important prognostic information so that an appropriate treatment plan can be instigated. It should be noted that the X-ray report should not be seen as a statement of absolute truth but rather as a specialist opinion.

Findings should be compared with the overall clinical picture. Even when X-rays are normal, if the physiotherapist is suspicious of underlying pathology, e.g. when a person has intractable night pain, weight loss or the pain is not behaving in a normal musculoskeletal pattern, the physiotherapist should consult with relevant specialists, including radiologists to ensure appropriate further investigation. On the other hand, findings on X-ray may be entirely unrelated to the person's symptoms. The relevance of any imaging findings will require careful correlation with the clinical findings.

Several different modalities for imaging the musculoskeletal system are now commonly utilized in day-to-day practice, from plain film radiography to the more powerful and sophisticated ultrasound, computed tomography (CT) and magnetic resonance imaging (MRI). We need to understand the clinical indications, the capabilities and limitations, possible adverse effects and, in these times of cost containment, the expense of these various imaging investigations. The specific information required by the clinician, the personal preference and expertise of the radiologist and the availability of the various imaging modalities will also have a part to play in the decision process.

Careful clinical evaluation is essential before choosing any imaging test. One must always ask: 'What useful information will this test provide?' and 'Will the result affect patient management?'.

It is recommended that physiotherapists utilize the services of a specialist radiology practice where there is radiologist supervision and a written report is provided by the radiologist. All requests for diagnostic imaging should have a clear clinical indication, and this should be stated on the request form. This will allow the radiologist to plan a suitable examination and provide an informed report. It is recommended that imaging techniques other than plain X-rays are requested in consultation with a radiologist or other relevant medical practitioner.

To maximize the benefit from X-ray examinations and to be able to recognize normal and abnormal findings, physiotherapists need to be knowledgeable about radiographic anatomy (see the Appendix) and terminology used in radiology reports. They should also understand common disease processes, their imaging correlation and also what are significant and clinically relevant findings versus normal variants or incidental findings of little clinical significance. The only way to improve X-ray interpretation skills is to look at as many films as possible. Most hospital radiology departments have a film library which can be utilized.

tion on the first consultation but if the problem does not respond in a predictable manner, radiography may be required to provide more information about the underlying pathology or to exclude unsuspected pathologies. Repeated examinations, particularly when they involve the radiosensitive organs (thyroid, bone marrow, female breast and gonads) (i.e. spine and pelvic examinations), should be avoided especially in close succession.

All radiographic examinations should be avoided throughout pregnancy especially during the first trimester, and generally are not performed at all when a woman has missed a period and early pregnancy is possible.

In the remainder of this chapter the basic physical principles involved in image formation with the different imaging modalities will be discussed along with their advantages and disadvantages and a current evaluation of their role in musculoskeletal imaging.

X-ray safety

Many of the imaging techniques described in this chapter use X-ray radiation as the basis of image formation. X-rays are a form of ionizing radiation and so there is a risk of cell damage. Especially of concern is the possibility of inducing malignancy or gene mutation which are both chance phenomena related to dose, but there is no safe dose below which these effects cannot occur. There is some uncertainty about the risks of inducing these effects with the low doses of radiation utilized in modern diagnostic radiology, but the risks are thought to be very small. The embryo and children are at greatest risk. The International Commission of Radiological Protection recommends that radiological examinations should be carried out only when the information obtained will be useful for the management of the patient. There should be no such thing as a routine X-ray examination; there should always be a clear clinical indication. A person, for example, who has severe pain arising from the cervical region following trauma will obviously require imaging for diagnosis. The person who is suffering from a mild strain of the gastrocnemius muscle does not routinely require an X-ray examination because diagnosis can be made satisfactorily on clinical examination. Sometimes the physiotherapist may not order an X-ray for a person with a minor musculoskeletal dysfunc-

Imaging techniques, their role in diagnosis and the advantages and disadvantages of their use

Some imaging techniques have specific clinical indications (e.g. ultrasound, CT, MRI) and each examination is tailored to answer a specific clinical question. Other techniques (e.g. plain film radiography) are used for more general imaging purposes.

Plain film radiography

X-rays generated in an X-ray tube pass through the body region of interest to form an image on photographic film, with contrast in the image reflecting differential absorption of the X-ray beam by the various tissues in the path of the beam (depending primarily upon atomic number and density of the tissues).

Role

Plain films are almost always the initial form of imaging. They are able to document the majority of fractures and other structural bony abnormalities such as arthritis, tumour, infection, metabolic bone disease (e.g. osteoporosis and Paget's disease) and developmental anomalies. In many instances no further imaging is required. However, when there are no relevant plain film findings and there is clinical suspicion of abnormality (e.g. stress fracture) or the plain films are not suitable for full evaluation of a suspected abnormality (e.g. disc herniation or rotator cuff tear) further assessment can be obtained by using other more sensitive and sophisticated imaging modalities.

Advantages

1. Very good spatial resolution. The structure of bone is well demonstrated as are soft tissue calcifications.
2. Good overall evaluation of the anatomy and alignment of the entire region.
3. Relatively cheap and widely available.

Disadvantages

1. Poor resolution of the soft tissue structures. At best, radiographs can only differentiate fat from all the other soft tissues and so are very limited in the evaluation of the articular and peri-articular soft tissue structures apart from demonstrating soft tissue calcification. However, soft tissue swelling and joint effusions can often be appreciated.
2. Planar images – superimposes all the structures in the body in the path of the X-ray beam and so difficulties may arise in evaluating abnormalities in regions with complex anatomy (e.g. pelvis). In general, a plain film examination of a region should always include two views at right angles to each other.
3. Utilizes ionizing radiation. Examinations of the spine and pelvis require the highest radiation doses.

Cross-sectional imaging

Being able to image only a selected thin slice of the body without the superimposition of other structures can have significant advantages in visualizing the various bony and soft tissue structures and their interfaces and for accurately localizing abnormalities.

Ultrasound, CT and MRI are all relatively new modalities which utilize state-of-the-art technology to produce cross-sectional (tomographic) images with superb detail. Their introduction has allowed musculoskeletal imaging to reach a very sophisticated level with the added benefit of decreasing the need for more invasive investigations such as myelography.

Because cross-sectional images view only a small area of the anatomy in one plane at a time, multiple images (scans) are required to evaluate a region of interest. In addition, images may be required in multiple planes as well (e.g. axial, sagittal, coronal or oblique) depending upon the orientation of the structure or abnormality in question.

Conventional tomography

This technique utilizes conventional X-ray tubes and image receptors which are capable of moving relative to each other so as to blur out all structures except those in a chosen focal plane. However, there is usually some unwanted blurring of the focal plane structures as well. Images can be obtained in multiple planes including the sagittal and coronal planes. The radiation dose is moderately high depending upon the number of scans required.

Before the widespread introduction of CT and MRI this technique was frequently employed in bone imaging (e.g. tibial plateau and vertebral column fractures, evaluation of the sternoclavicular and temporomandibular joints and in the assessment of chronic osteomyelitis searching for a sequestrum and/or cortical disruption). Nowadays, tomography has been largely superseded by CT and MRI as they can provide images of superior detail, especially with regard to the soft tissues, and utilize less or no ionizing radiation.

However, tomography can still be useful in certain circumstances mainly in the spine where tomograms can evaluate multiple segments in the sagittal plane on one image (e.g. to visualize more clearly the craniocervical junction and upper cervical spine, and the lower cervical and upper thoracic spine). Tomography is also useful when metal implants preclude useful CT imaging or there is a contraindication to an MRI examination.

Ultrasound

Ultra high frequency sound waves (ultrasound) are propagated into the tissues via a probe (transducer) placed upon the skin surface. The sound waves are both reflected and transmitted at interfaces between the different tissues, and by calculating the time it takes an echo to return to the transducer the depth of a structure can be determined and an image formed. Each individual tissue has a characteristic echotexture which relates to its own unique internal structure.

Musculoskeletal imaging is performed with a high-resolution (5–10 MHz) probe and images can be obtained of the various soft tissue structures including tendons, ligaments, bursae and muscles.

Role

Diagnostic ultrasound is now well established in musculoskeletal imaging, and clinical applications include:

1. Evaluation of:
   (a) tendons:
      (i)   tendinitis
      (ii) tenosynovitis
      (iii) tendon rupture (e.g. rotator cuff, Achilles tendon, patellar tendon, tibialis posterior tendon)
      (iv) tendon dislocation (e.g. long head of biceps, flexor and extensor tendons of the hand)
      (v)   tendon impingement (e.g. impingement of the rotator cuff tendons beneath the coraco-acromial arch with shoulder abduction)
   (b) ligaments (e.g. rupture of collateral ligaments of the knee)
   (c) muscles (e.g. rupture)
2. Characterizing the location and nature (e.g. solid or cystic) of palpable soft tissue masses [e.g. popliteal (Baker's) cyst, ganglion]. Neoplastic soft tissue masses are better evaluated with MRI.
3. Identifying joint and bursal effusions (e.g. transient synovitis of the hip, subacromial bursitis).
4. Assessing congenital hip dislocation in infants.

Good results require considerable experience in a practice where a special interest is taken in this particular branch of ultrasonic imaging.

Advantages

1. Very good image detail (can visualize the fibrillar structure of tendons).
2. Cross-sectional images in a variety of planes.
3. Real-time (dynamic) imaging – structures can be visualized as they move through their physiological range of motion.
4. Interactive – any area of tenderness or a palpable mass can be precisely localized with the transducer.
5. Side to side comparison – facilitates detection of any abnormality.
6. No harmful biological effects have been identified to date (does not utilize ionizing radiation).
7. Low to moderate cost.
8. Widely available.

Disadvantages

1. Ultrasound cannot penetrate bone and therefore cannot be used to image:
   (a) the internal structure of bone, although the surface contour of bone can be seen;
   (b) structures covered by bone (e.g. cruciate ligaments).
2. Limited depth penetration – cannot image deep structures.
3. Small field of view.
4. Contrast resolution is limited.
5. Alterations in echogenicity may lack specificity.
6. Images are difficult to interpret by the novice.
7. Difficult learning curve – quality of images is operator dependent. It is important that the radiologist has correlated his or her results with surgical findings to enhance accuracy of diagnosis.

Computed tomography (CT)

Initially, a scout image (digital radiograph) is obtained to plan where the scans will be taken. Cross-sectional images are produced by rotating a thin X-ray beam and detector array around the outside of the body through the region of interest. The X-ray transmission data are digitized and then reconstructed with high-speed computers into a 2-D image of the internal body structures. As this is a digital imaging process, contrast in the image can be manipulated to emphasize bony or soft tissue structures. Section thickness can be as small as 1.5 mm when high-resolution detail of the bone or joints is required.

Role

CT is now frequently utilized in musculoskeletal imaging. Clinical applications include evaluation of:

1. Intervertebral disc herniation, spinal stenosis and associated compression of neural structures. In the lumbar spine a modern CT scanner is usually able to discriminate disc, bone, nerve roots and thecal sac and has a high accuracy in visualizing disc herniations and also the cause(s) and severity of spinal stenosis. CT is less reliable in the cervical spine without intrathecal contrast. Thin section axial scans are obtained at the clinically involved level(s) and the adjacent levels both above and below.
2. Complex fractures and dislocations, especially when they involve joints (e.g. acetabulum, vertebral column, tibial plateau, calcaneus, proximal humerus, radial head, distal radius, ankle, carpus and tarsus) where CT is very helpful in determining the need for surgical intervention. Subluxation or dislocation of the sternoclavicular and distal radio-ulnar joints are best assessed with CT as plain films are unreliable.
3. Shoulder instability – performed in conjunction with arthrography.
4. Suspected fractures with negative plain films (e.g. femoral neck, hook of the hamate and stress fractures of the sacrum and navicular) and evaluation of fracture union (e.g. scaphoid).
5. Evaluation of joint problems (e.g. subtalar joints when tarsal coalition is suspected, osteochondral lesions and loose bodies of the ankle, knee and elbow joints).
6. Evaluation of patellofemoral alignment and tracking with knee flexion.
7. Measurement of true leg length discrepancy (determined from scout images).
8. Osteonecrosis – useful in staging (but not early detection) of osteonecrosis of the femoral head.
9. Assessment of bone tumours.
10. Evaluation of chronic osteomyelitis (searching for a sequestrum and/or cortical disruption).

Advantages

1. Excellent detail of bony architecture. Occasionally, 3-D reconstruction can be helpful in allowing a single image to show the entire region (e.g. fractures of the acetabulum).
2. Good resolution of soft tissue structures.
3. Non-invasive.
4. Fairly widely available.

Disadvantages

1. Limited scanning planes. Depending on the region of the body anatomic restrictions may limit scanning to only the axial plane (e.g. spine and shoulder). This limits the use of CT in the spine to processes that are localized to a single or a few segments. Images can be computer reformatted in any plane but multiple thin sections are required; however, the results are never as good as direct images.
2. Artifact sensitivity – streak artifacts may be caused by metal implants or superficial bony structures (e.g. shoulders when scanning the lower cervical segments) which may preclude any useful imaging of that region. Plaster casts do not degrade images.
3. Soft tissue resolution degraded in obese persons (e.g. when possible disc herniation is evaluated). This is especially a problem with older model scanners.
4. Utilize ionizing radiation. However, the dose is considerably less than conventional tomography, and CT doses are similar to an equivalent plain film examination of the same region.
5. Cost – moderately expensive.

Magnetic resonance imaging (MRI)

This is based upon the rather complex principle of nuclear magnetic resonance. The hydrogen nucleus (a single proton), largely contained in tissue water molecules, is utilized for imaging. The body is placed in a very high strength magnetic field (0.5–1.5 T) which magnetizes the hydrogen protons, and coils around the body part to emit a sequence of radiofrequency waves which excite the hydrogen protons to a resonance state. When the hydrogen protons return to the ground state a MR signal is emitted ('echo'), the intensity of which reflects the proton density and relaxation properties of the hydrogen protons in a particular tissue. Different sequences are utilized to emphasize anatomic detail (T1-weighted) or contrast between normal and abnormal soft tissues (T2-weighted).

Role

MRI can offer an accurate and comprehensive non-invasive evaluation of many musculoskeletal problems including:

1. Intervertebral disc degeneration, disc prolapse, spinal stenosis and associated compression of neural structures. The high intrinsic contrast resolution of MRI allows direct visualization of the thecal sac, spinal cord, nerve roots, discs, bone and bone marrow. Disc degeneration can be assessed by the reduced water content (dehydration) of the nucleus pulposus. A modern MRI unit utilizing dedicated surface coils and the ability to produce high-resolution thin sections can obtain a very high degree of accuracy in the assessment of disc herniations and spinal stenosis in both the cervical and lumbar regions. MRI is the only reliable imaging method that can differentiate post-operative scarring from recurrent disc herniation in the failed back syndrome. This is achieved with intravenous gadolinium (a para-magnetic contrast agent) which enhances fibrosis but not avascular disc material.
2. Intrinsic spinal cord disease including spinal cord injury.
3. Knee:
    (a) Trauma – meniscal and ligamentous tears, osteochondral lesions and trabecular microfractures. Accuracy is as good as arthroscopy.
    (b) Patellofemoral tracking.
4. Shoulder – impingement, rotator cuff tear and instability.
5. Osteonecrosis – very sensitive and specific in the early detection of osteonecrosis. MRI is very important in the assessment of possible osteonecrosis of the hip in being able to detect osteonecrosis before femoral head collapse and also showing the size and position of any osteonecrotic segment. Surgical intervention may be considered in the early stages to help prevent articular collapse.
6. Ankle – osteochondral lesions. Tendon (e.g. Achilles and tibialis posterior) and ligament injuries.
7. Wrist – tears of the triangular fibrocartilage complex and intercarpal ligaments. Evaluation of the carpal tunnel. Assessment of osteonecrosis of the lunate.
8. Temporo-mandibular joints – evaluation of internal disc derangements. MRI is considered to be the current procedure of choice to image the temporomandibular joint.
9. Occult fractures [e.g. femoral neck, stress fractures and trabecular microfractures (bone 'bruise')].
10. Evaluation of bony and soft tissue tumours and marrow infiltrating disorders. Very important in the staging of bone tumours.

The very high cost of this technology has limited the widespread use of MRI.

MRI competes with arthroscopy in the evaluation of internal derangements of the joints especially the knee, and to a lesser extent the shoulder. Arthroscopy is invasive and requires a general anaesthetic but has the potential advantage that certain therapeutic procedures (e.g. repair of a torn knee meniscus) can be performed at the same time.

Advantages

1. Superb anatomic detail because of the high intrinsic contrast resolution, especially of soft tissue structures, allowing visualization of all the articular and periarticular structures such as cartilage, tendons, ligaments and bone marrow as well as the spinal cord and nerve roots. MRI has the best overall soft tissue resolution of any imaging modality.
2. Very sensitive in the detection of disease.
3. Can image directly in any plane (multiplanar). Sagittal images are very useful in the spine.
4. Non-invasive.
5. No known harmful biological effect (does not utilize ionizing radiation).

Disadvantages

1. High cost.
2. Limited availability at present.
3. Bony abnormality and small areas of calcification may not be as well shown as with plain films or CT.
4. Abnormalities may lack specificity for a particular disease process (e.g. tendinitis versus a partial tendon tear).
5. Metallic objects in the body may present a hazard. Persons with:
    (a) clips on a cerebral aneurysm (may twist off), or
    (b) cardiac pacemakers, or

(c) metallic foreign bodies in the eyes must never undergo an MRI examination. The metal implants used in orthopaedics (e.g. prosthetic joints and internal fixation devices) are safe as they are solidly fixed to bone; they cause focal signal loss, but generally less artifact than with CT.

6. Can cause claustrophobia – the person has to lie in a narrow tunnel.
7. Clinicians may be unfamiliar with MRI images and radiologist expertise may be limited as MRI is a relatively new imaging modality.

Myelography

Myelography involves injecting water-soluble contrast into the subarachnoid space via a spinal puncture (lumbar or cervical). Contrast fills the subarachnoid space of the thecal sac and nerve root sleeves and so outlines the contour of the thecal sac, nerve roots and spinal cord. Standard radiographs are then taken and any displacement or compression of these neural structures can be assessed. Compressed nerve roots often appear swollen.

Advantages

1. Moderately high accuracy in diagnosis of compression of the spinal cord and/or nerve roots. However, the accuracy of lumbosacral disc herniation is not as good as at other levels as the nerve roots are separated from the disc by plentiful epidural fat.
2. Very good spatial resolution, and a single image covers the entire region showing all of the neural structures at once, facilitating comparison.
3. Image format is familiar to clinicians and the images are usually straightforward to interpret.

Disadvantages

1. Invasive procedure. With modern contrast agents and fine-gauge needles significant adverse reactions such as headache, nausea, vomiting, seizures and arachnoiditis are rare. However, overnight hospitalization is usually required.
2. Lacks some specificity. It can be difficult to tell the exact nature of a compressing structure (e.g. disc or bone). Post-myelography CT is often utilized to make this distinction. Also, after back surgery, it is difficult to differentiate epidural fibrosis versus recurrent disc herniation. MRI (with gadolinium) can be very helpful in these circumstances.
3. Nerve root sleeves may not fill with contrast (e.g. arachnoiditis after prior surgery) and so assessment of nerve root compression is very difficult. CT and MRI are useful in these circumstances.
4. Far lateral disc herniations are not usually shown. These make up approximately 12% of disc herniations. Nerve root compression occurs at the exit foramen or just beyond and as the nerve root sleeve does not extend out this far myelography often fails to demonstrate these foraminal disc herniations. However, they are well demonstrated by CT (Figure 3.3) and MRI.

To improve the diagnostic accuracy of myelography, CT is frequently performed shortly after the myelogram.

Discography

This invasive procedure uses X-ray guidance to place a needle directly into the nucleus pulposus of the disc (lumbar or cervical) and then a small volume of contrast is injected directly into the disc. Usually two or three discs are evaluated. There are two parts to the examination:

1. An image (plain film or CT) of the disc architecture to show (a) any disruption of the nucleus pulposus or (b) ruptures of the annulus fibrosis where disc herniations can occur.
2. Provocative – to see if the person's usual symptoms are reproduced when the disc volume is increased by the contrast injection.

With the advent of non-invasive methods to assess disc degeneration and herniation such as MRI and CT, discography is only infrequently performed now although the procedure has a small but enthusiastic following mainly for the value of the provocative part of the study. Discography can be helpful in localizing the symptomatic disc herniation before surgery when there is herniation at more than one level.

Radionuclide bone scan

This involves an intravenous injection of a radioactively tagged substance (tracer) which localizes in bony tissue (usually Technetium-99m-labelled methyl diphosphonate). The scan detects altered physiology by concentrating in areas of increased vascularity and areas of increased bone turnover. The emitted radiation is recorded by a gamma camera adjacent to the body. The whole body is imaged with spot views of the regions of interest. Cross-sectional images (SPECT – single photon emission computed tomography) are possible with a special rotating gamma camera device. This allows more exact localization of abnormalities in the bone [e.g. vertebral pedicle (suggests malignancy) versus facet joint (suggests degenerative disease) versus pars defect (suggests symptomatic spondylolysis)].

The modern technique, which improves specificity, involves a 'triple phase' study with (1) images immediately after injection showing blood flow, (2) blood pool images at 10 min detecting areas of abnormal vascularity in the soft tissues and (3) delayed images (2–3 h after injection) demonstrating areas of increased bone uptake ('hot') or occasionally areas of decreased bone uptake ('cold') when a lesion fails to stimulate osteoblastic activity (e.g. myeloma) or the blood supply is compromised (e.g. osteonecrosis).

Role

Clinical applications include:

1. Evaluation of bone pain when plain films are normal (e.g. stress fractures, shin splints, infection, tumour).
2. Infection:
   (a) to detect early osteomyelitis – plain films may take up to 10 days to show any abnormality;
   (b) cellulitis versus osteomyelitis – delayed images do not show increased bony uptake with cellulitis alone;
   (c) re-activation of chronic osteomyelitis.
3. To screen for bony metastases – can demonstrate metastases before any plain film changes. Unreliable in multiple myeloma as the lesions may not stimulate osteoblastic activity.
4. To help characterize bone tumours. A lesion without increased uptake is usually considered benign. However, some benign lesions can show increased uptake.
5. Evaluation of the painful joint prosthesis – helping to differentiate mechanical loosening from infective loosening. Indium labelled leucocytes or gallium may be used in addition to

methyl diphosphonate as they are more specific for infection.
6. To assess the activity and distribution of arthritis (e.g. rheumatoid arthritis) and metabolic bone disease (e.g. Paget's disease).
7. Assessment of osteonecrosis – useful in early detection to help identify areas of vascular compromise ('cold'). However, MRI is superior in this respect. Increased tracer uptake occurs in the repair and revascularization stages.

Advantages

1. High sensitivity – will detect bony abnormalities before any plain film changes.
2. Whole body imaged.
3. Widely available.
4. Low to moderate cost.

Disadvantages

1. Relatively non-specific. The bone scan is good for localizing an abnormality but further imaging is usually required to define the exact nature of the abnormality.
2. Spatial resolution not as good as other modalities.
3. May be difficult to detect abnormalities in regions with a normally high bone turnover (e.g. growing epiphyses, sacroiliac joints).
4. Moderate radiation dose.

Arthrography

This specialized procedure evaluates internal derangements of joints by injecting a contrast agent into a joint followed by a radiographic examination. The contrast may be either (1) positive (water-soluble iodine-containing compound), (2) negative (air) or more commonly (3) a combination of both (double contrast). Using X-ray guidance (fluoroscopy) a needle is placed into the joint followed by injection of the contrast agent(s). In experienced hands the procedure is relatively straightforward and minimally invasive with few adverse effects. The most common complaint is aggravation of joint pain.

The radiographic examination to follow can involve plain films, CT or digital subtraction techniques. Currently, MR arthrography is being evaluated, especially in the shoulder. The MR contrast agent gadolinium is injected into the joint followed by a MRI examination. Its role is yet to be fully defined, but the multiplanar capability and superb soft tissue resolution may be distinct advantages.

With the introduction of sophisticated non-invasive and radiation-free imaging techniques such as ultrasound and MRI, and the widespread use of arthroscopy (especially in the knee), there has been a substantial decrease in the utilization of arthrography. However, arthrography still has a place in certain clinical situations and is often the 'gold standard' against which the accuracy of other imaging techniques is measured.

Role

Clinical indications could include:

1. ***Shoulder***
   (a) evaluation of instability (performed in conjunction with CT);
   (b) rotator cuff tears;
   (c) adhesive capsulitis (frozen shoulder).
2. ***Knee***
   (a) meniscal tears – high accuracy in the diagnosis of meniscal tears but now has been largely replaced by MRI and arthroscopy which are able to make a more comprehensive evaluation of the knee joint;
   (b) cystic masses about the knee – to determine if they communicate with the knee joint [e.g. popliteal (Baker's) cyst];
   (c) osteochondral lesions and intra-articular loose bodies;
   (d) to evaluate possible loosening of a knee joint arthroplasty.
3. ***Wrist***
   (a) to evaluate tears of the (i) triangular fibrocartilage and (ii) intercarpal and capsular ligaments.
4. ***Hip***
   (a) evaluation of a painful prosthesis for possible loosening – when loose, contrast tracks down in the interface between the prosthesis or cement and the bone (subtraction technique required);
   (b) congential hip dislocation – to show (i) the exact position of the unossified femoral head within the acetabulum and (ii) whether the limbus is everted, preventing reduction; largely replaced by ultrasound now.
5. ***Ankle***
   (a) osteochondral lesions;
   (b) loose bodies within the joint cavity;
   (c) ligamentous tears.
6. ***Elbow***
   (a) osteochondral lesions;
   (b) intra-articular loose bodies (often in conjunction with CT).
7. ***Temporomandibular joints***
   (a) to evaluate disc dysfunction (e.g. dislocating disc) – dynamic assessment of disc dysfunction with opening and closing of the mouth can be provided with videofluorography.

Many of the different imaging modalities give complementary information and the imaging evaluation of some problems may require multiple modalities (e.g. suspected rotator cuff tear and disc prolapse). However, in most cases the plain film will be the initial examination.

Examination by plain film radiography – standard and supplementary views

We will now discuss the plain film examination of the spine, pelvis and peripheral joints. The various projections included in a standard radiographic examination of each region will be discussed. The standard views will provide an adequate evaluation in the large majority of cases. Supplementary views are also discussed which are performed only on request to evaluate a specific clinical problem.

Cervical spine

Standard views

Frontal (AP)

● Demonstrates C3 to C7: C1 and C2 are obscured by overlying structures.

Shows the vertebral bodies, disc spaces, uncovertebral joints, spinous processes (in profile), any supernumerary (cervical) rib (Figure 3.1) and frontal alignment.

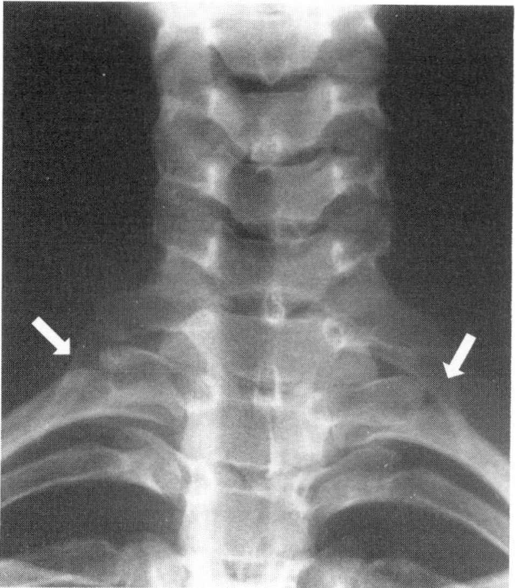

Figure 3.1 Cervical ribs. Cervical spine – frontal view. Miniature ribs (arrows) articulate with enlarged transverse processes of C7 bilaterally. They may compress the neurovascular structures of the thoracic outlet

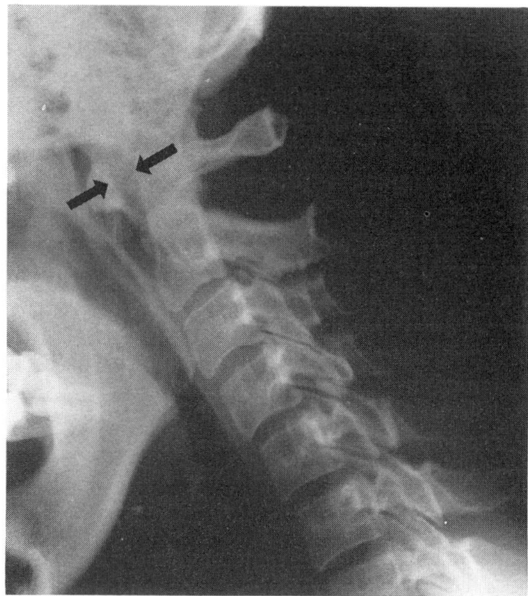

Figure 3.2 Atlantoaxial subluxation (rheumatoid arthritis). Lateral view of the cervical spine with flexion shows an abnormally widened pre-dens space (arrows). This narrows the spinal canal and cord compression may occur

Lateral (neutral position)

- Shows the vertebral bodies, disc spaces, spinal canal, spinous processes and lateral alignment (normally a mild lordosis is present). The cervicothoracic junction may not be adequately seen due to the overlapping shoulders.

Oblique (left and right at 45°)

- The intervertebral foramina (where the nerve roots exit) are profiled. The articular pillars, facet joints and pedicles are well shown.

Note: The labelling of oblique films refers only to the side of the body. The neuroforamina in profile are the same as the side of the occiput.

Supplementary views

Flexion and extension (lateral)

- To assess motion between the segments.

Useful when instability is suspected [e.g. after trauma or in rheumatoid arthritis where important

atlantoaxial subluxation may occur (Figure 3.2)]. The space between the back of the anterior arch of the atlas and the front of the dens (pre-dens space) on the lateral view should not be greater than 2.5 mm. Any subluxation will be accentuated on the flexion view.

Odontoid ('peg') view

- Frontal view of C1 and C2 with the mouth open. Utilized mainly in trauma to show any fracture of the odontoid process (dens) of C2 and to assess alignment between the lateral masses of C1 and C2 (Figure 3.3). Also used when checking for erosion of the dens in rheumatoid arthritis.

'Swimmer's' view

- To show the cervicothoracic junction when this is not adequately demonstrated on the standard lateral view.

Note: The atlanto-occipital joint is not ideally shown with plain films because of overlapping

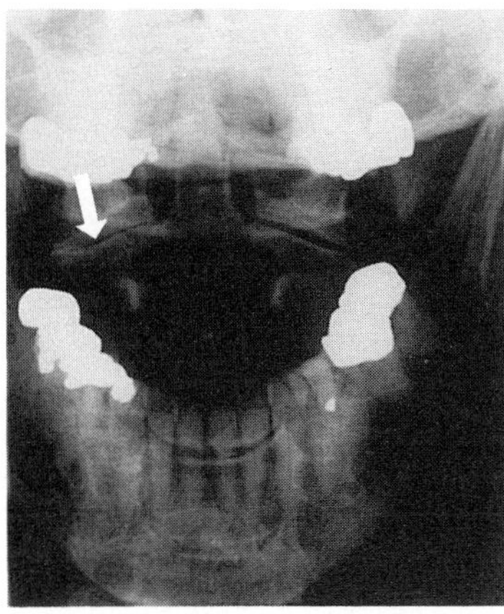

Figure 3.3 Osteoarthritis–atlantoaxial joint. Frontal view of C1 and C2 ('peg' view) showing loss of joint space, subchondral sclerosis and marginal osteophytes

structures and when specific evaluation of this joint is required MRI, CT or conventional tomography may be utilized.

Thoracic spine

Standard views

Frontal (AP)

- Shows the vertebral bodies, disc spaces and frontal alignment. The pedicles and spinous processes are shown in profile.

Lateral

- Shows the vertebral bodies, disc spaces, posterior elements and lateral alignment (normally a mild kyphosis is present). The cervicothoracic junction and upper thoracic vertebrae are usually not well shown because of the overlying shoulders. When assessment of this area is required a 'swimmer's' view or conventional tomography may be utilized. If the thoracolumbar junction is of particular interest (e.g. ankylosing spondylitis), frontal and lateral views centred to this region are helpful.

Lumbosacral spine

Standard views

Frontal (AP)

- Shows the vertebral bodies, disc spaces, transverse processes and frontal alignment. The pedicles, spinous processes and often the facet joints are all shown in profile.

Lateral

- Shows the disc spaces, vertebral bodies, spinal canal, spinous processes and lateral alignment (normally a mild lordosis is present). In addition, a coned view of the lumbosacral junction is performed.

Oblique (left and right at 45°)

Supplementary views

- To optimize the evaluation of the posterior elements, especially the pars regions and facet joints (e.g. suspected spondylolisthesis).

Functional views (standing)

- To demonstrate abnormal spinal movement (e.g. segmental instability as may occur with degenerative disease of the spine).
  1. Lateral views with flexion and extension. Checked for:
     (a) forward or backward displacement of one vertebra upon another;
     (b) abrupt change in the length of the pedicles;
     (c) foraminal narrowing;
     (d) loss of disc height.
  2. Optional – frontal views with lateral bending to the left and then to the right. Checked for:
     (a) asymmetry in bending;
     (b) loss of normal vertebral rotation and tilt;
     (c) abnormal opening or closure of disc spaces;
     (d) lateral translation;
     (e) malalignment of spinous processes and pedicles.

There is some controversy regarding the clinical utility of these views. They should be ordered with discretion as the radiation dose is moderate.

Note: Plain films of the spinal region may be performed either recumbent or erect. Spinal curvatures should be assessed with erect views.

Pelvis

Standard view

Frontal (AP)

- Centred to include the lumbosacral junction and hip joints.

Supplementary view

'Flamingo' views for instability

- To demonstrate ligamentous instability of the symphysis publis – sacroiliac joint complex as can occur in athletes. Frontal views are obtained with the patient standing on one leg then the other leg. A difference in the height between the superior pubic rami of greater than 2 mm or widening of the symphysis beyond 10 mm is considered abnormal (Figure 3.4).

Sacrum and coccyx

Standard views

Frontal (angulated)

- The sacrum may not be ideally visualized on a frontal view of the pelvis and a coned angled view is useful when the sacrum is of clinical interest.

Lateral

- Provides a lateral view of the sacrum and coccyx.

Sacroiliac joints

Standard views

Frontal pelvis

- As described above.

Frontal pelvis (AP with angulation)

- X-ray beam is angulated 30° towards the head which provides a better profile of the joints. Both joints are included on a single view to facilitate comparison.

Note: Oblique views of the sacroiliac joints are not recommended as they are technically difficult to perform and do not usually contribute to an assessment of sacroiliitis.

Hip

Standard views

Frontal pelvis (AP)

- Allows comparison with opposite hip (Figure 3.29).

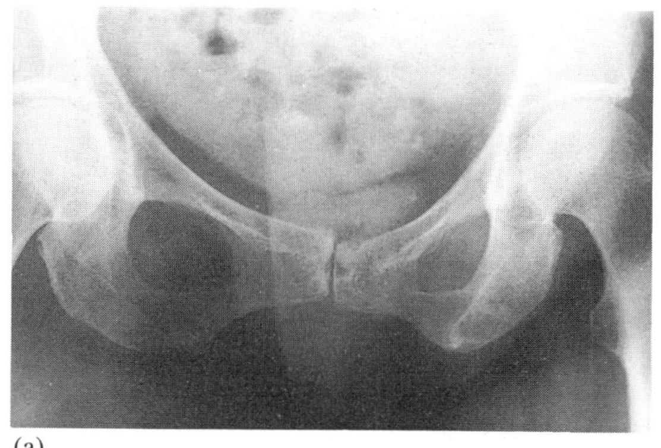
(a)

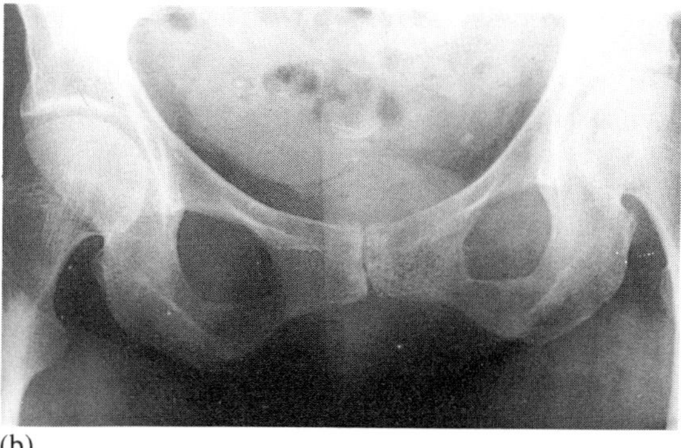
(b)

Figure 3.4 Osteitis pubis–'Flamingo' views. (a) Standing on left leg and (b) standing on right leg. There is subchondral erosion and sclerosis of the symphysis pubis. Instability is demonstrated when standing on the right leg where there is a greater than 2 mm difference in height between the superior pubic rami

Lateral hip ('frog leg' position)

- Provides a true lateral view of the femoral head and neck, but not of the acetabulum. In trauma, when the hip cannot be comfortably moved, a true lateral view (cross-table) of the femoral head and acetabulum is performed.

Supplementary views

Orthopaedic pelvis

- Before and after hip joint replacement a low centred frontal view of the pelvis is performed so that the entire prosthesis is included on a single film. An assessment of any leg length discrepancy can also be made.

Oblique (anterior and posterior at 45° – 'Judet')

- Visualizes the bony columns of the pelvis and the anterior and posterior acetabular rims. These views may be useful after fracture/dislocation of the acetabulum although CT is superior in this respect.

Knee

Standard views

Frontal (AP with knee fully extended)

- Shows the distal femur, patella, proximal tibia, joint space in the lateral and medial compartments, and femorotibial alignment.

Lateral (20–35° of knee flexion)

- Assesses patellar height and shows any joint effusions. A cross table (decubitus) lateral view is performed in acute trauma to show the presence of any fat–fluid level which would suggest intra-articular fracture.

Patella (axial view – 'skyline')

- Profiles the patellofemoral joint. Shows the morphology of the joint surfaces and patellar alignment. The preferred technique is that of Merchant with 40° of knee flexion. Skyline views of the patellofemoral joint with 30°, 60° and 90° of knee flexion for assessment of patellar tracking are not recommended as most abnormalities occur with knee flexion of 30° or less. CT and MRI are far superior in the assessment of patellar tracking.

Supplementary views

Frontal (weight-bearing)

- Utilized in the evaluation of osteoarthritis of the femorotibial compartments of the knee joint. Weight-bearing on the affected side allows a more accurate assessment of the loss of cartilage space and resulting angular (usually varus) deformity (Figure 3.5). Alternatively, a long film with weight-bearing which includes the hip and ankle joints may be utilized to allow

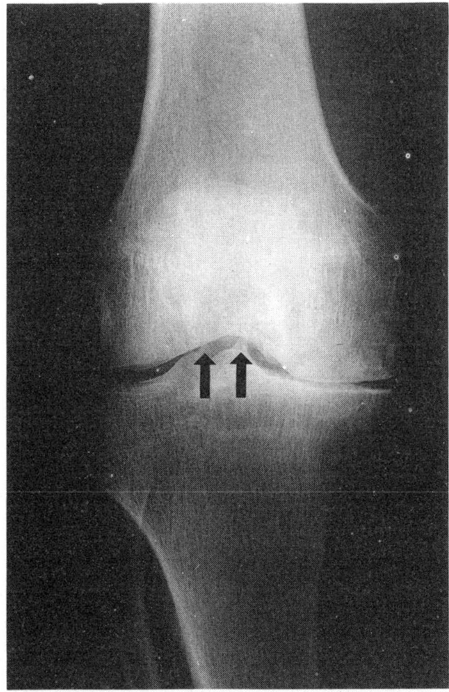

Figure 3.5 Osteoarthritis – knee joint. Frontal view with weight-bearing. The weight-bearing medial femorotibial compartment demonstrates almost complete loss of articular space with subchondral sclerosis and there is osteophytic enlargement of the tibial spines (arrows). There is moderate loss of bone stock of the medial tibial plateau and a mild varus deformity

measurement of the angular deformity along the mechanical axis of the leg as part of the preoperative work-up before osteotomy or total knee joint arthroplasty.

Oblique (left and right at 45°)

- Useful in trauma when the standard views are normal and a joint effusion is present to help show subtle fractures of the tibial plateaus and femoral condyles. Also allows evaluation of the proximal fibula and superior tibiofibular joint.

Intercondylar ('tunnel') view

- To show the intercondylar notch. Gives a better view of the joint surfaces of the femoral condyles, tibial plateaus and the tibial spines. Useful in demonstrating osteochondral lesions of femoral condyles and cruciate avulsion fractures.

Stress views

- Infrequently utilized. Can demonstrate ligamentous instability – medial, lateral, anterior or posterior – by applying manual stress in the appropriate direction.

Ankle

Standard views

Frontal (AP)

- Shows the joint surfaces (tibial plafond and talar dome), joint spaces and the malleoli.

Oblique ('Mortise' view – with 15–20° of internal rotation of the foot)

- Opens up the joint space to give a better profile of the ankle joint, especially medially, the inferior tibiofibular syndesmosis and the inferior tip of the lateral malleolus.

Lateral

- To show the distal tibia, talus, calcaneus and Achilles tendon. Allows assessment of any joint effusion.

Supplementary views

Stress views

- With acute twisting injuries of the ankle when plain films have excluded a fracture, and ligament or tendon injury is suspected, stress views may help to demonstrate instability. Stress views may also be helpful in cases of chronic instability as well. Comparison is made between the injured and normal sides as the degree of ankle joint laxity is variable. For medial (deltoid) and lateral ligament injuries frontal views are taken with manually applied eversion or inversion stress respectively. Any abnormal widening (greater than 5°) of the ankle joint mortise compared with the normal side suggests instability. Stress views are contraindicated in children with open growth plates.

Weight-bearing views

- Utilized in congenital hindfoot deformities (e.g. club foot) and chronic instability as positional relationships may change dramatically when weight-bearing.

Impingement view

- A weight-bearing view of the ankle taken with maximum dorsiflexion ('demi-plie') is useful when assessing for anterior impingement.

Axial view of calcaneus

- Useful in suspected calcaneal fractures.
CT is utilized for the assessment of intra-articular calcaneal fractures.

Subtalar joints

Not ideally assessed by plain film radiography

Note: These joints are best assessed with coronal CT (e.g. talo-calcaneal fusion).

Shoulder

Standard views

Frontal (external and internal rotation)

- To evaluate the glenohumeral and acromioclavicular joints. The external rotation view is performed obliquely so as to give a true frontal profile of the glenohumeral joint and a true frontal view of the scapula. This view also profiles the greater tuberosity and is useful for detecting calcification in the supraspinatus tendon (Figure 3.6). The internal rotation view is useful for detecting calcification in the remaining cuff tendons and viewing the acromioclavicular joint.

Lateral (trans-scapular 'Y' view)

- To assess alignment of the humeral head in the glenoid fossa and so is important in trauma. Does not profile the glenohumeral joint but demonstrates the coracoacromial arch.

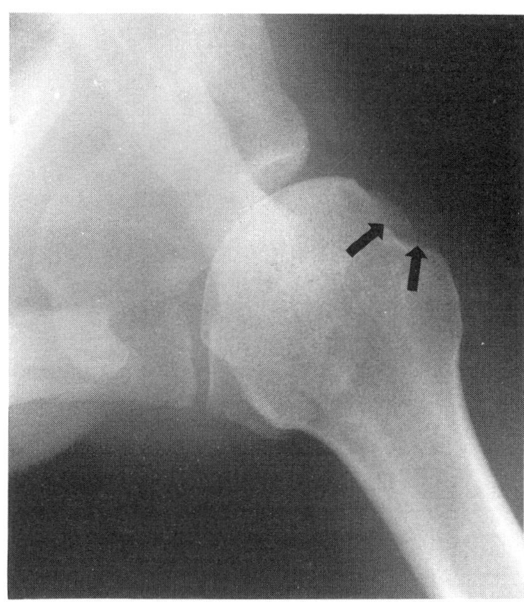

Figure 3.7 Hill–Sachs lesion. Shoulder – Stryker notch view. There is a large osteochondral defect from the posterolateral aspect of the humeral head (arrow) which is hatchet shaped – proof of prior anterior dislocation

Lateral (axillary projection)

- Gives a true lateral view of the glenohumeral joint and shows glenohumeral alignment, but is difficult to obtain with acute trauma as some shoulder abduction is required.

Supplementary views

Supplementary views are generally indicated to identify anterior instability or impingement/rotator cuff problems.

1. Instability – two traumatic chondro-osseous lesions which are not reliably shown on standard views are a marker for anterior instability (proof of prior anterior dislocation).

   (a) ***Stryker notch view*** gives the best view of a Hill–Sachs lesion – an osteochondral impaction fracture of the posterolateral humeral head (Figure 3.8).
   (b) ***WestPoint axillary view*** gives the best view of a Bankart lesion (osseous type) – an osteochondral fracture or periostitis of the anteroinferior glenoid rim.

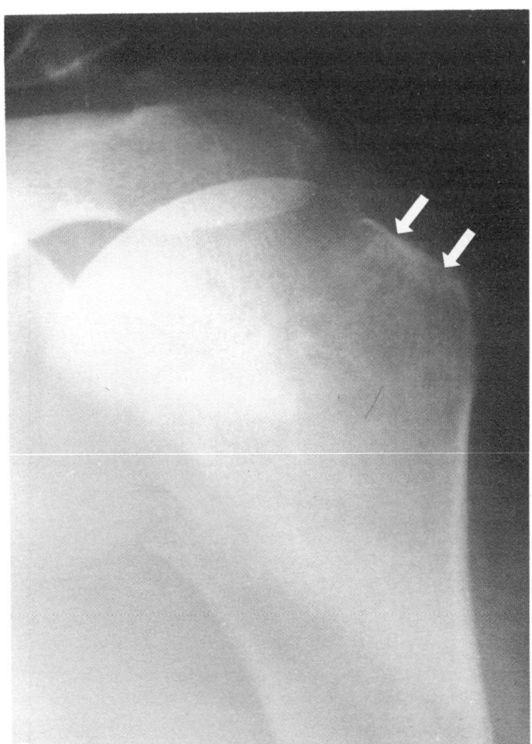

Figure 3.6 Calcific tendinitis. Shoulder – frontal view with external rotation. Calcification is present in the distal portion of the supraspinatus tendon (arrows) adjacent to the greater tuberosity of the humerus

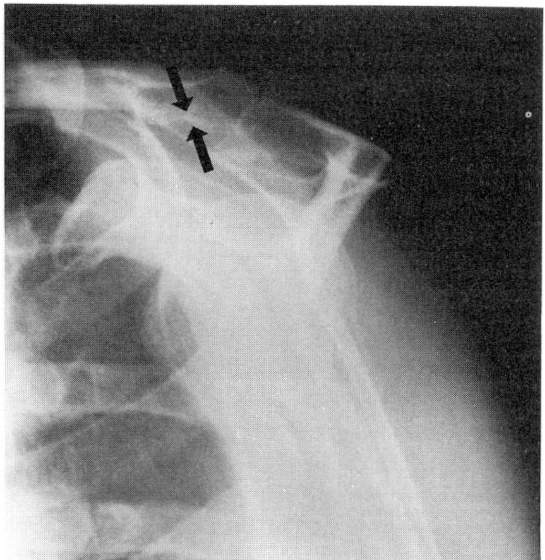

Figure 3.8 Subacromial spur. Supraspinatus outlet view. There is a traction spur (arrows) on the undersurface of the anterior acromion which can impinge upon the supraspinatus tendon leading to tendinitis and cuff tear

2. Impingement views – to demonstrate anterior subacromial and acromioclavicular joint spurs.

   (a) ***Supraspinatus outlet view*** – profiles the coracoacromial arch ('Y' view with 20° caudal angulation and weight-bearing) showing the morphology and presence of any spurs from the anterior undersurface of the acromion (Figure 3.8).
   (b) ***Frontal view with 30° caudal angulation*** – to show spurs projecting inferiorly from the undersurface of the anterior acromion and acromioclavicular joint.

Acromioclavicular joint

Standard views

Frontal (angulated)

● The standard frontal view of the shoulder shows the acromioclavicular joint, but a better profile of the joint is obtained with the X-ray beam angulated 15° towards the head.

Supplementary views

Stress views (weight-bearing)

● These may be necessary to diagnose and grade traumatic separation of the acromioclavicular – coracoclavicular complex when the standard view is normal. Weights are hung from both wrists (not held in the hands) and a single film is taken to demonstrate both joints to facilitate comparison. Assessment is made of (1) the width of the acromioclavicular joint and (2) the distance between the upper tip of the coracoid process and the adjacent undersurface of the clavicle which is indicative of coracoclavicular ligament disruption when there is a 5 mm or greater increase in coracoclavicular distance.

Sternoclavicular joints

● Adequate plain film views are difficult to obtain and they are often non-diagnostic. CT is the preferred examination to assess subluxation, dislocation, erosion and hyperostosis.

Elbow

Standard views

Frontal (AP with the elbow joint extended and the hand in full supination)

● Shows the distal humerus including the epicondyles, proximal radius and ulna, and the joint spaces.

Lateral (90° of elbow flexion)

● Provides a lateral view of the distal humerus and proximal forearm. The olecranon process is well shown. Joint effusion can be assessed by displacement of fat pads.

Supplementary views

1. Trauma – in the case of trauma when a joint effusion is demonstrated but no fracture is seen on the standard views the following views may be helpful to show minimally displaced

fractures of the radial head, capitellum and coranoid process;

(a) *oblique (lateral and medial)*
(b) *radial head – capitellum view* – eliminates overlap of the humero-ulnar and humero-radial joints (radial head is projected anterior to coronoid process).

Axial view (elbow flexed 45°)

● Provides an axial view of the olecranon process and profiles the epicondyles. This view may be helpful in showing osteophytes from the humero-ulnar joint, loose bodies in the space between the olecranon process and capitellum, and periarticular calcifications.

Wrist

Standard views

Frontal (PA)

● Shows the radiocarpal and intercarpal joints, carpal arcs (proximal and distal rows of carpal bones) and any ulnar variance (ulna shorter or longer than the radius).

Lateral (neutral position)

● Important in assessing axial alignment for various instability patterns that can follow ligamentous injury.

Oblique (semipronated and semisupinated)

● To show the ulnar and radial aspects respectively of the carpus.

Supplementary views

Scaphoid views

● To enhance fracture detection.

Stress views

● May be useful when carpal instability is suspected following ligamentous injury (e.g. scapholunate dissociation or dorsal and volar instability).

1. **frontal views** with ulnar and radial deviation;
2. **lateral views** with palmarflexion and dorsiflexion;
3. **frontal view with a clenched fist ('grip' view)** – accentuates potential scapholunate dissociation by loading the capitate on to the proximal carpal row.

Carpal tunnel view

● To demonstrate the osseous structures of the carpal tunnel, including the hook of the hamate.

Note: The soft tissue structures of the carpal tunnel are much better evaluated with ultrasound or MRI.

Distal radio-ulnar joint

● Subluxation or dislocation of this joint is not reliably demonstrated on plain films and, when indicated, CT should be used to assess alignment or instability.

Clinical problems and their evaluation using imaging techniques

We have chosen to discuss topics which are both common and likely to be of interest to the physiotherapist. The clinical background is presented along with the various imaging modalities that may be utilized, a description of the imaging findings and, finally, clinical correlation with signs and symptoms.

Spinal and pelvic problems

The taking of spinal and pelvic radiographs using the views described is only one aspect of a clinical examination. In isolation, standard radiographs are rarely indicative of appropriate management. They do, however, serve a very useful role in excluding unsuspected important disease and mechanical deformity. Most persons attending for physiotherapy for spinal pain have normal films or ones that show degenerative disease of the spine. It is important for the practitioner to have an appreciation of some of the more common abnormalities of the axial skeleton seen on imaging studies.

Degenerative disease of the spine

Also referred to as osteoarthritis or spondylosis, degenerative disease of the spine encompasses a variety of distinct and separate disease processes of the spine. Most commonly it is primary (or idiopathic), but it may be secondary to trauma, an underlying arthritis (e.g. rheumatoid arthritis) or infection.

Degeneration of the intervertebral disc

This involves two separate entities:

1. *Intervertebral osteochondrosis* – where the chondromucoid elements of the nucleus pulposus decrease with resultant dehydration and loss of viscoelasticity of the disc. The radiographic changes include (Figure 3.9):

   (a) loss of disc height;
   (b) gas within the disc space – the so-called vacuum phenomenon – due to gas (approximately 90% nitrogen) collecting within the clefts of a degenerating disc (Figure 3.10);
   (c) sclerosis of the vertebral body endplates adjacent to the disc;
   (d) loss of the normal cervical or lumbar lordosis;
   (e) disc calcification – usually localized to one or two discs in the mid-thoracic and upper lumbar spine.

2. *Spondylosis deformans* – the formation of bony outgrowths (osteophytes) from the vertebral body margin at the site of the ligamentous attachment of the disc (Figure 3.9). This is thought to result from the breakdown of the outer fibres of the annulus fibrosis which allows disc material to stress the ligamentous attachment. Radiographically, the osteophytes first appear horizontally from the vertebral body margin and then tend to curve vertically and may eventually bridge the disc space in an attempt to stabilize the spine. In the cervical spine osteophytes from the posterior vertebral margin can form a bony ridge which may compress the adjacent spinal cord.

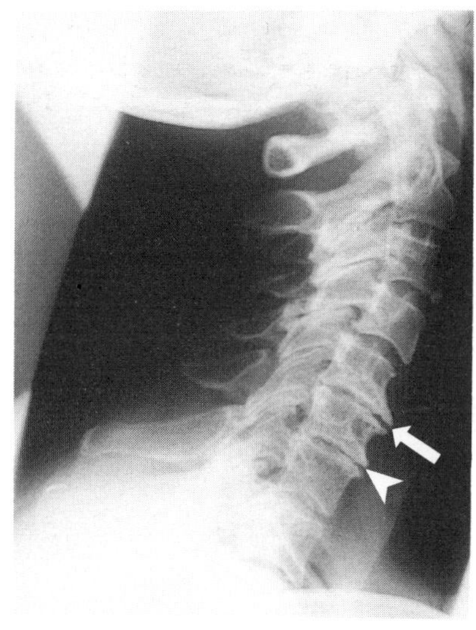

(a)

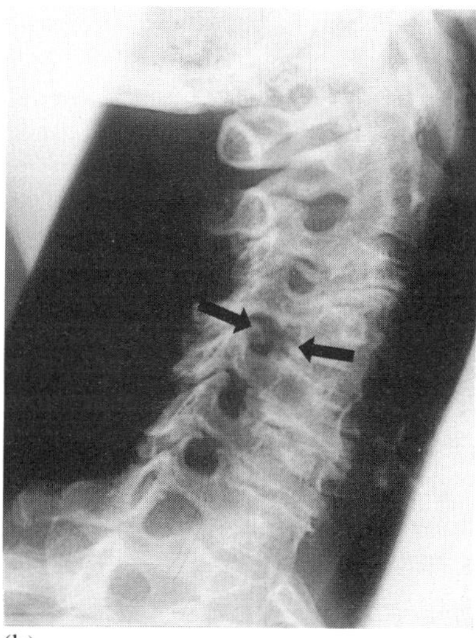

(b)

Figure 3.9 Degenerative disease of the cervical spine. Cervical spine; (a) lateral and (b) oblique views. The C5–6 (arrow) and C6–7 (arrowhead) discovertebral joints are narrowed with subchondral sclerosis and osteophytes at the vertebral body margin. There is also involvement of the corresponding facet joints and uncovertebral joints. The oblique view shows osteophytes projecting into the C5–6 (arrow) and C6–7 neuroforamina from the front and back where they may cause nerve root compression

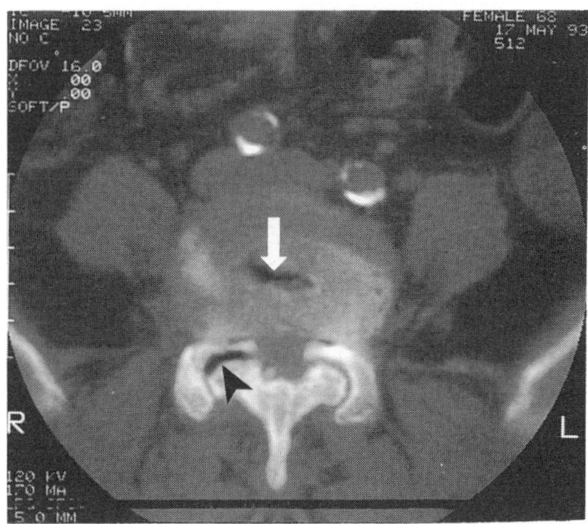

Figure 3.10 Degenerative spinal stenosis. Axial CT scan through the L4–5 disc space. The central spinal canal is narrowed as a result of a bulging disc, osteophytic facet joint hypertrophy and ligamentum flava hypertrophy. Compression of the nerve roots lying within the thecal sac may occur. Note the gas (vacuum phenomenon) in the degenerative disc (arrow) and right facet joint (arrowhead)

Osteoarthritis of the zygapophyseal (facet) joints

This is often a sequela of degeneration of the disc which allows excessive stress of these joints but occasionally osteoarthritis can predominate in these joints with little or no radiographic change in the discs. Clinical features of facet joint disease include local pain on palpation over the facet joint and back pain which may radiate and mimic sciatica. Radiographic features include (Figures 3.9 and 3.10):

1. joint space narrowing,
2. subchondral sclerosis,
3. osteophytosis.

The osteophytes may be of clinical importance as they may:

1. hypertrophy the facet joints and contribute to stenosis in the central spinal canal (Figure 3.10);
2. project into the nerve root canals [lateral recess (Figure 3.11) or exit foramen (Figure 3.12)] where they may impinge upon spinal nerves or nerve roots;
3. project into the foramen transversarium (cervical spine only) where they may impinge upon the vertebral artery. This is rare.

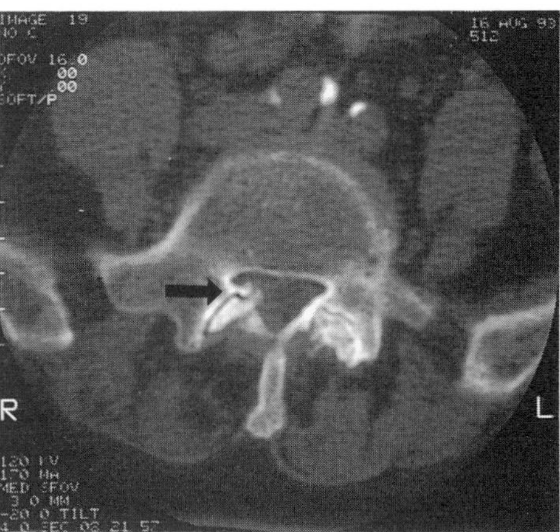

Figure 3.11 Lateral recess stenosis. Axial CT scan through the pedicles of L5. Osteophytes from the facet joint project into the lateral recess (the entrance zone of the nerve root canal) where they may compress the right L5 nerve root (arrow)

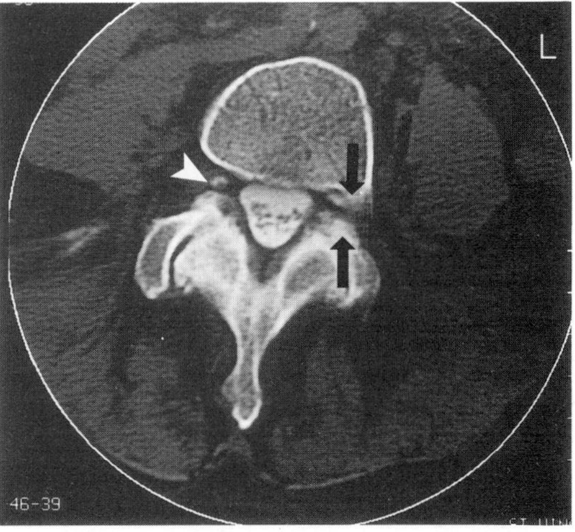

Figure 3.12 Foraminal stenosis. CT-myelogram – axial section just above the L4–5 disc space. The left L4 exit foramen (the exit zone of the nerve root canal) is narrowed by osteophytes from the front and back (arrows) and compression of the L4 spinal nerve or nerve root may occur. The right L4 nerve root can be seen normally (arrowhead) at its exit foramen

Uncovertebral (neurocentral) joint arthrosis

These are small synovial joints located at the posterolateral margins of the vertebral bodies C3 to C7 which commonly degenerate when they are impacted with the loss of disc height that occurs

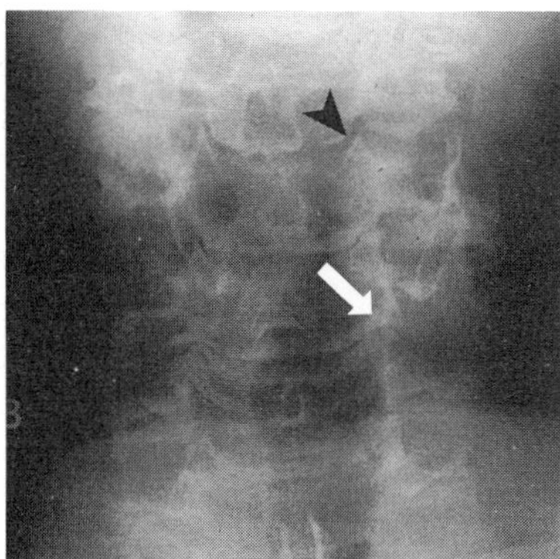

Figure 3.13 Unconvertebral joint osteoarthrosis.
There is loss of joint space, rounding off and
osteophytic enlargement of the unconvertebral joints
(arrow). A normal joint (arrowhead) is shown for
comparison

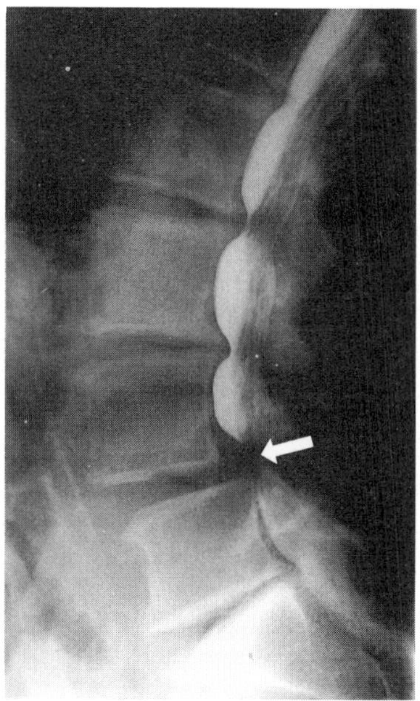

Figure 3.14 Degenerative spinal stenosis.
Myelogram – lateral view. There is multilevel spinal
stenosis compressing the thecal sac. This is most
marked at the L4–5 level where a degenerative
spondylolisthesis further narrows the spinal canal
(arrow)

with disc degeneration. X-rays show (Figure
3.13):

1. rounding off of the uncinate process;
2. narrowing of joint space;
3. osteophytes which may project into the neuroforamina and cause nerve root compression
   (assessed on the oblique views) (Figure 3.9). It
   is thought that the neuroforamina need to be
   narrowed by at least 50% to be clinically
   significant.

Complications of degenerative spinal disease

Alterations of vertebral alignment

1. *Segmental instability* – see discussion under
   functional views of lumbar spine;
2. *Degenerative spondylolisthesis* – slippage of
   one vertebra upon another (spondylolisthesis) is
   commonly seen in the degenerative spine. It is
   due to subluxation of osteoarthritic facet joints
   and is most commonly seen in the mobile
   segments of the cervical and lumbar spine (e.g.
   C5–6, C6–7, L3–4, L4–5). Two patterns occur:
   (1) anterolisthesis, due to anterior slippage of
   the upper vertebrae (Figure 3.14) or, (2) retro-
   listhesis, due to posterior slippage of the upper
   vertebra. In both instances the spinal canal is
   narrowed as a result, contributing to spinal
   stenosis, but in many instances the slip is

asymptomatic. This is to be contrasted with the
situation of spondylolisthesis associated with
pars defects (lytic spondylolisthesis) where the
spinal canal is widened and stretching of the
nerve roots can occur.

Intervertebral disc herniation and spinal stenosis

Plain films cannot directly show the spinal cord,
CSF, thecal sac, nerve roots or herniated discs
(except in the rare instance of a calcified disc
herniation). Owing to the very close anatomic
relationships, disc herniation and spinal stenosis
may cause spinal cord compression (myelopathy)
or nerve root compression (radiculopathy) and
when this is suspected clinically on the basis of
symptoms and objective neurological findings
other imaging modalities such as CT (Figure 3.15),
MRI (Figure 3.16) and myelography (Figure 3.17)
are utilized. Surgical intervention may be considered in these patients and accurate radiological
diagnosis is mandatory.

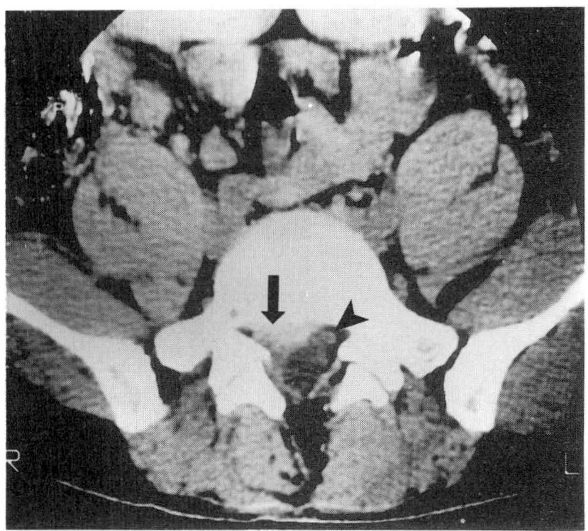

Figure 3.15 Intervertebral disc herniation. Axial CT scan just below the L5–1 disc shows focal right sided paracentral herniation where it can compress the right S1 nerve root as it leaves the thecal sac. The normal left sided S1 nerve root is shown (arrowhead)

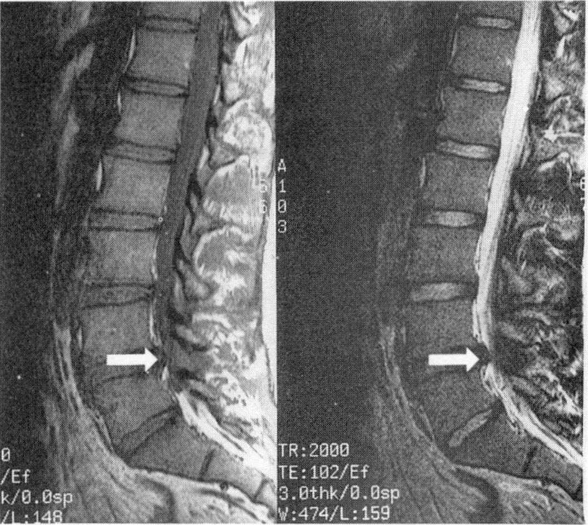

Figure 3.16 Lumbar disc herniation. MRI scan – sagittal section, T_1-weighted (left) and T_2-weighted (right) images. There is a paracentral herniation of the L4–5 disc (arrows) compressing the L5 nerve root as it leaves the thecal sac. The loss of signal in the L4–5 disc on the T_2 image reflects the dehydration seen with disc degeneration

Intervertebral disc herniation

Disc material which is displaced posteriorly, posterolaterally or laterally can be very important clinically because of potential compression of the spinal cord and/or nerve roots. The extent of the disc displacement is described by the following terms:

1. Bulging annulus – here the annular fibres remain intact but protrude in a diffuse pattern into the spinal canal.
2. Disc protrusion (or prolapse) – the nucleus pulposus protrudes focally through some of the fibres of the annulus fibrosis but is still contained by intact outer fibres.
3. Disc extrusion – when the nucleus pulposus extrudes through all the fibres of the annulus fibrosis, but remains confined by the posterior longitudinal ligament.
4. Disc sequestration – where (i) the herniated disc material penetrates the posterior longitudinal ligament and lies free in the epidural space or (ii) a separated disc fragment migrates superiorly or inferiorly beyond the disc space beneath the posterior longitudinal ligament.

Disc protrusion, extrusion and sequestration are all types of herniation of the nucleus pulposus. Imaging cannot usually distinguish disc protrusion versus extrusion. Posterolateral (or paracentral)

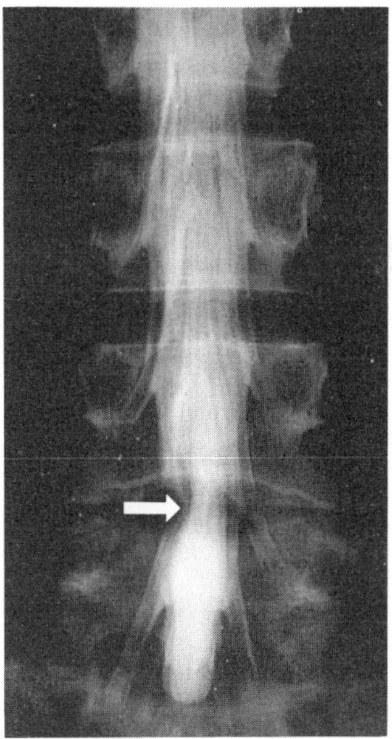

Figure 3.17 Lumbar disc herniation. Lumbar myelogram – frontal view. There is an extradural defect on the thecal sac in a right paracentral location due to disc herniation (arrow). The right L5 nerve root is compressed as it leaves the thecal sac with abrupt cut off ('amputation') in contrast filling the nerve root sleeve (compare with normal left sided L5 nerve root)

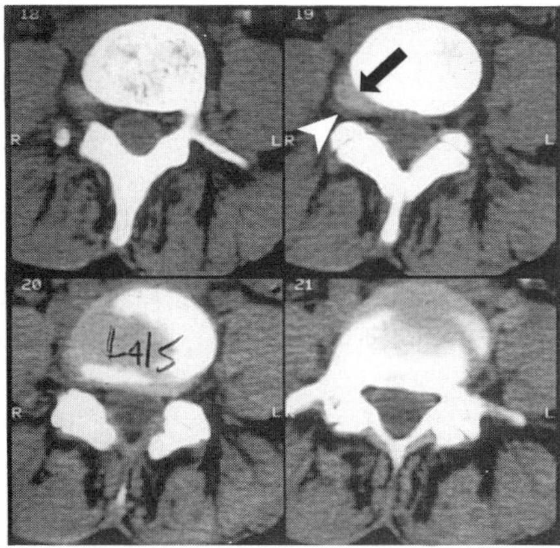

Figure 3.18 Foraminal disc herniation. Axial CT scans show a right-sided far lateral herniation of the L4–5 intervertebral disc (arrow) which has migrated upwards into the exit foramen where it displaces the L4 nerve root (arrowhead)

disc herniation is the most common pattern (Figure 3.15) which is thought to be due to the fewer and weaker annular fibres in this region. Less commonly, spinal nerve or nerve root compression may occur at the exit foramen (foraminal disc herniation) when a far lateral disc herniation migrates upwards (Figure 3.18). A combination of paracentral and lateral disc herniation can compress two separate nerve roots.

Spinal stenosis
Stenosis in the central spinal canal is due to a combination of bony and soft tissue factors such as disc bulging, osteophytes from the posterior vertebral body margin, facet joint and ligamentum flavum hypertrophy and spondylolisthesis (Figures 3.10 and 3.14), often on a background of a developmentally small canal. It often occurs at multiple levels and can produce significant compression of the thecal sac and its contents. In the lumbar spine, spinal stenosis can produce the clinical syndrome of intermittent neurogenic claudication (activity-related pain and weakness in the legs) whereas, in the cervical spine, limb weakness and hyper-reflexia may occur.

Stenosis may also occur in (i) the lateral recess (Figure 3.11) or exit foramen (Figure 3.12) of the nerve root canals of the lumbar spine, usually due to adjacent facet joint osteophytes, or (ii) the nerve root canal in the cervical spine, usually due to uncovertebral joint osteophytes (Figure 3.9). In

both instances compression or entrapment of the nerve roots may occur.

Degenerative disease of the spine predominates in the weight-bearing mid and lower segments of the cervical, thoracic and lumbar spine. Degenerative changes in the thoracic segments are seldom of clinical significance as compression of the neural structures at this site is unusual.

The diagnostic accuracy of MRI and CT and myelography for disc herniation and spinal stenosis are about equal. Individual practice will vary with the preference and experience of the radiologist and the availability of MRI. Most patients with suspected disc herniation or spinal stenosis will be screened non-invasively with CT or MRI. When surgery is being considered, myelography, often with post-myelography CT, may be performed as an additional means to support the diagnosis and to help plan the surgical approach.

Clinical correlation

The radiographic demonstration of degenerative changes in the spine is age related – commonly seen after the age of 40, rising to 70% of people greater than 70 years of age – and equally present in both asymptomatic and symptomatic persons. Therefore, the clinical severity of degenerative disease correlates poorly with the severity of radiographic changes. The main role of plain films is to confirm degenerative disease in symptomatic persons and to exclude unsuspected pathology.

In addition, asymptomatic disc herniation and spinal stenosis are not uncommon, so any imaging abnormality must be carefully correlated with the person's symptoms and findings on clinical examination. If a person on clinical examination has clear findings of spinal nerve or nerve root compression and a demonstrable disc herniation on imaging, physiotherapy treatment may still be given but the extent of the herniation and the severity or chronicity of the symptoms will all affect treatment outcome and raise the possibility of surgical intervention. The majority of persons who have disc herniation settle with conservative management.

Persons who have severe intermittent neurogenic claudication and clear radiological evidence of canal stenosis usually respond poorly to physiotherapeutic measures. Conservative management involves rest, anti-inflammatory drugs and facet joint or epidural injection. The aim of the conservative therapy is to reduce the inflammatory response in neural tissue as one cannot affect the bony entrapment. If this fails and the patient is severely disabled, surgical decompression is required and is usually successful in relieving the claudicant symptoms.

Anatomical anomalies of the vertebral column

Anomalies of the bony configuration of the spine are commonly seen. Minor asymmetries and even malformations are frequently seen, especially in the cervical and lumbar spine on plain films. Most of these anomalies are of no clinical significance and they are no more prevalent in persons with spinal pain. However, spondylolysis, spondylolisthesis or a transitional vertebra may render a spine more vulnerable to back pain.

Spondylolysis and spondylolisthesis

Spondyloysis (pars defect) is a bony defect in the pars interarticularis (the part between the superior and inferior articular process) of a vertebra. This is a fairly common entity which may be unilateral or bilateral. The usual site of involvement is a mid or lower lumbar vertebra especially L5 (Figure 3.19). Spondylolysis may cause back and/or radicular pain, but it is often asymptomatic. The aetiology of this condition is thought to be an acquired fracture

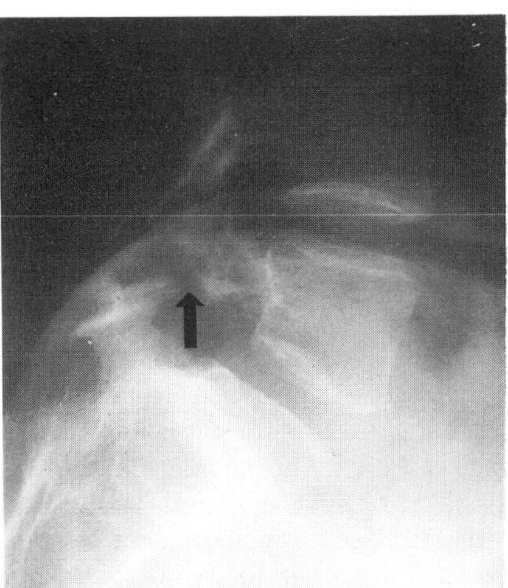

Figure 3.19 Lytic spondylolisthesis. Lumbar spine – lateral view. There are lytic defects through the pars interarticulares of L5 (arrow). There is an associated minor forward slip of L5 on S1

occurring in infancy or early adult life often with an underlying congenital predisposition. Most often this is a stress-type fracture following repeated trauma. These defects tend to persist and unlike other stress fractures tend to heal with fibrous union (with or without pseudoarthrosis). If pseudoarthrosis occurs, hypertrophic change may develop around the pars defect which can entrap the nerve root or spinal nerve as it runs under its pedicle.

Spondylolysis when bilateral may be associated with displacement of one vertebral body on to the adjacent one (spondylolisthesis); the vertebra with the pars defect slipping forward on the vertebra below (Figure 3.19). This is referred to as a lytic spondylolisthesis and should be distinguished from the more commonly seen degenerative spondylolisthesis. The magnitude of the slip is usually small (less than 1 cm) and progression is not usually seen beyond skeletal maturity. The slip is usually not symptomatic but surgical decompression and fusion may be necessary in some cases.

Radiographic features of spondylolysis

A lucent line is demonstrated through the pars region. This is often visible on the lateral view (Figure 3.19), but is seen to best advantage on the oblique view (as a break through the neck of the 'scottie dog'). If there is any doubt, CT can provide further evaluation. If there is a unilateral pars defect, hypertrophy and reactive sclerosis of contralateral pedicle may be seen.

Radiographic features of spondylolisthesis.

Spondylolisthesis when present is measured. There may be tilt as well as a slip. The vertebra below the slip can tilt forward and narrow the neuroforamina and this may cause entrapment of the nerve roots at the exit foramen. A radionuclide bone scan may be helpful (i) in detecting early defects when plain films are normal and (ii) to ascertain whether a discovered defect is symptomatic.

Clinical correlation

Spondylolisthesis is a good example where radiographs will greatly help in the diagnosis and management of spinal pain. If on clinical grounds the therapist feels that the person's pain is related to a radiographically demonstrated slip, then this pain may be due to instability at the defect, entrapment of a spinal nerve or nerve root or an incidental disc prolapse. Careful evaluation of the signs and symptoms will establish what structures are involved and the appropriate management.

Transitional vertebrae at the lumbosacral junction

It is not uncommon to find congenital transitional vertebrae at the lumbosacral junction. A wide variety of patterns exist including sacralization of L5 and lumbarization of S1, which may be complete or incomplete. A true joint may exist between an enlarged transverse process of L5 and the adjacent ala of the sacrum which can be unilateral (Figure 3.20) or bilateral. Degenerative changes can occur in these joints due to the altered mechanics and this may progress to bony ankylosis. There is also an increased incidence of pars defects. The relationship between low back pain and transitional vertebrae at the lumbosacral junction is the subject of debate. It has been suggested

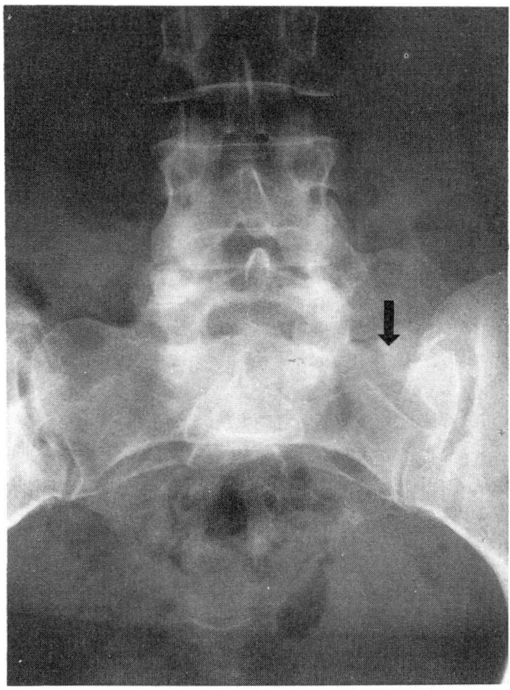

Figure 3.20 Transitional vertebra. Lumbosacral spine – frontal view. An enlarged left sided transverse process of L5 (arrow) forms a true joint with the adjacent ala of the sacrum

that a unilateral joint between the transverse process of L5 and the sacrum is more likely to be symptomatic.

Cartilaginous nodes

Also commonly known as Schmorl's nodes, cartilaginous nodes represent disc material that has been displaced either superiorly or inferiorly through the cartilaginous and vertebral body endplates into the spongy bone of the vertebral body. They occur in a variety of conditions that can weaken the cartilaginous endplate of the disc or the subchondral bone plate of the vertebral body including trauma, disc degeneration and rheumatoid arthritis and Scheuermann's disease (juvenile kyphosis). Cartilaginous nodes are not synonymous with Scheuermann's disease.

Radiographic features of cartilaginous nodes are characteristic; a rounded radiolucent area of variable size with the vertebral body immediately adjacent to the endplate surrounded by a cap of sclerosis. Mild endplate irregularity and cartilaginous node formation are frequently seen around the thoracolumbar junction, without kyphosis. These findings are not likely to be symptomatic and are of doubtful clinical significance.

Avulsion of the ring apophysis

A related condition is avulsion of the ring apophysis. This occurs in the skeletally immature before apophyseal fusion when the cartilaginous growthplate is a point of weakness. Disc material may herniate through this area isolating a small wedge-shaped segment of the apophysis. This usually occurs at the anterosuperior corner of a lumbar vertebral body (limbus vertebrae) (Figure 3.21). However, the avulsed ring apophysis occasionally can occur from the posterior corner of the vertebral body when it could potentially compress neural structures in the spinal canal.

Spinal alignment

Slight malalignments of spinal curvature on erect radiographs are quite common and are mainly asymptomatic. Some practitioners place great emphasis on these findings but any abnormal finding must be carefully correlated with the person's symptoms and objective clinical findings. Two common alignment problems in the spine are scoliosis and kyphosis.

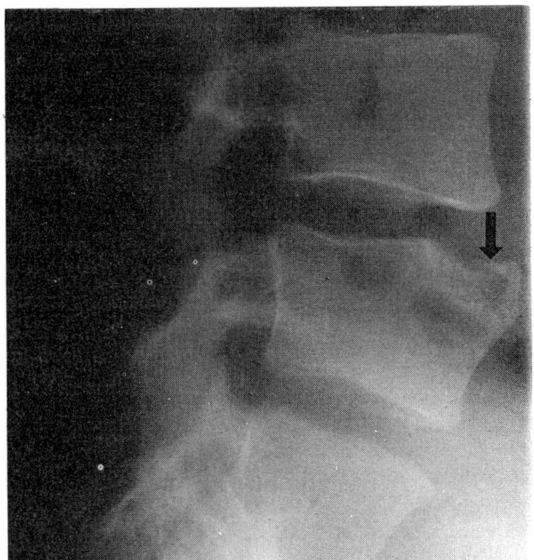

Figure 3.21 Avulsion of the ring apophysis (limbus vertebra). Lumbar spine – lateral view. A triangular fragment of bone (arrow) is separated from the anterosuperior aspect of the L5 vertebral body

Scoliosis

The cause of scoliosis may be structural, postural or protective, and imaging can clearly help in this differentiation. Many scolioses cause no trouble for years but as age advances symptoms are thought to develop because of increased mechanical strains on joints and soft tissues. Some people develop a scoliosis in response to a short leg. The scoliosis develops as a compensatory mechanism and usually the convexity in the lumbar area is on the side of the short leg.

Idiopathic scoliosis in adolescents and young adults is a common finding. However, symptoms are rare and if back pain is present, it is likely to be unrelated. The large majority of persons with a postural scoliosis do not have any underlying structural abnormality and do not require an X-ray examination. If there is significant back pain associated with scoliosis a radiological work-up using special long films with the person standing and bending in various directions may be indicated, but this should only be requested by a specialist orthopaedic surgeon.

Scoliosis may appear in the lumbar spine of elderly persons which may progress. It is uncertain whether this condition is a significant source of symptoms or not. The exact cause is unclear but it is not usually the result of degenerative disease of the spine. However, complicating degenerative change can occur and this is most marked along the concavity of the curve.

Thoracic kyphosis

In the younger person increased thoracic kyphosis can be postural or structural, and if the latter, the likely cause is Scheuermann's disease. Although definitions vary, the essential feature of Scheuermann's disease is a fixed lower thoracic kyphosis in an adolescent person. Cartilaginous node formation, endplate irregularity and anterior wedging of the vertebral bodies are seen involving at least three contiguous vertebrae. It is thought to be the result of trauma during the vulnerable stage of rapid growth on a background of congenital endplate weakness.

An exaggerated thoracic kyphosis is common in elderly patients. This can result from one of two processes or a combination of both:

1. Osteoporotic kyphosis – the osteoporotic vertebrae collapse anteriorly and so become wedge shaped. Changes predominate in the middle and upper thoracic spine, especially T6 and T7.
2. Senile kyphosis – related to degeneration of the anterior aspect of the discs. Radiographs show narrowing of the disc space, endplate sclerosis and osteophytes in the anterior aspect of the disc. Eventually, bony ankylosis occurs at this site.

Diffuse idiopathic skeletal hyperostosis (DISH)

The essential feature of this skeletal disorder is an excessive bone-forming tendency at entheses (where the ligaments and tendons attach to bone) which are sites of stress. This is a fairly common entity seen in middle aged and older persons, is more frequent in males, and the cause is unknown. The radiographic changes are often quite striking with exuberant new bone formation and large irregular bony outgrowths. The majority of patients have symptoms, but these are generally mild.

Spinal manifestations of DISH

Radiographic changes are most commonly seen in the middle and lower thoracic segments where there is flowing ossification along the anterolateral

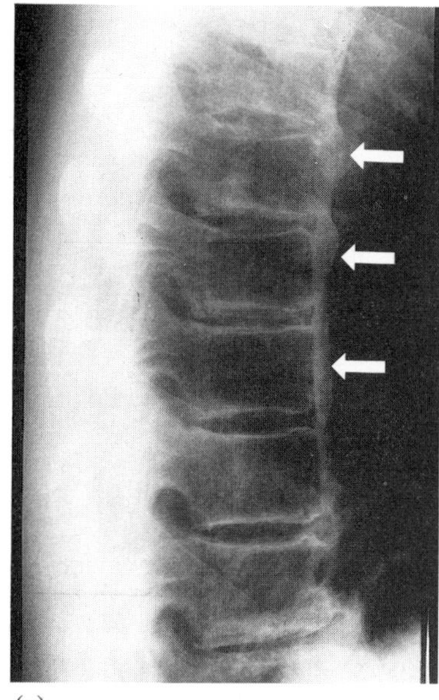

(a)

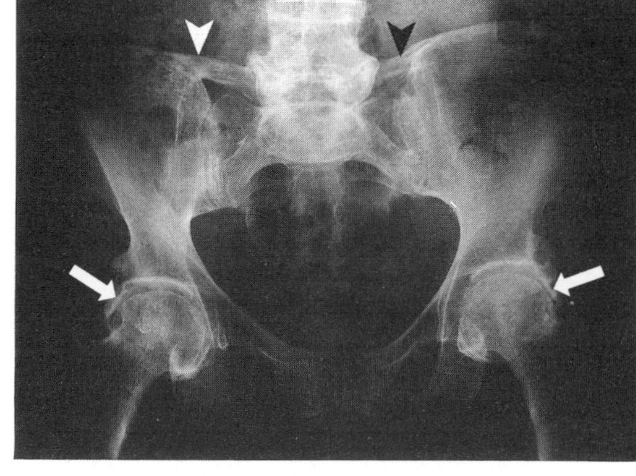

(b)

Figure 3.22 DISH. (a) Thoracic spine – lateral view. There is thick flowing ossification adjacent to the anterior vertebral body margin (arrows). The discovertebral joints are normal. (b) Pelvis – frontal view. Prominent pararticular ossification of the hip joints (joint space is normal) which effectively ankyloses the hip joints. In addition, there is ossification of the iliolumbar ligaments (arrowhead)

aspect of the vertebral bodies in the anterior longitudinal ligament and annulus fibrosis which is often quite thick and often has an undulating contour. There are often lucent gaps where it crosses the disc spaces (Figure 3.22(a)).

It is not unusual to see progressive involvement into the upper lumbar and mid and lower cervical segments. The most common symptoms are spinal stiffness and mild non-radiating back or neck pain. In the cervical spine the ossification may also occur at the posterior vertebral body margin and so may cause spinal stenosis.

DISH in the spine is differentiated from degenerative disc disease by the absence of (1) loss of disc height, (2) vacuum phenomena and (3) subchondral sclerosis, from ankylosing spondylitis by absence of (1) vertebral body erosion and (2) ankylosis of the facet joints, and from acromegaly by the absence of soft tissue thickening.

Extraspinal manifestations of DISH

Extraspinal manifestations are also frequent and distinctive. Radiographic changes include:

1. Pelvis:

   (a) well-defined bony proliferation, without erosion, at the iliac crest, ischial tuberosity and trochanters. This often has a 'whiskering' configuration.

   (b) ligamentous ossification [e.g. iliolumbar (Figure 3.22(b)) and sacrotuberous].

   (c) para-articular osteophytes in relation to the inferior aspect of the sacroiliac joints and acetabulum which may progress to para-articular osseous bridging (Figure 3.22(b)).

2. Heel and elbow – well-defined spurs which are often quite large arising from the superior (Achilles tendon attachment) or inferior surface (plantar aponeurosis attachment) of the calcaneal tuberosity (Figure 3.23), or the olecranon process (triceps tendon attachment). Clinically, there may be non-inflammatory tendinitis and palpable spurs.

3. Knee – cortical thickening of the anterior surface of the patellar and large bony spurs arising from the inferior and superior margins of the patella, extending into the adjacent ligaments.

Osteitis pubis

This clinical entity is a potential cause of pubic pain in athletes (e.g. soccer players and runners) and can also be seen in women after childbirth or other pelvic operations. The exact cause in athletes is not clear but it is thought to result from repetitive minor trauma during activities that excessively

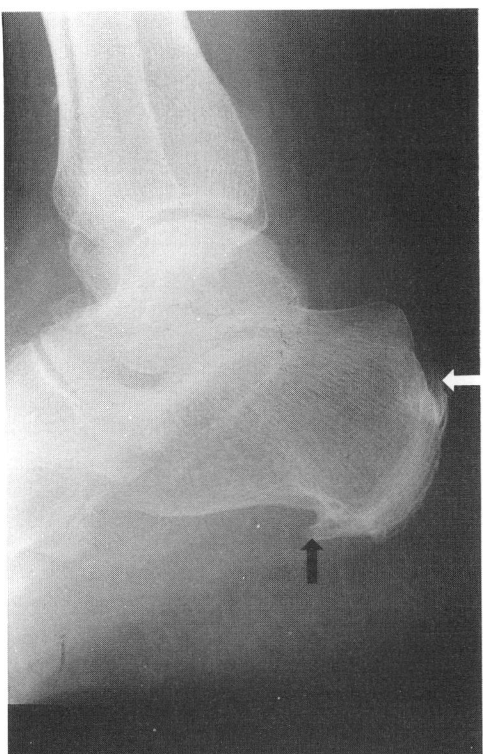

Figure 3.23 Calcaneal traction spurs. There are well defined bony spurs at the attachment of the plantar aponeurosis (black arrow) and Achilles tendon (white arrow) to the calcaneal tuberosity

stress the symphysis and sacroiliac joint complex (e.g. running, jumping and kicking). Tension from the adductors and rectus abdominus may also be a factor.

Clinical features include localized pubic pain and tenderness, muscle spasm and an antalgic limp which can mimic adductor muscle strain, but muscle stretching will aggravate the pain. In addition, a clicking sensation may be present indicating instability.

Radiographic features include:

1. symmetrical bony resorption at the medial ends of the pubic bones with cortical irregularity and sclerosis (Figure 3.4);
2. widening of the symphysis pubis;
3. stress sclerosis on the iliac side of the sacroiliac joints – this is usually triangular in shape, localized to the inferior aspect of the joint and symmetrical (osteitis condensans ilii);
4. instability of the symphysis pubis – sacroiliac joint complex (demonstrated on 'flamingo' views) (Figure 3.4).

Peripheral joint problems

Three musculoskeletal syndromes have been chosen to illustrate the application of modern imaging technology in the evaluation of bony and soft tissue problems of the shoulder and knee. These syndromes are; impingement and rotator cuff tears, glenohumeral instability and disorders of patello-femoral alignment and tracking. Newer imaging modalities can detect soft tissue lesions with increased accuracy. It may be argued that a careful clinical examination can accurately assess the state of the soft tissues but imaging technology can be utilized when necessary to confirm a clinical impression and to document soft tissue abnormalities more accurately. A physiotherapist may occasionally treat a person with shoulder pain that is resistant to all forms of therapy, and detailed imaging can be of great assistance in further management. The request for these investigations comes best from the person's primary-care medical practitioner or a specialist.

Impingement and rotator cuff tears

The impingement (painful arc) syndrome is a common shoulder complaint that relates to obstruction to gliding of the subacromial tissues under the coracoacromial arch. It is associated with bursitis, rotator cuff tendinitis and tear, and also bicipital tendinitis. The large majority of cuff tears are thought to be primarily the result of chronic impingement, although tears may occur in older persons without impingement as a result of age-related degeneration of the tendons and also with a single episode of acute trauma. Impingement most commonly occurs at the site between the anterior third of the acromion and the underlying tendons (supraspinatus outlet impingement).

Evaluation of impingement by imaging techniques

Impingement is primarily a clinical diagnosis but there are anatomic findings which can contribute to impingement and subsequent cuff disease. Various imaging modalities are used, including plain films, ultrasound and MRI.

Plain films

The following findings can be identified on plain films:

1. anterior subacromial spurs (traction spur resulting from stressing of the coracoacromial ligament) (Figure 3.8);
2. hooked configuration of the undersurface of the anterior acromion (developmental in nature);
3. degenerative disease of the acromioclavicular joint producing inferiorly pointing osteophytic spurs and/or joint hypertrophy.

The two supplementary impingement views (supraspinatus outlet view and frontal view with caudal angulation) are useful in documenting impingement anatomy as acromioplasty may be considered. Acromioplasty, ideally, should be performed at a stage before a full thickness cuff tear develops.

Later findings of impingement observed on plain films include:

1. A greater tuberosity which shows flattening, sclerosis and cystic change (the result of mechanical impaction) (Figure 3.24) and this is usually associated with insertional damage to the cuff tendon.
2. A decrease in acromiohumeral space (between the top of the humeral head and inferior surface of the acromion). The acromiohumeral space is largely occupied by the supraspinatus tendon and should normally meaure more than 7 mm. At this stage there is usually a full thickness cuff tear.
3. Subacromial erosion. Eventually this process may progress to allow the humeral head to migrate proximally and articulate upon the undersurface of the acromion where it produces a concave pressure erosion. At this stage a massive cuff tear is usually present. Secondary osteoarthritis can then occur in the glenohumeral joint and this endstage of impingement is known as 'cuff tear arthropathy' (Figure 3.24).

Calcification may be associated with impingement syndromes. The calcification is usually the result of inflammation and subsequent degeneration of the rotator cuff tendons from chronic impingement and can be acutely painful. Periarticular calcification is identified on plain films and may be seen in:

1. The rotator cuff tendons – most commonly adjacent to the greater tuberosity in the supraspinatus tendon (Figure 3.6).
2. The subacromial–subdeltoid bursa. Often this is the result of tendinous calcification rupturing into the adjacent bursa.

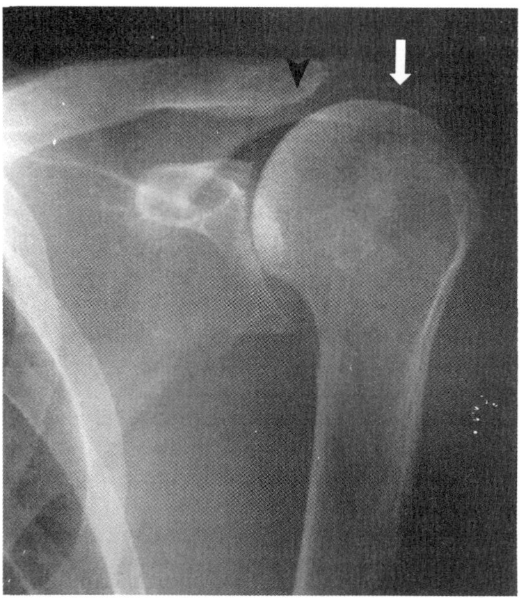

Figure 3.24 Cuff tear arthropathy. Shoulder – frontal view. A full-thickness tear of the rotator cuff can allow upward subluxation of the humeral head with erosion of the undersurface of the acromion (arrow) and outer end of the clavicle (arrowhead). There is secondary osteoarthritis of the glenohumeral joint (loss of joint space and subchondral sclerosis)

Ultrasound

Ultrasonic visualization in real-time of the cuff tendons gliding under the coracoacromial arch is valuable in the assessment of impingement. Any buckling or hesitancy of the cuff beneath the arch which corresponds with the person's pain is highly suggestive of clinically relevant impingement.

MRI

MRI can provide an accurate and comprehensive evaluation of impingement. The osseous, bursal and tendinous manifestations of mechanical impingement can all be detected simultaneously.

Evaluation of rotator cuff tears by imaging techniques

Cuff tears can be accurately diagnosed with ultrasound, arthrography and MRI. The majority of cuff tears occur in the supraspinatus tendon about 2 cm proximal to its insertion on the greater tuberosity where the impingement process most commonly occurs. Determining whether a full-thickness cuff tear is present may be useful in management as surgical repair may be considered.

Ultrasound

In experienced hands ultrasound has a high accuracy in the diagnosis of cuff tears, especially full-thickness tears. Full-thickness tears appear as a localized area of focal thinning in the cuff with an associated contour abnormality of the adjacent deep surface of the deltoid muscle (Figure 3.25). With large tears there is complete absence of the cuff as the torn edge is retracted under the acromion. Assessment can also be made of the status of the cuff muscles, the biceps tendon in both its intra-and extra-articular portions and the presence of any bursal or biceps tendon sheath effusions. Fluid in the biceps tendon sheath is a non-specific finding that is most commonly seen with cuff tears but can also be seen with the

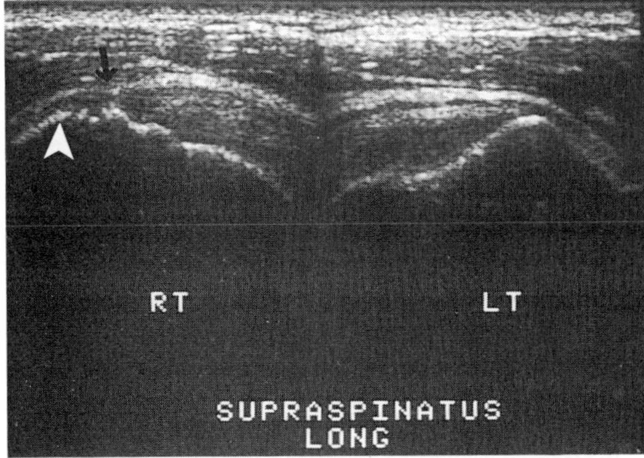

Figure 3.25 Rotator cuff tear. Ultrasound images showing the distal portion of supraspinatus tendon in longitudinal (a) and transverse (b) sections. There is focal thinning and flattening of the upper surface (arrow) of the right supraspinatus tendon a short distance before it inserts onto the greater tuberosity of the humerus (arrowhead). A normal left-sided tendon is shown for comparison

impingement syndrome, adhesive capsulitis, labral tears and primary biceps tendinitis.

Arthrography

This minimally invasive technique has a high accuracy for the diagnosis of full-thickness cuff tears and partial thickness tears involving the humeral side of the cuff. Contrast enters the subacromial bursa from the joint space through the defect in the torn cuff. Evaluation of the characteristics of the tear is limited. Arthrography is a useful alternative where ultrasonic expertise is not available.

MRI

As well as a high accuracy in the diagnosis of full-thickness cuff tears MRI can provide an evaluation superior to ultrasound or arthrography in estimating the size of a tear, degree of proximal retraction, whether there are degenerative changes in the torn edges and the degree of atrophy of the cuff muscles. Some clinicians find this extra information useful to aid identification of cases where surgical repair is less likely to be successful. MRI has limited ability to differentiate partial cuff tears from tendon degeneration.

Clinical correlation

Cuff tears are one cause of pain and/or weakness of the shoulder. However, cuff tears may be asymptomatic especially in the elderly population.

Glenohumeral instability

This clinical entity is usually seen in the younger athletic population with recurrent subluxation or dislocation of the shoulder and may present as an impingement syndrome. Imaging is useful in confirming a clinical impression of instability, documenting the direction of the instability (anterior, posterior or multidirectional) and helping to decide the need for and type of surgery (e.g. open versus arthroscopic).

The soft tissue abnormalities associated with instability include:

1. tears and detachment of the glenohumeral ligament–labral complex (Figure 3.26); when this occurs at the glenoid insertion it is known as a Bankart lesion;

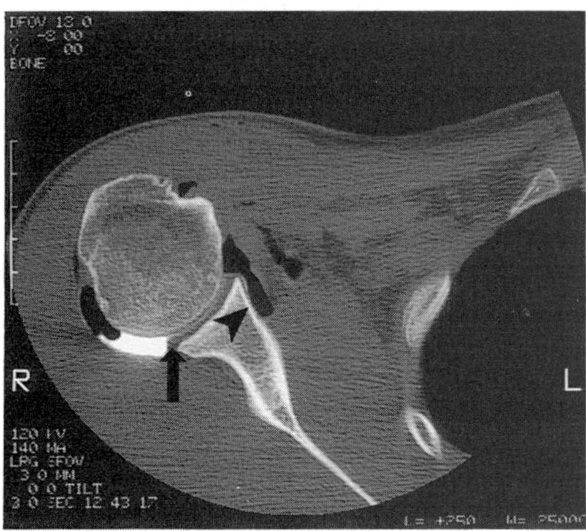

Figure 3.26 Anterior instability. CT arthrogram – axial section at the level of the subscapularis tendon. The anterior glenoid labrum is detached from the glenoid rim [compared with normal posterior labrum (arrow)]. In addition, there is capsular stripping along the anterior scapular neck (arrowhead)

2. capsular redundancy (intrasubstance ligament failure);
3. capsular stripping from the scapular neck (Figure 3.26).

The bony lesions associated with instability (Hill–Sachs and bony Bankart lesion) can be demonstrated on plain films.

CT arthrography, which distends the joint capsule and allows evaluation of labral, ligamentous and capsular attachments, is currently the most accurate imaging means for documenting these lesions of instability (Figure 3.26). The role of MR-arthrography is currently under investigation with benefits of multiplanar imaging and better visualization of the glenohumeral ligaments and labrobiceps complex, but the cost is very high.

Disorders of patellofemoral alignment and tracking

CT and MRI are very useful in the evaluation of disorders of patellar alignment and tracking. A kinematic study is performed by taking axial scans through the mid portion of both patellae with the knee in different degrees of flexion throughout the range 5–40° (Figure 3.27).

Assessment is made of the morphology and congruence of the articular facets of the patella and the apposing femoral trochlear groove [e.g. a

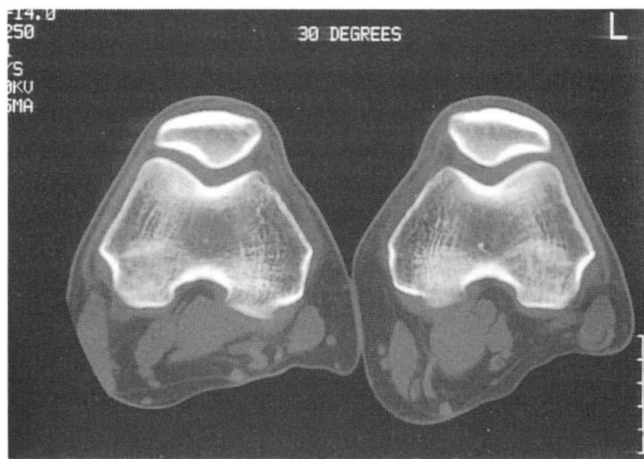

Figure 3.27 Patellofemoral CT. Axial section through the patellar equator at 30° of knee flexion. Normal examination showing normal morphology of the joint surfaces and normal alignment with the patellar ridge centered in the femoral trochlear groove

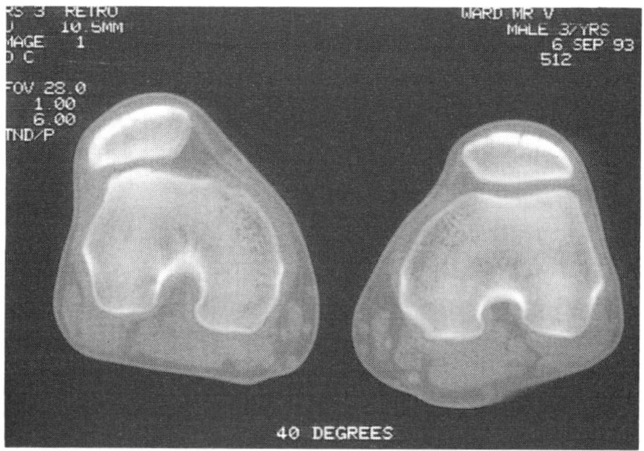

Figure 3.28 Patello-femoral dysplasia. Axial CT section at 40° of knee flexion. The articular surface of the patellae show dominant lateral facets which are flat with a poorly developed interfacetal ridge. The femoral trochlear groove is very shallow with hypoplastic lateral trochlears. On the right there is malalignment – the patella is laterally subluxed with tilt and there is irregularity and sclerosis of the lateral bony joint surfaces from mechanical impaction

dominant lateral facet of the patella, small lateral femoral trochlea and a shallow femoral trochlear groove all tend to be associated with patellar malalignment and subluxation (Figure 3.28) as are patellae which are positioned too high (patella alta), or too low (patella baja) in the trochlear groove].

Patellar tracking with knee flexion is then evaluated. Normally during knee flexion the ridge between the lateral and medial patellar facets

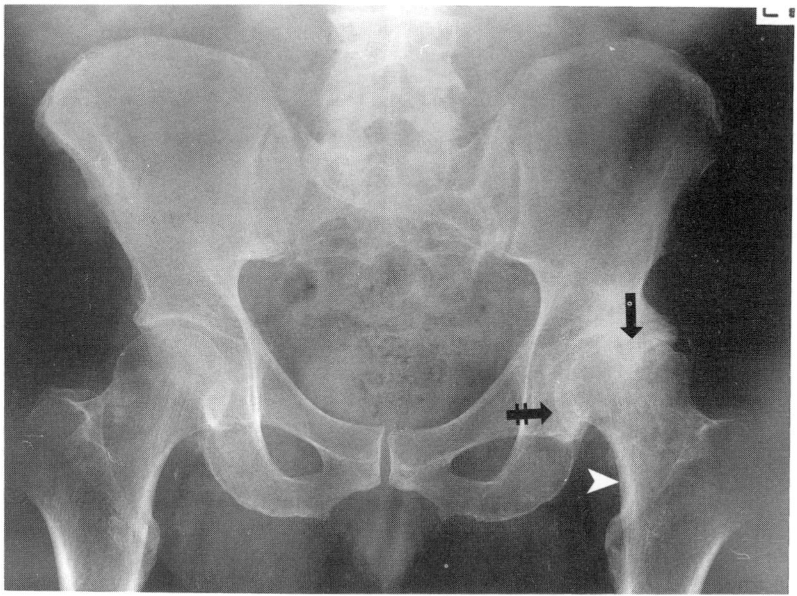

Figure 3.29 Osteoarthritis – hip joint. Pelvis-frontal view. The left hip joint shows complete loss of joint space in the weight-bearing superolateral portion of the joint with subchondral sclerosis and cyst formation and flattening and irregularity of the bony joint surfaces (arrow). There are prominent osteophytes at the joint margins and in addition, there is a large central osteophyte arising from the femoral head (hatched arrow) – these can form when there is lateral subluxation of the femoral head. Note also the buttressing of the medial cortex of the femoral neck (arrowhead)

should travel in a vertical plane centred in the trochlear groove without transverse displacement or tilt of the patella.

The common malalignment syndromes are:

1. Lateral subluxation of the patella – the ridge of the patella is displaced laterally relative to the trochlear groove. The subluxation tends to improve with increasing knee flexion with the patella normally centred by 40° of knee flexion. Lateral subluxation may be combined with lateral tilting of the patella, usually when the lateral femoral trochlea is hypoplastic (Figure 3.28). In addition, a cartilage defect is often seen at the point of impact between the lateral patellar facet and lateral femoral trochlea. Deficient medial stabilizers are thought to be responsible and a redundant lateral patellar retinaculum is often seen.
2. Excessive lateral pressure syndrome (ELPS) – this clinicoradiological entity is characterized by lateral tilting of the patella without significant lateral subluxation. The tilt tends to increase with increasing knee flexion. The lateral patellar facet is usually dominant and will often show stress-related change with a thickened subchrondral bone plate and a traction spur at its lateral margin. Excessively taut lateral structures are thought to be responsible and a tight, shortened lateral retinaculum is usually shown.

CT and MRI are helpful in confirming patellofemoral malalignment, characterizing its type and severity and also in planning corrective treatment.

Conclusions

A plain film radiographic examination will be the initial and often the only form of imaging investigation required with musculoskeletal problems. When imaging beyond plain films is considered necessary there is a wide and often confusing range of more sophisticated imaging modalities available each with their own individual advantages and disadvantages. Many factors are involved in selecting the appropriate modality, including the particular information required by the clinician, the preference and expertise of the radiologist, availability, cost and whether the investigation is invasive or utilizes ionizing radiation. Arthroscopy is a competing force in the evaluation of internal derangements of joints, especially the knee. Imaging pathways are in a constant state of flux as further advances in imaging technology become available.

It has not been the aim of this chapter to cover any one particular area of diagnostic imaging in depth or to review recent radiological literature, but rather to stimulate and interest the physiotherapist in this area. For this reason further suggested reading has been included. The physiotherapist has an important part to play in the diagnosis of musculoskeletal pain and dysfunction. In some countries the responsibility of ordering imaging investigations has been accepted both at a professional and government level, and it serves the physiotherapist well to keep abreast of current imaging practices to ensure optimum patient care.

Further reading

Normal anatomy

Agur, A. and Lee, M. (1991) *Grant's Atlas of Anatomy* (9th edn). London: Williams and Wilkins. (An atlas with imaging correlation)

Johnson, W.H. and Kennedy, J.A. (1982). *Radiographic Skeletal Anatomy* (2nd edn). London: Churchill Livingstone (Labelled standard radiographs with anatomic correlation)

Imaging of musculoskeletal disorders

Resnick, D. and Niwayama, G. (1988). *Diagnosis of Bone and Joint Disorders* (2nd edn). London: W.B. Saunders Co, [A standard reference book (6 volumes superbly illustrated and excellent radiological–pathological correlation)]

Resnick, D. (1989). *Bone and Joint Imaging.* London: W.B. Saunders Co. (A condensed single volume version of the above reference. Highly recommended as reference)

Stoller, D. (1993). *Magnetic Resonance Imaging in Orthopaedics and Sports Medicine.* Philadelphia: J.B. Lippincott Co. (A comprehensive text of musculoskeletal MRI with excellent illustrations including normal MRI anatomy)

Orthopedic physical assessment

Magee, D.J. (1987). *Orthopedic Physical Assessment.* London: W.B. Saunders Co.

Chapter 4

Principles of examination and measurement

E.M. Gass

The role of the physiotherapist has changed significantly since early in the twentieth century when members of groups such as The Australian Massage Society and the Chartered Society of Massage and Medical Gymnastics in the United Kingdom began working with medical practitioners in physical rehabilitation. Of critical importance to the present role definition is the way physiotherapists examine patients, decide a clinical diagnosis, and, in combination with the patient's needs and goals, implement an effective dose of appropriate treatment to cause a favourable adaptation or outcome. The process of diagnosis in physiotherapy has been the subject of several articles in professional journals (Rose, 1988; Sahrmann, 1988; Jette, 1989; Guccione, 1991). There is not yet consensus on what constitutes a diagnosis made by physiotherapists; however, it is generally agreed that this diagnosis will be complementary to the diagnosis of the medical practitioner (Rose, 1988; Sahrmann, 1988). As direct-access practice by physiotherapists has increased, so has the need for the physiotherapist to make a diagnosis.

Changes in medical referrals to an outpatient physiotherapy department of a large teaching hospital in a major city of Australia have been recently analysed (Wong *et al.*, 1994). Using randomly selected medical referral forms from 1982 and 1989 these authors were able to categorize diagnostic inclusion and referral mode. The majority of referrals in both years included a formal diagnosis, but significantly more in 1982. In 1989 the medical referrals were less likely to specify the type of physiotherapy treatment, rather

asking for physiotherapy in general as a treatment and indicating expected patient outcomes. This study concluded that the differences in medical referral in 1982 and 1989 suggested a trend toward an expectation by medical practitioners of greater autonomy by physiotherapists in making decisions in clinical practice. A decline in prescriptive referral to physiotherapists in Britain has been previously reported (Williams, 1983), but 74% of referring physicians in North America are reported to have indicated a preference for prescriptive referral (Uili *et al.*, 1984). These latter findings are of some concern because it has also been established that medical practitioners are familiar with traditional technical physiotherapy procedures or modalities, and less familiar with the current approach of prescribing a variety of management strategies based upon a sound examination (Uili *et al.*, 1984; Stanton *et al.*, 1985).

In a study investigating decisions made by physiotherapists (Dennis, 1987), patient referrals to physiotherapists from medical practitioners accounted for 67% of the total, 19% presented with no referral, 12% presented at the recommendation of a lay person and 2% were referred by other health professionals. Some form of treatment was prescribed in 45% of the referrals from medical practitioners and other health professionals, with electrotherapy being the most frequently requested modality. Overall this study provided evidence that prescriptive referral occurred in less than 25% of all referrals, and that most referrals left the management decisions to the physiotherapist (Dennis, 1987). This study supported the assertion that medical practitioners are, on the whole, unaware of the range and extent of current physiotherapy practice (Twomey, 1983; Uili *et al.*, 1984). These findings reinforce the necessity for physiotherapists to make a full clinical diagnosis to enable treatment selection and progress evaluation.

Purpose and aims of examination

The physiotherapist must be clear about the purpose of the clinical examination in order to collect the most relevant information. If the physiotherapist is unclear about the purpose and aims of the examination, then the procedures and tests selected, and subsequent interpretation made from the information gathered during the clinical examination, are likely to be muddled and inconclusive.

The aims of the physiotherapy examination of a patient with a musculoskeletal disorder are to:

1. establish a sound therapeutic relationship with the patient;
2. make a clinical diagnosis;
3. identify the goals or outcome of physiotherapy management;
4. establish a set of baseline data and measurement procedures that can be used to judge treatment outcome;
5. establish the presence of any contraindications or precautions to treatment;
6. identify the most appropriate intervention strategy to achieve the goals;
7. decide upon the dose of the specific strategies or treatments that will be effective in achieving the goals or outcomes.

To achieve these aims the clinical examination must include all procedures necessary to collect data relevant to the patient's presenting clinical picture. The methods of acquiring the data should be reliable and valid. Data interpretation and treatment selection will involve analysis of the collected data using the clinician's theoretical knowledge and previous clinical experience.

It is important to remember that the physiotherapy examination involves at least two key participants – the physiotherapist and the patient. On some occasions other health care professionals or friends or relatives of the patient are involved. The clinical examination process is an interactive one with possibilities for error and misinterpretation of information from all the participants. The examination is usually the first interaction between the patient and the physiotherapist and sets the scene for the therapeutic relationship that is to follow. In order to maximize reliability and validity of information collected, and to establish an appropriate therapeutic relationship, the physiotherapist must be sensitive to the patient, and their needs and goals of treatment. The physiotherapist must also instil a sense of trust in the patient, especially concerning confidentiality and privacy.

What is meant by a clinical diagnosis?

The term diagnosis is commonly used by many health professionals. It can be defined as the process of determining, by examination of the patient, the nature and identity of a disease condition or the decision reached from such an examination (Delbridge, 1988). A medical dictionary suggests diagnosis is the term denoting the name of the disease a person has or is believed to have and the value of establishing a diagnosis is to provide a logical basis for treatment and prognosis (Taber, 1970). Such medical definitions often describe different types of diagnosis namely cytological, differential, pathological and clinical. These different terms denote the method by which the diagnosis was made (Taber, 1970).

In the medical model, distinction is usually made between a pathological and a clinical diagnosis. Feinstein (1967) suggests that the main diagnostic taxonomy used by medical practitioners is that of pathological diagnosis based upon the nomenclature of morbid anatomy used by pathologists. Examples of pathological diagnoses are myocardial infarction, duodenal ulcer, multiple sclerosis and nephritis. None of these diagnoses represent any entity that is seen, heard, or touched in the observations made by the average clinician. These disorders are abnormalities of internal anatomic structure accessible in the main only to pathologists, hence the term pathological diagnosis.

This type of diagnosis is inadequate; instead the medical clinician should classify the patient's abnormalities in physiological, biomechanical and clinical function in addition to naming the structural or pathological disorder (Feinstein, 1967). This point can be illustrated with the example of myocardial infarction – a clinician will infer or clinically diagnose myocardial infarction by observation of clinical signs and symptoms such as presence or absence of chest pain, shock, dyspnoea and arrhythmias. The clinician may see an abnormal electrocardiograph or results of other laboratory tests, but only the pathologist or surgeon will see the myocardial infarction. The pathologist would make the diagnosis of myocardial infarction by examining the heart. The major ingredients of clinical diagnosis are recognition of the clinical features of the illness, and the personal and environmental features of the patient, as well as the pathological diagnosis of the disease. A clinical diagnosis could be defined as the set of history, symptoms and signs which clearly and distinctly identify an individual patient. It may be possible to arrive at a pathological or structural diagnosis on the basis of the clinical diagnosis; however, successful treatment will usually be based upon the clinical diagnosis, not the pathological diagnosis. The pathological diagnosis is an important subset of the clinical diagnosis. The former provides the framework, prognosis and guidance for treatment, whereas the latter is usually the basis for the specific treatment and dose of treatment used.

In medicine there are two types of clinical decisions – explicatory and interventional. Explicatory decisions relate to the intellectual process of giving a name, cause or mechanism to the patient's signs and symptoms. Interventional decisions relate to choice of treatment to remedy or prevent the signs and symptoms (Feinstein, 1975). The explicatory decisions are traditionally regarded as the science of medicine whereas the interventional decisions are often regarded as the art. Unfortunately along with this convention goes the thinking that there is no scientific challenge in the clinical management of the patient. A flaw in this thinking is that choice of treatment depends on diagnostic naming. Of course diagnosis is an important step; however, scientific selection and evaluation of the clinical intervention requires much more intricate analysis of the data than simply identifying a diagnosis (Feinstein, 1975).

In physiotherapy there has traditionally been less emphasis on the diagnosis (or the science) and more emphasis on the treatment (or the art) than in medicine. Physiotherapists have a major role in delivering treatment and initiating prevention strategies, therefore care must be taken to structure the type of diagnosis that best suits physiotherapy practice and not to unthinkingly stereotype 'science' and 'art'. When Maitland (1986) separated the term diagnosis from the history, symptoms and signs with the brick wall analogy, he implied that the history, symptoms and signs were different from a pathological diagnosis. History, symptoms and signs cannot reliably provide an uncontestable pathological diagnosis but conversely the pathological diagnosis cannot provide history, symptoms and signs. The clinical diagnosis is the basis for specific treatment and outcome decisions in most musculoskeletal disorders seen by physiotherapists. In some circumstances the pathological diagnosis does direct treatment, for example when a bone is fractured or when a ligament is ruptured. In other instances the pathological diagnosis provides guidance regarding prognosis and the overall treatment strategy, for example, a compressed spinal nerve/nerve root or gross spondylosis of the cervical spine. In such situations, however, the clinical diagnosis will direct aims of treatment, treatment strategies and choice of outcome measures. In other situations a pathological or structural diagnosis is not possible, and the clinical diagnosis will direct treatment and prognosis. Identification of both pathological and clinical diagnoses, in combination with referral to a sound theory base and appropriate referral to other health professionals, should ensure the most effective treatment prescription for each patient.

The concept of clinical diagnosis is important to current physiotherapy practice. With growing autonomy and accountability comes a need to justify procedures and process in physiotherapy. The community, health professional colleagues, and the variety of bodies who pay for physiotherapy services, expect that a physiotherapy service will include a diagnosis. The recognition that one of the responsibilities of a physiotherapist is to make a clinical diagnosis encourages focused physiotherapy examination procedures and evaluative clinical decision making. It should also be remembered that diagnosis is not an end in itself, rather a 'mental resting place for prognostic considerations and therapeutic decisions' (Wulff, 1976). The parameters of the clinical diagnosis need careful thought and definition. Physiotherapists have moved from the stage of hypothesis-oriented algorithms (Rothstein and Echternach, 1986) and models of evaluation and dysfunction Harris and Dyrek, 1989; Schenkman and Butler, 1989) to the challenge of specific diagnosis and diagnostic classification or taxonomy (Rose, 1988; Sahrmann, 1988; Jette, 1989). These challenges need urgent attention, not only because of the autonomy of physiotherapists but because it will remain difficult to investigate effectiveness of physiotherapy intervention if conditions being treated cannot be clearly delineated. It would indeed lead to a unifying paradigm of musculoskeletal physiotherapy (Guccione, 1991) if diagnostic classification or the taxonomy of musculoskeletal disorders could be developed and validated.

How do physiotherapists make a clinical diagnosis?

When the patient presents to the physiotherapist with a probable musculoskeletal disorder, the physiotherapist must systematically gather the information that will be the basis for the clinical diagnosis. First the physiotherapist asks the patient a series of questions. The responses to these questions, integrated with any other information available from laboratory tests or the medical practitioner, will provide the physiotherapist with a number of likely and unlikely possible or provisional diagnoses. The physiotherapist will refer to the knowledge base to then decide which tests should be carried out in the physical examination to clarify the clinical diagnosis. Some of these tests will aim to gain more information to enable a complete clinical diagnosis, while other tests will check that unlikely diagnoses identified from the history are, indeed, unlikely. The clinical diagnosis is made after thorough data gathering and an analysis of these data. Reference to the existing knowledge base and previous clinical experience is necessary to allow formulation of the clinical diagnosis. The process by which the data are gathered is the physiotherapy examination. The important concepts underlying this examination and the commonly used components are described in detail in Chapters 5 and 6.

It has been said of the diagnostic process that it has no set starting point, no rules of evidence, information is often gained in an unorganized way and the clinician has the difficult task of translating the patients' language to clinical concepts (Grant, 1989). To make it more difficult there are no pre-prepared pathways to take nor does one necessarily know when one has finished (Grant, 1989). It could be suggested that the clinical examination provides the pathways and helps determine the end point. Some of the difficulties arise because of the complexity and confused nature of the information about how clinicians reason. Grant (1989) has suggested that diagnostic skill can be best improved by helping clinicians and students develop self-awareness and self-monitoring of their thinking rather than by teachers imposing

forms of diagnosis. This suggestion is based upon the four key features identified in diagnostic thinking namely:

1. organization of clinical memory,
2. individuality of thinking,
3. ways of gaining access to memory,
4. response to clinical information (Grant, 1989).

These concepts should be considered when planning the most effective way to examine a patient and make a clinical diagnosis. Teaching and learning in this area often concentrate on retaining large amounts of knowledge. However, it is important to organize this knowledge in a way that is clinically important and speedily retrievable. If this is done, the physiotherapist will be able to plan an appropriate examination confidently and achieve the desired aims, one of which is to make a clinical diagnosis.

Principles of measurement in physiotherapy practice

To make a diagnosis to provide a sound basis and justification for treatment selection, and to be able to demonstrate clinical efficacy, it is imperative that physiotherapists confront the issue of measurement in clinical practice. The importance of measurement in research, and the importance of research for professional growth is acknowledged by most. The role of measurement in clinical practice is less recognized. Without sound measurement practices it is difficult to demonstrate the outcome of treatment. If the outcome cannot be demonstrated, then effective treatments may be ignored and ineffective treatments continued.

Outcome can be thought of as the result or visible effect of a certain event. In the context of health, outcome is often defined in terms of achievement of or failure to achieve certain goals. Outcome and need are related terms and the same instrument can usually be used to measure both. In physiotherapy practice we are increasingly concerned with outcome following our intervention. When attempting to measure outcome we need to be aware of a number of issues that can affect this variable, in addition to the treatment strategy. These include the natural history and progress of the disorder; the objectives or goals against which the outcome will be measured; a clear recognition and description of any inputs which can affect the outcome; and the desirability of specifying the hypothesized relationship between input and outcome. These issues are of more obvious importance in research but also need consideration in clinical practice to help maximize applicability and generalizability of outcome measures.

Knowledge of the natural history of a disorder is important because if one knows the time course of the problem without intervention, then this can provide a baseline against which outcomes are measured. In musculoskeletal physiotherapy there are some disorders where the natural history may be known, for example, a sprained ankle or acute low back disorder, but there are many disorders for which natural history is unknown. The best strategy under these circumstances is to use the history of the disorder under the existing pattern of physiotherapy treatment as a baseline. New treatment strategies can then be evaluated against the outcomes associated with the existing pattern.

Definition of the objectives or aims of physiotherapy intervention can occur at a number of levels. Global objectives such as restoration of function or increased functional capacity are not particularly helpful when evaluating the effectiveness of a specific treatment. There is an advantage in having specific aims such as the ability to walk up two flights of stairs with even weight bearing or the ability to hang out one load of washing. Sometimes the objectives and aims are assumed and not stated after a physiotherapy examination, or, if formulated, the objectives only reflect the priorities of the physiotherapist. Involvement of the patient, and where appropriate family, friends and other health professionals, may result in more relevant and encompassing objectives. This is turn means more realistic and valid outcome measures.

It is almost impossible to describe outcomes unless there is careful definition of inputs. It is, however, not easy to account for all inputs in the therapeutic setting. Some recognition of the majority of inputs is necessary, however, before the physiotherapist can ascribe a favourable outcome to a particular intervention.

If physiotherapists wish to extrapolate and build upon outcomes of clinical practice, then it is also important to specify the relationship between inputs and outcomes. For example, a physiotherapist may have data to support the use of active exercise programmes in those who have chronic low back pain. Before other physiotherapists start using this treatment they would probably ask questions like:

1. Could it have been the attention given to these patients that caused the change?
2. Could the fact that these patients had something to do each day have caused the outcome?
3. Could it be that mixing with other people with a similar condition caused the outcome?

If the physiotherapist had identified the possible relationships between these inputs and the outcome at the start, then some, or all, could have been accounted for in the way the trial was conducted and the data were collected. The data could then provide guidance to other physiotherapists about the role of an exercise programme for people with chronic low back pain.

Basic to these issues concerning input and outcome, and definition and achievement of objectives is the concept of measurement.

What do we mean by measurement?

Measurement is the process by which one can obtain answers to questions such as 'how many?' and 'how much?'. Measurement has been linked to the belief that if something is measured, it must be scientific (Feinstein, 1967). It is reported (Feinstein, 1967) that Kelvin stated that measurement was a prerequisite to science, setting the scene for biologists and other scientists to try to measure, and for clinicians to feel lost. Medical clinicians could measure height, blood pressure and cardiac output but were unable to measure headache, angina pectoris, dyspnoea or anxiety. As science clearly depends on dimensional measurement, then this logic would suggest a clinician could never attain science because so much of the information gathered at the bedside has no dimensional expression (Feinstein, 1967). An interesting solution to this dilemma was proposed by suggesting that there are two types of measurement, mensuration and enumeration (Feinstein, 1967). Mensuration is the use of a scale to determine a dimension that represents the amount of some substance whereas enumeration is the counting of a group of entities that have been categorized as single units. A counted number is a sum of individual units whereas a dimensional number is a proportional amount of some unit demarcated on a scale. A dimensional number answers the question 'how much?', whereas a counted number will answer the question 'how many?'.

In dimensional measurement the item must first be identified or extracted in some way from a collection of items and then this item is given dimension by comparing its value on a calibrated scale. In enumerational measurement the item to be tested is already a unit and the measurement consists of finding a particular category in which the unit can be counted. Mensurated variables are isolated and related to a calibrated scale whereas enumerated variables are observed and classified according to criteria. Reliability is assured if the isolation and calibration are adequate and if the observation and criteria for classification are accurate. It is worth noting that there is no ordinary method of dimensionally measuring the locations, qualities and other characteristics of the different types of pain produced by toothache, migraine, pleurisy, abdominal cramps or angina pectoris yet each of these pains can be uniquely characterized by verbal description (Feinstein, 1967).

It has been suggested (Wilkin *et al.*, 1992) that measurement can be divided into three broad categories: discrimination, prediction and evaluation. Discrimination involves measurement of differences between groups or individuals and is necessary if differences in health experience or areas of need are to be described. Prediction, or measurement as a basis for foretelling, is useful in health because individuals who may have a certain condition or outcome in the future can be identified. If predictive measures are sound then preventive strategies or intervention can be instituted at an early stage. Evaluation involves ascertaining the amount of something, appraising or assessing. Increasingly researchers, clinicians and policy makers are using measurement to evaluate or monitor the impact of health phenomena. Measures are needed to pick up changes between groups of patients. These changes or outcomes can then be attributed to certain interventions or treatments.

The level of precision of these categories of measurement will depend upon the context of use. The physiotherapy clinician is usually interested in differences within an individual and thus needs measures that can do this. The researcher may require a lower level of precision as they are examining differences in groups of individuals. Another factor that influences the level of precision is knowledge of the expected magnitude of the differences. If the magnitude of clinically important differences is small, then the measure chosen needs to be quite precise.

Measurement and related terms

Certain terms are integral to an understanding of measurement, in particular *methods, reliability, validity, sensitivity* and *specificity*. An understanding of these terms will enable the physiotherapist to design and implement sound measurement procedures in their clinical practice.

Methods

Methods is a term with which most physiotherapists will be familiar, particularly from reading research papers. Methods is the section where all procedures to be used are explained. This practice is based on the premise that in order to measure any particular item it is first necessary to describe and define exactly what it is that is to be measured. Rothstein when writing about measurement in clinical practice (Rothstein, 1985) suggests the use of the term *operational definition* instead of methods, noting that this term means specification of the procedures or operations to be used in taking the measurement. Further, he suggests that for an operational definition to have value in clinical practice it must have some generalized applicability and sound theoretical assumptions. This term is useful because it specifies its purpose; however, it seems redundant to use a different term, *operational definition*, from that commonly used in the scientific community, *methods*. The issue at point is that whenever a physiotherapist wishes to measure something the measurement procedure should be carefully described. Succinct definition or description of the variable to be measured is essential. Such a definition or description should be acceptable to most physiotherapists and should reflect current theoretical knowledge.

In physiotherapy practice there is widespread usage of descriptive terms such as muscle weakness, muscle tightness, decreased movement, and joint stiffness. When speaking with colleagues and when reading or writing clinical notes we tend to assume that the definitions of such terms are obvious and that all physiotherapists will quantify or measure these clinical phenomena in the same way. Observation for a short time would make it obvious that there is a great variety in the way physiotherapists evaluate or measure such variables. This variation is based partly on an inadequate knowledge base and partly on the unwillingness of physiotherapists to access and integrate such knowledge into their clinical practice even when it is available.

Whenever clinical measurements are made the methodology must be clearly documented. This could be by written description, a diagram or photograph or a videotape. The exact definition of the variable to be measured should be provided, e.g. muscle strength might be defined as the absolute force produced during one maximal contraction, or it might be the number of steps a person can climb in a certain time period. It is important that justification can be provided for any definition of the variable being measured and that the definition is stated clearly. Physiotherapists should feel confident in deciding on a definition.

Reliability

Reliability is a term commonly encountered in scientific literature. Definitions of the term abound with a useful definition stating that the reliability of a measure is the extent to which it yields the same results in repeated applications on an unchanged population or phenomenon (Wilkin *et al.*, 1992). Thus the reliability of a measurement or observation is its repeatability, i.e. providing all conditions remain the same, if the test or observation is repeated, the likelihood that the same result will be obtained. Reliability is related to terms such as stability, dependability, predictability and accuracy or the amount of measurement error (Kerlinger, 1964). One of the aims of any measurement should be to reduce random and non-random error. The more reliable a measure is, the lower the element of random error, i.e. error which follows no systematic pattern (Wilkin *et al.*, 1992). Non-random error or bias is assessed by testing validity.

The concept of reliability depends on whether one is operating from the basis of classical measurement or generalizability theory. The former theory suggests that every measurement will consist of a true score and an error component whereas generalizability theory recognizes that there are different sources of variability for any measurement made. Under this latter theory measurement error can be divided into sources of variability of interest to the measurer. The advantage of the generalizability approach is that it provides a way to quantify many sources of variability, a common situation in physiotherapy clinical practice (Roebroek *et al.*, 1993). For a review of measurement theory in general and these concepts in particular the reader is directed towards Domholdt (1993).

If a measurement procedure is not reliable and will not give similar results when repeated under similar conditions, or if the reliability is unknown, then it becomes difficult to interpret the results obtained by such a measure. If it were to be established that a certain clinical test, when repeated under identical conditions, gave a result that varied by 10% in either a positive or negative direction, then the physiotherapist using this test would need to demonstrate changes of more than $\pm 10\%$ to be able to have confidence that there had been a change in the measured variable. There are many factors that can affect the reliability of a measure, particularly the clinician, the instrument and the patient. Texts commonly discuss instrument, intra-rater (in the same individual), inter-rater (between individuals) and intra-subject (within the same subject) reliability. Of course even if there is high inter-observer and/or intra-observer reliability this does not necessarily imply that the observations or measurements are accurate – observers or raters can be reliably wrong!

Intra-rater reliability can be defined as the consistency with which a rater assigns scores to a single set of scores on two occasions (Waltz *et al.*, 1984). This is sometimes difficult to ascertain as the subject being repeatedly measured can change, this change being difficult to distinguish from an error on the part of the rater.

Inter-rater reliability is defined as consistency between different observers or users of the instrument (Wilkin *et al.*, 1992). This is easier to ascertain as multiple raters can measure a subject at the same or closely related time. If measurements are not possible at the same time then the same difficulty of partitioning out subject variability arises as did with testing intra-rater reliability.

Instrument reliability is sometimes known as *test–retest reliability*. Given that such testing occurs on two different occasions, the issue as to whether the subject being tested has changed or the instrument has changed is still present. [For more discussion on the types of instruments used by physiotherapists and methods to measure their reliability see Domholdt (1993).]

Intra-subject reliability is difficult to estimate. If one were confident that both tester and instrument were perfectly reliable, then measuring the subject on two occasions could provide intra-subject reliability.

Measurement of reliability

It is possible to quantify reliability either by examining the relationship between two or more sets of repeated measures, or by examining the variability of the scores from measurement to measurement. [For discussion on this point see Domholdt (1993) or Kerlinger (1964).] Reliability is usually calculated by use of procedures such as Pearson product–moment correlation coefficient, intra-class correlation coefficient, or coefficient of variation. Each of these analyses gives slightly different information. Any statistical text will explain the assumptions underlying these tests and the circumstances for which they are appropriate. Most of these tests are based on the concept that, when two variables are correlated, the value an individual achieves on one variable relates to the value achieved on another variable (Domholdt, 1993). It is important to remember that these correlations describe relationships between variables and cannot be used to ascribe causality. Statistical or research texts should be consulted for the formulae for calculation of the common correlation procedures. It should be remembered that a number of assumptions underlie these reliability measures, e.g. there needs to be a linear relationship between sets of scores in order to be able to use the Pearson product–moment correlation coefficient. Before using these tests ensure that the data meet the assumptions.

To decide that a real change or adaptation has occurred, it is important to know the magnitude of change that needs to be measured in a patient that reflects true change and not a measurement error. This issue is of importance in both clinical practice and research. It is tempting, particularly when one has access to measuring devices that give results in numbers, to assume that such numbers are always true. The issue of reliability relates to how confident the physiotherapist can be that the numbers have meaning and can be used to monitor progress and prescribe treatment. Physiotherapists should be aware of the basic principles of operation of these instruments and be able to go back to 'first principles' to check the numbers being generated. Manufacturers of instruments such as goniometers, tape measures or force transducers normally provide information about the accuracy of the instrument, for example ± 5° for a goniometer or ± 0.1% for a force transducer. Instruments should be calibrated against a known standard at regular intervals to ascertain the degree of accuracy. If drift of the instrument has occurred then, depending on the instrument, adjustments can often be made to 'reset' the instrument according to the known standard. When physiotherapists evaluate or purchase measuring or therapeutic equipment it is good practice to read the specifications of the equipment carefully in order to be sure the accuracy is appropriate to the task to be performed.

The issue of reliability is an important one for physiotherapy for, unless reliable measurements are possible, the correct diagnosis, treatment selection and evaluation of treatment effects becomes difficult. In order to demonstrate clinical efficacy and respond to challenges of role definition for physiotherapy, reliable measurement must be the cornerstone of clinical practice.

Validity

Validity is a more complex concept than reliability. Validity is a term sometimes confused with reliability because it has a related, but quite different, meaning. Simply stated a valid measurement is one that actually measures what it is supposed to measure. The validity of an instrument relates to the non-random or systematic error (Wilkin *et al.*, 1992). A valid measurement procedure therefore allows legitimate judgement or inference (Rothstein, 1985). One of the reasons validity is a more complex concept than reliability is that validity usually necessitates some inquiry into the nature and meaning of the variables (Kerlinger, 1964). For example, a thermometer is routinely used to measure temperature. It has been pointed out that the reason a patient's temperature is measured is not to infer something about the kinetic energy of molecules, rather, on the basis that an elevated temperature can infer presence of infection, the patient's elevated temperature can infer the presence of disorder or disease (Rothstein, 1985). Another example is the use of the test of bending forwards trying to reach fingertips to the floor. It is valid to infer something about the person's flexibility through flexion, from this test; however, it would not be valid to infer the amount of lumbar flexion as so many other factors such as range of hip movement and length of hamstrings muscles can contribute to the forward flexion range.

A number of different types of validity have been identified, most importantly content, concurrent, predictive and construct validity (Cronbach and Meehl, 1955).

Content validity is concerned with how representative the content of the measure is of the universe of content of the property being measured. To ascertain content validity one could ask whether the choice of, and relative importance given to, each component of the index is appropriate for the domains they are supposed to measure (Wilkin *et al.*, 1992). An example is functional ability, a broad term with a large number of subsets such as activities of daily living, grooming activities, mobility activities, leisure activities and work activities. A test high in content validity would theoretically be a representative subset of the universe of functional ability. In reality, however, the universe of content only exists as a theoretical concept. To decide whether a test has sufficient content validity, a judgement is made by deciding how representative the tests to be used are of the item under consideration. Careful definition and description of test items is necessary to allow the judgement to be made. Content validity is particularly relevant to questionnaire or observational measuring instruments. The Functional Status Index test (FSI), for example, was designed to measure the degree of dependence, pain and difficulty experienced by people with arthritis living in the community (Wilkin *et al.*, 1992), and it has been tested for inter-observer and test–retest reliability with satisfactory results (Harris *et al.*, 1986). Content validity is claimed to be better with this instrument than other measures of function; however, comparisons between FSI scores, patient self ratings and staff ratings have produced varied results (Denniston and Jette, 1980). When designing such measuring instruments it is useful to evaluate the content validity or spend time researching content validity of existing similar instruments. Content validity should be evaluated both by experts in the area and representatives of the community to be measured.

Concurrent and predictive validity are similar to each other as both relate to prediction against an outside criterion, and both are characterized by checking the measuring instrument against some outcome (Kerlinger, 1964). When a measurement tool, such as manual ligament testing of the ankle, is compared with a measurement standard, such as arthroscopy or radiological testing, then concurrent validity is being determined. Predictive validity is more concerned with tests that measure performance in a certain way and predict what the status will be in the future. Many health-screening programmes are based on predictive validity.

Construct validity is concerned with the underlying explanation or meaning of the test. This type of validity is different from the others because there is a preoccupation with theory, the theoretical constructs and testing of hypothesized relations (Kerlinger, 1964). The question that defines construct validity is: do the results obtained confirm the expected pattern of relationships or hypotheses derived from the theoretical constructs on which the measure is based (Wilkin *et al.*, 1992)?

Construct validation and empirical scientific inquiry are closely allied. In order to determine construct validity Cronbach (1960) has suggested three key steps:

1. identifying any constructs that might account for test performance;
2. deriving hypotheses from the theory involving the construct;
3. testing the hypotheses empirically.

Strength is a poorly delineated construct in physiotherapy literature (Domholdt, 1993). The term strength can mean a variety of things and, before construct validity can be maximized, the basic concepts underlying the measures must be very clear. First one must decide, for example, whether the underlying construct is isometric, functional or eccentric strength. Once this decision is made, the construct must be clearly defined and delineated to allow measurement. Careful definition or delineation will not only help ensure construct validity but other physiotherapists are then able to evaluate such definitions and form their own opinion of the construct (Domholdt, 1993). Ultimately this process will provide a strong basis for refinement and improvement of testing procedures. Clear and careful definition of constructs in physiotherapy in the public domain is the first step towards a coherent research effort and outcome oriented clinical practice.

Specificity and sensitivity

Specificity and sensitivity are terms used to describe the likelihood that test results are able to delineate those people without or with a disease or disorder.

The *specificity* of a finding is an indication of how often someone without a particular disease or disorder in the population will have a truly negative finding for the test (Balla, 1985). The answer to the question 'if the disease is not present what is the likelihood that the result will be normal (negative)?' addresses the specificity of a test. Another way of thinking of specificity is to relate it to the term 'true negative'. A highly specific test would mean that very few healthy people would have an abnormal result. *Sensitivity* is an indication of how often a positive test result occurs in the presence of disease. If a test has high sensitivity and the result is negative, then one can feel confident that a particular disease or disorder has been excluded because a high percentage of people with the disease would have a positive test. If the question is asked 'if the disease is present what is the likelihood that the test result will be abnormal (positive)?' then the answer indicates the sensitivity of the test. Sensitivity is a term related to 'true positive', thus if a test is highly sensitive then a negative result is a good predictor of the absence of disease (Balla, 1985).

Specificity and sensitivity can be depicted as equations:

$$\text{Specificity (\%)} = \frac{\text{True negative}}{\text{True negative + false positive}} \times 100$$

$$\text{Sensitivity (\%)} = \frac{\text{True positive}}{\text{True positive + false negative}} \times 100$$

A table could be constructed to help determine sensitivity and specificity (Table 4.1).

Table 4.1 Relationship between predictor and 'gold standard' tests

Predictor test	'Gold standard' test	
	Abnormal	*Normal*
Abnormal	True positive	False positive
Normal	False negative	True negative

An example may clarify the use of these terms. The results of exercise tolerance tests (ETT) have been compared among subjects with and without coronary artery disease (Weiner *et al.*, 1979). Luminal narrowing of at least 70% of one or more major coronary vessels defined those with coronary artery disease. This angiographic testing was the 'gold standard' or best measure of the true incidence of coronary artery disease. A positive exercise test was defined as one in which there was more than 1 mm horizontal or downward displacement of the ST segment, or elevation for at least 0.08 s compared with the resting baseline record.

The *sensitivity* of the ETT for the presence of coronary artery disease in this example is 80% and the *specificity* is 74%. Thus in those men with proven coronary artery disease the exercise tolerance test demonstrated the disease 80% of the time (using ST segment changes as the criterion). In those men with no evidence of coronary artery disease the exercise tolerance test was normal in 74%. Another way of stating these results is that the test did not identify the disease in those who had it 20% of the time (false negative) and the test suggested that healthy people had the disease 26% of the time (false positive). Tests rarely possess 100% sensitivity and 100% specificity. Knowledge of these attributes of a test simply gives an indication of the likelihood or probability that the disease is present.

A term related to sensitivity and specificity is *prevalence*. The prevalence or incidence of a disease or disorder is simply the range of occurrence or number of cases present in a specified population at a given time. Given that clinicians are interested in the predictive value of tests, it is important to understand that the predictive value is affected not only by sensitivity and specificity, but also by the prevalence of the disorder in the population. The lower the prevalence of a condition or disorder in the population, the less the predictive value of a positive result. These concepts are presented in more detail in other sources (Benson and Rubin, 1978; Lundberg, 1983; Griner *et al.*, 1986).

Terms such as specificity, sensitivity, true positive and true negative are common in medical literature and the sensitivity and specificity can be calculated for many procedures. Incidence rates of many diseases have been established to such an extent that mathematical calculations can be used to estimate the likelihood of a disease being present or not. Such predictive ability assists in diagnosis and prognosis and hence ultimately assists in selection of the appropriate treatment for the patient.

Weighting of clinical information

The process of arriving at a clinical diagnosis relies heavily on how we weight the importance of the data gathered. The weight attached to a piece of information refers to the significance assigned to this piece of information by the clinician. This in turn will affect the decisions made by the clinician. It is usually difficult for clinicians to explicitly state what weighting was assigned to different pieces of information gathered during the examination; however, they intuitively know that different weights are being assigned.

The physiotherapist must assess the significance or importance of information as it is acquired, as a basis for the decisions that are made in order to weight according to importance. The significance of the presence and the absence of clinical features needs to be known. Importance of data gathered may vary depending on what other symptoms or signs are present (or absent) in the patient.

Research in medical literature would suggest that different specialty groups attach different weights to the same information (Balla, 1982). Cardiologists, neurologists and medical students were provided with brief case histories in one study (Balla, 1982). One patient had olfactory sensations and déjà vu, both strong cues for epilepsy but all other signs and symptoms of epilepsy were noted as being absent. Most of the participants diagnosed epilepsy, but preference for this diagnosis increased with expertise. When additional information was provided that this patient had been drinking and felt ill before he collapsed then the students and cardiologists diagnosed this as an epileptic fit but the neurologists did not. This seemed to suggest that this additional information had more weight for the expert than those less experienced in neurological diagnosis.

Another point about weighting of information is that the same symptoms and signs in different settings can have different weights. For example a study was conducted with medical students, cardiologists and neurologists (Balla, 1982). Brief case histories of three patients were presented. All patients had typical fainting spells. Patient A was a young girl who 'blacked out' in church, patient B was a much older person who fainted and no information about age or gender was provided about patient C. All respondents were confident to diagnose that patient A was experiencing vasovagal episodes because of their knowledge that such a cause is common in young females. The respondents were much less confident about a vasovagal diagnosis for patient B because this is a much less common cause of fainting in older people. No accurate diagnosis was possible for patient C. This study showed how the same signs and symptoms in three different settings had completely different weighting and how this was related to prior knowledge. Interestingly it has been shown that negative information is difficult to handle, even if it contains critical information.

Negative information is frequently ignored by inexperienced clinicians, although experts may regard it highly. If a young male has headaches there are many possible diagnoses. Given that temporal arteritis and polymyalgia rheumatica are diseases of the elderly (Balla, 1985) then, as this information is absent or negative in this example, these diagnoses should be unlikely. Similarly a blackout in a child could be caused by petit mal but if the patient is 50 years old and suffers his first blackout, then it cannot be petit mal (Balla, 1985).

Other chapters in this book (Chapters 5 and 6) will discuss specific aspects of making a clinical diagnosis. In general, however, in order to make a diagnosis and clinical decisions, the physiotherapist must collect and process information. This process involves both the patient and the physiotherapist receiving, providing and interpreting information in relation to their own experience and knowledge. Related concepts important in the context of information gathering include reliability, validity, specificity, sensitivity and prevalence. These concepts need to be applied in order that the physiotherapist can make a sound judgement about the data being gathered and be reasonably certain about the diagnosis made and plan of action proposed.

It is important to recognize explicitly that one of the purposes of the physiotherapy examination procedure for those with musculoskeletal disorders is to diagnose. This recognition will help physiotherapists structure and interpret the examination and may lead to the development of a taxonomy or classification of musculoskeletal clinical diagnoses. This would improve patient management and form the basis for continued questioning, discussion and research.

Reliability and validity when taking a history and performing the physical examination

Identification of the clinical diagnosis and selection of treatment depend on gathering reliable and valid data in the clinical examination. Whenever evaluating reliability the physiotherapist should know the normal response to a test so that responses outside the normal range can be analysed systematically for their clinical relevance. This could involve measurement of many people of different ages and characteristics, possibly outside the usual clinical setting. The data obtained in the physical examination should correlate with the data obtained in the history. This correlation is often difficult for students to recognize because their main concern is to complete the history or the physical examination without missing out 'relevant' procedures. Repetition with patients and practice with colleagues will help overcome this problem so that the more important concept of internal consistency of the examination can be mastered. Internal consistency means that the data collected are homogeneous and accurate. If one were to inter-correlate samples of the data there would be high reliability. If inconsistent data appear then either the information gathering and testing procedures need modification, or alternative diagnoses need to be entertained, or both.

Laboratory and radiographic investigations are all too often assumed to be highly reliable. Reading of X-rays and electrocardiographs shows large individual variation, and errors also occur with laboratory investigations. Such test results should be seen as part of the information gathering towards the clinical diagnosis proposed by the physiotherapist. Physiotherapists need to be aware of sensitivity and specificity of laboratory and radiography tests and to have some idea whether the test results are useful for confirming a diagnosis (sensitivity) or excluding a diagnosis (specificity). Such information can be found in text books describing laboratory and radiographic tests or can be ascertained by enquiry to the laboratory or medical practitioner concerned. This information is important to be able to weight information appropriately.

Reliability of information collected during history taking can be affected by the source method of collection of the data. When questioned the patient must interpret their own signs and symptoms and convey this interpretation to the physiotherapist. This can be a source of confusion and possibly error. The patient may have inadequate verbal skills to describe symptoms in any detail, simply stating that he or she feels unwell and has great pain. The history of any precipitating incident and subsequent development of symptoms often provides strong evidence for a particular diagnosis yet the patient's memory can be unreliable and hence provide inaccurate or conflicting information.

The skill of the physiotherapist comes from recognizing that this information is unreliable, despite trying different questioning strategies and manoeuvres, and then putting less weight on this information when it comes to making a diagnosis. Inaccurate history taking on the part of the physiotherapist can also lead to unrealiable data. Balla and Iansek (1979) suggest that the major problem is lack of data clarification whereby instead of being absolutely sure of the detail of what the patient is reporting the physiotherapist may assume they know what is meant and not seek to establish the actual details.

References

Balla, J.L. (1982). The use of critical cues and prior probability in decision making. *Methods Information Med.*, **19**, 88–92. Also in *The Diagnostic Process* (1985) (J. Balla, ed.), Cambridge: Cambridge University Press.

Balla, J.L. (1985). *The Diagnostic Process*. Cambridge: Cambridge University Press.

Balla, J.I. and Iansek, R. (1979). The neurological diagnostic process. In *Proceedings of the 5th Asian and Oceanian Congress of Neurology* (G.L. Gamez, ed.) Excerpta Medica. Manila: Also in *The Diagnostic Process* (1985) (Balla, J.L. ed.) Cambridge: Cambridge University Press.

Benson, E.S. and Rubin, M. (eds) (1978). *Logic and Economics of Clinical Laboratory Use*. New York: Elsevier.

Cronbach, L. (1960). *Essentials of Psychological Testing*. (2nd edn). New York: Harper and Row.

Cronbach, L. and Meel, P. (1955). Construct validity of psychological tests. *Psychol. Bull.*, **LII**, 281–302.

Delbridge, A. (ed.) (1988). *The Macquarie Dictionary*, (2nd revision) The Macquarie Library Pty.

Dennis, J.K. (1987). Decisions made by physiotherapists: a study of private practitioners in Australia. *Austr. J. Physiother.*, **33**, 181–91.

Denniston, O.L. and Jette, A.M. (1980). A functional status assessment instrument: Validation in an elderly population. *Hlth Serv. Res.*, **15**, 21–34. Also in *Measures of Need and Outcome for Primary Health Care* (1992) (D. Wilkin, L. Hallam and M.A. Dogget, eds.), pp. 56–7, Oxford: Oxford University Press.

Domholdt, E (1993). *Physical Therapy Research. Principles and Applications* pp. 143–61, Philadelphia: W.B. Saunders.

Feinstein, A.R. (1967). *Clinical Judgement*. New York: Robert Ekrieger Publishing Company.

Feinstein, A.R. (1975). Science, clinical medicine and the spectrum of disease. In *Textbook of Medicine* (P.B. Beeson and W. McDermott, eds), pp. 3–6, Philadelphia: W.B. Saunders.

Grant, J. (1989). Clinical decision making – rational principles, clinical intuition or clinical thinking? In *Learning in Medical School* (J.L. Balla, ed.), Hong Kong: Hong Kong University Press.

Griner, P.F., Panzer, R.J. and Greenland, P. (1986). *Clinical Diagnosis and the Laboratory.* Chicago: Year Book Medical Publishers Inc.

Guccione, A. (1991). Physical therapy diagnosis and the relationship between impairments and function. *Phys. Ther.*, **71**, 499–503.

Harris, B.A. and Dyrek, D.A. (1989). A model of orthopaedic dysfunction for clinical decision making in physical therapy practice. *Phys. Ther.*, **69**, 548–53.

Harris, B.A., Jette, A.M., Campion, E.W. and Cleary, P.D. (1986). Validity of self report measures of functional disability. *Top. Geriatr. Rehabil.*, **1**, 31–41. Also in *Measures of Need and Outcome for Primary Health Care* (1992) (D. Wilkin, L. Hallam and M.A. Doggett, eds) pp. 56–7, Oxford: Oxford University Press.

Jette, A.M. (1989). Diagnosis and classification by physical therapists: a special communication. *Phys. Ther.*, **69**, 87–9.

Kerlinger, F.N. (1964) *Foundations of Behavioural Research*, pp. 429–53. New York: Holt Rinehart and Winston Inc.

Lundberg, G.D. (ed.) (1983). *Using the Clinical Laboratory in Medical Decision Making*, pp. 229–33. Chicago: American Society of Clinical Pathologists Press.

Maitland, G.D. (1986). *Vertebral Manipulation* (5th edn). London: Butterworths.

Roebroek, M.E., Harlaar, J. and Lankhorst, G.J. (1993). The application of generalisability theory to reliability assessment: an illustration using isometric force measurements. *Phys. Ther.*, **73**, 386–95.

Rose, S.J. (1988). Musing on diagnosis – editorial. *Phys. Ther.*, **68**, 1665.

Rothstein, J.M. (1985). Measurement and clinical practice: theory and application. In *Measurement in Physical Therapy* (J.M. Rothstein, ed.), New York: Churchill Livingstone.

Rothstein, J.M. and Echternach, J.L. (1986). Hypothesis-oriented algorithm for clinicians. *Phys. Ther.*, **66**, 1388–94.

Sahrmann, S.A. (1988). Diagnosis by the physical therapist – prerequisite for treatment. *Phys. Ther.*, **68**, 1703–6.

Schenkman, M. and Butler, R.B. (1989). A model for multisystem evaluation, interpretation and treatment of individuals with neurologic dysfunction. *Phys. Ther.*, **69**, 538–47.

Stanton, P.E., Fox, K., Frangos, K.M. *et al.* (1985). Assessment of resident physicians knowledge of physical therapy. *Phys. Ther.*, **65**, 27–30.

Taber, C.W. (ed.) (1970). *Tabers Cyclopaedic Medical Dictionary*, Philadelphia: F.A. Davis Company.

Twomey, L.T. (1983). The physiotherapist. *Med. J. Austr.*, **1**, 422–4.

Uili, R.M., Shepard, K. and Savinar, E. (1984). Physician knowledge and utilization of physical therapy procedures. *Phys. Ther.*, **64**, 1523–30.

Waltz, C.F., Strickland, O.L. and Lenz, E.R. (1984). *Measurement in Nursing Research*, Philadelphia: F.A. Davis Company.

Weiner, M.D., Ryan, T.J., McCabe, C.H. *et al.* (1979). Correlations among history of angina, ST-segment response and prevalence of coronary-artery disease in the coronary artery surgery study (CASS). *N. Engl. J. Med.*, **301**, 230–8.

Wilkin, D., Hallam, L. and Doggett, M.A. (1992). *Measures of Need and Outcome for Primary Health Care*, pp. 56–7. Oxford: Oxford University Press.

Williams, J.L. (1983). The three times a week syndrome. *Physiotherapy*, **69**, 235–7.

Wong, W.P., Galley, P. and Sheehan, M. (1994). Changes in medical referrals to an outpatient physiotherapy department. *Austr. J. Physiother.*, **40**, 9–14.

Wulff, H.R. (1976). *Rational Diagnosis and Treatment*. Oxford: Blackwell Scientific Publications.

Chapter 5

The history

K.M. Refshauge and J. Latimer

The history is arguably the most important part of the whole examination, because it is from this that we decide the nature of the patient's problem and the possible treatments that might consequently be used. From the history we develop general ideas about the probable location and type of pathology, the clinical symptoms to be treated, possible strategies to manage the problem, contraindications or precautions to examination and treatment procedures, and likely prognosis. We rarely gain completely new ideas from the physical examination. Rather we test the hypotheses we derived from the history, confirming some and rejecting others. This process is not unlike the practice of all who are engaged in problem-solving. Consider the car mechanic who asks questions to establish that the problem is a rattle, the type and location of the rattle and any other symptoms the car has. In this way the mechanic narrows the problem to a few likely sources, and then tests each of these possibilities. The management of the car rattle follows from the identification of its cause. Likewise lawyers, accountants and medical practitioners must be informed by the client about the nature of the presenting problem and any associated problems so that appropriate action can be instituted. Obviously, good management is extremely difficult without interaction with the client.

A further important function of the history is to establish the patient's expectations of treatment. The physiotherapist should discuss these expectations with the patient rather than make assumptions, and ensure that expectations are realistic and achievable. In this way the patient and the physiotherapist work together to maximize the benefit from treatment. This avoids the scenario where a patient is disappointed because return to work or golf, for example, is not yet possible, yet the physiotherapist believes that the patient is progressing satisfactorily because a small increase in range of spinal movement has been achieved. If a patient believes that the treatment is ineffective or misdirected, compliance with home programmes is also likely to be reduced (see Chapter 9).

Clearly, then, taking an effective history is fundamental to good management. An effective history is designed to gain information about all aspects of the patient's problem including any impact on the patient's daily life. The value of information acquired from the patient can be maximized by employing strategies known to enhance reliability and validity of patient report data. Therefore, before proceeding with details about taking a history from a patient with a musculoskeletal disorder, a discussion about patient report data is essential.

Patient report data

Introduction

Patient report data is the term used to describe any information that is supplied by patients during their assessment. This information may include a description of their symptoms, how their disease has developed, the effect of the disorder on their daily function, and most importantly their expectations of treatment. The importance of this information should never be undervalued as it is the patient's own reporting of their condition, rather than the physiotherapist's interpretation, that is likely to be more reliable and valid.

These data provided by the patient form the basis of our clinical decisions, not only to establish a diagnosis, but to help plan the physical examination, to help select and evaluate treatment, to document patient progress and to establish patient prognosis. While there has been extensive research into the reliability of physical examination procedures used by physiotherapists, there has been little investigation of the quality of the information obtained from the patient during history taking. This section will consider the quality of this patient reported data and how best to obtain and use this information.

Occasionally physiotherapists will use the term 'subjective' to describe the data obtained by the therapist during the patient interview. The term 'subjective', however, should not be used to infer that patient reported information is of an inferior quality to the data obtained by the physiotherapist in the physical examination. The use of the term 'subjective' in this manner may serve to devalue the patient, throwing suspicion on his or her ability to provide reliable information. It may also suggest that in this patient/therapist relationship the therapist is the authoritarian figure, the patient assuming a submissive passive role. Consequently it is recommended that the term 'history' be used to describe the interview of the patient, and the term 'physical examination' be used to describe the assessment of the patient's physical signs.

How are these data obtained?

When the patient presents for physiotherapy treatment an extensive clinical history is taken, documenting the area, quality and intensity of pain, the degree of functional disability, the onset and progression of the disorder, the presence of contraindications or precautions to treatment and the patients expectations of treatment. These data are obtained by interviewing the patient, asking them to complete a questionnaire, or using a combination of both.

An interview structure allows collection of a large amount of data, some of which may have originally fallen outside the physiotherapist's frame of reference. An interview is often preferred by the patient because of the necessary patient/ therapist interaction. The therapist may employ a variety of questioning styles to obtain the information including dichotomous questions requiring a simple yes/no answer, forced choice questions requiring the patient to choose one of the answers offered, e.g. is your pain better, worse or the same?, or open-ended questions, e.g. could you describe the quality of your pain? Interviews usually contain a combination of these various questioning styles. Dichotomous questions will provide reliable information, but the information gained is severely limited and may provide little insight into the patient's problem (Waddell *et al.*, 1982). Forced choice questions should be used judiciously, for example, when a patient is unable to answer a specific question. In this instance providing the patient with several options may help. For example, if a patient, when asked to describe their pain, appears at a loss, the therapist may ask *'Is the pain deep or superficial?' 'Is the pain sharp or dull?'* The patient, once supplied with the possible options, may find it very easy to choose between these or may spontaneously supply their own choice.

Open-ended questions provide reliable and valid information (Waddell *et al.*, 1982) and are often used when asking the patient about the distribution of the symptoms and the onset and duration of their condition. Sometimes the reply may be complex, rambling and difficult to categorize, thus making it difficult to compare the patient's responses at subsequent treatments (French, 1988). In patients who appear reluctant to talk about their condition, open-ended questions may be used to encourage them to talk further. The physiotherapist must also reassure the patient that by talking about their symptoms they are not complaining but rather informing the physiotherapist, and hence assisting in determining the best choice of treatment. Also the therapist should stress to the patient that the information they provide will be held in the strictest confidence and not disclosed without first obtaining the patient's consent.

Although interviews are widely used to obtain much information from the patient, their time-consuming nature, combined with the difficulty in categorizing the patient's responses for subsequent comparison and the difficulty in accurately establishing the reliability of this information, could be substantially overcome by asking the patient to complete a structured questionnaire before or after the interview.

Questionnaires are less labour intensive thus having a high cost/benefit ratio, and are standardized to enable comparison of results. Many of the questionnaires used in the assessment of patients with low back pain have demonstrated high reliability and validity in their measurement of pain and disability (Melzack, 1975; Fairbank *et al.*, 1980; Waddell *et al.*, 1982; Gilson *et al.*, 1985). These questionnaires have also been shown to be sensitive to change, a patient's score on the questionnaire improving as his or her condition improves (Melzack, 1975; Fox and Melzack, 1976; Fairbank *et al.*, 1980; Linton and Gotestam, 1983). The main disadvantages of a questionnaire are that they may limit the response of the patient by using closed or forced choice questions, they may not be useful in patients with poor English (although the McGill pain questionnaire has been successfully translated into several different languages), and some questionnaires may be complex to score. Consideration of these advantages and disadvantages suggests that a combination of both interview and questionnaire formats will be most successful in obtaining high-quality data from the patient.

Questionnaire

After the initial greeting of the patient many physiotherapists ask a general question regarding the patient's main reason for attending physiotherapy. The response provided indicates the measurement that the therapist needs to perform. For example, if a patient with chronic low back pain tells you that their main reason for attending physiotherapy is to enable them to return to work, we must measure their disability. Commonly used low back pain disability questionnaires include:

- Roland and Morris disability questionnaire (Roland and Morris, 1983)
- Functional assessment screening questionnaire (Millard, 1989)
- Oswestry low back disability questionnaire (Fairbank *et al.*, 1980)
- Pain disability index (Pollard, 1984; Tait *et al.*, 1987)

One of these questionnaires may be given to the patient before the physical examination or after the initial assessment and treatment. The results will provide a reliable and valid measure of the patient's presenting level of disability and can be used to reflect changes in disability after treatment and over time. Although these questionnaires are

designed for patients with back pain they may also be used for those with neck dysfunction. In these instances the questions may be modified to ascertain whether or not specific disruptions (e.g. lying down, poor appetite, sleep disturbances, lack of concentration etc.) occur because of neck pain rather than back pain. Disability questionnaires are likely to be most useful for patients with chronic musculoskeletal conditions who may require several months of treatment. It is unlikely that disability needs to be measured in patients presenting with acute musculoskeletal conditions such as an acute wry neck where rapid recovery is predicted and any disability is temporary.

If, like the majority of patients with musculoskeletal conditions, the patient is seeking treatment for the relief of pain, then adequate measurement of pain must be performed. Several studies have demonstrated that there is little correlation between measures of disability and direct measures of pain, although disability may be related to attitudes and beliefs about pain (Meade *et al.*, 1990; Strong *et al.*, 1990). Therefore a disability measure cannot be used to infer information regarding pain or vice versa. Pain may be measured both directly and indirectly. Indirect measures include measures of analgesic intake or demand, and measures of the number of times a patient engages in pain behaviours such as moaning, contortion, facial expressions etc. Direct pain measures commonly used by physiotherapists include spatial measures such as completion of a body chart, and sensory measures such as numerical rating scales, where the patient is asked to select a number from 1 to 10 which best describes their pain (Murphy *et al.*, 1988). Absolute visual analogue scales may also be used, where the patient is asked to mark on a line, anchored at either end by descriptive terms such as 'no pain' and 'the worst possible pain', the level of pain that they are experiencing (Scott and Huskinson, 1976).

These latter two pain scales have been shown to provide reliable measures of pain and are probably most useful in patients with acute and subacute conditions. These pain-rating scales assume pain to be a unidimensional experience varying only in intensity. However, the experience or perception of pain is influenced by many other factors including affective factors. Affective factors are emotional factors that may influence our perception of pain. The degree of anxiety of the patient or the significance of the pain in patients with a terminal disease may greatly alter their experience of pain. Some treatments used by physiotherapists (such as relaxation classes) may lessen the affective components of pain, without altering the sensation of pain, thereby diminishing the overall pain experience for the patient. It is necessary therefore, particularly in patients with chronic pain where there may be a large affective or emotional component, that all dimensions of the pain experience are measured. Only then can we be aware of the total effect of our treatments on pain.

The McGill pain questionnaire has been designed to measure not only the sensory dimension of pain but also the affective and evaluative dimensions. It is viewed as one of the most comprehensive measures of pain, with many authors reporting it to be a highly reliable and valid measure (Melzack, 1975). This pain questionnaire may be completed by the patient in about 10 min and includes:

1. a list of adjectives to describe pain;
2. a body chart indicating the spatial distribution of the pain;
3. a verbal rating scale to measure the intensity of the present pain.

It is recommended that a McGill questionnaire be completed by patients:

1. with subacute or chronic conditions likely to be receiving treatment for longer than 1 month;
2. thought to have a high affective component to their pain;
3. who are receiving treatment thought to influence the affective component of pain (e.g. relaxation classes for pain, education classes for pain, back school).

These patients should complete a McGill pain questionnaire early in their course of treatment, and then be reassessed after several weeks or at the end of their course.

Interview

After charting the area of pain and rating its intensity, physiotherapists generally proceed to interview patients with acute or subacute musculoskeletal conditions regarding many other aspects of the pain and resultant disability such as the quality of the pain, the extent of the patient's functional disability (although in patients with chronic conditions a disability questionnaire will be used), the onset and progression of the disorder and the presence of contraindications or precautions to treatment. Hypotheses regarding injured

structures, useful treatments, expected prognosis are generated based on the information obtained from the interview. It is essential therefore that this information be as accurate and reliable as possible.

It is necessary to state first of all, that the sometimes poor reliability of information gained from the patient is often not due to patient error, but is more frequently due to error incurred by the therapist when collecting and interpreting patient information.

Factors affecting reliability and validity

The most common reason for the sometimes poor reliability of patient reported data is problems in verbal communication. In the therapist–patient relationship many encoding and decoding errors may occur (Gerrard *et al.*, 1980). Encoding errors occur when the message formed in the mind of the sender is not translated (encoded) correctly, i.e. the question sent to the receiver is ambiguous or unclear. A decoding error occurs when the receiver incorrectly translates or decodes the question they have heard to determine its exact meaning. Successful communication occurs when the message formed = the message sent = the message received.

Sometimes the patient may be tired and appear uncooperative because of severe musculoskeletal pain, and therefore be increasingly reluctant to give much consideration to a barrage of difficult questions. This factor may be minimized by ensuring that the patient is as pain-free and undistracted as possible before commencing the interview. For patients with severe low back pain this may involve lying them on the bed in a position of comfort before commencing the interview. Patients with severe neck pain may also feel more comfortable lying with the head comfortably supported on a pillow before commencement of questioning.

Chamberlain and Johnstone (1975) discuss the problem of poor memory or recall and how this may reduce the reliability of the information provided by the patient. It is important that the physiotherapist avoids coercing the patient to supply an answer to a question that the patient is not able to answer, for example *'Was the back pain you experienced 15 years ago similar to this episode of back pain?'* If the patient is unable to recall the first episode in detail the therapist should reassure them that it is okay to respond with *'I can't remember.'* To improve patient recall, patients commencing treatment should be encouraged to keep a small diary noting any significant changes in symptoms after treatment. This should help improve data unreliability due to memory difficulties, although it will be of more benefit on subsequent treatment occasions than at the initial interview.

Occasionally patient reporting may be influenced by strong motivational factors, for example, desire to please or desire to appear stoic. Several authors have commented on the influence of financial compensation on pain reporting, suggesting that in some circumstances there is potential monetary reinforcement for a high pain report (Kremer *et al.*, 1981). Hence in these patients, responses may appear evasive or exaggerated. Patient reporting may also be influenced by the non-verbal cues they receive from the physiotherapist. If the physiotherapist appears tired and disinterested, or judgemental, then this may affect how the patient responds. The therapist needs to be positioned at the same level and facing the patient so they can best convey their interest in the patient's problems. The therapist should shake hands or smile to welcome the patient. During the interview, maintaining appropriate eye contact with the patient and nodding in affirmation of what the patient says helps to reassure the patient that the therapist is interested in their problem and helps to promote a relationship of trust.

Strategies to increase reliability and validity

In an attempt to prevent communication errors, therapists should avoid the use of jargon in their discussions with patients. Physiotherapists like other health professionals may often resort to physiotherapy jargon when attempting to explain the clinical problem or the most suitable treatment to the patient. This may involve the physiotherapist saying, for example, *'I think your lumbar pain would respond well to some mobilization and traction'*. This may mean little to the patient, and consequently anxiety about the unexplained pending treatment may influence the patient's subsequent responses. Patients may also use jargon such as *'My back feels like it's out'* or *'My leg feels funny'*. Physiotherapists must ensure that they fully understand the meaning of the patient's answer by

paraphrasing the patient's response and then clarifying this with the patient.

Questions that encourage the patient to respond in a specific way should, as a general rule, be avoided because they decrease validity. These questions are referred to as leading questions because they tend to influence the direction of the patient's reply. For example the following leading question, *'Is your back pain much better since your last treatment?'* makes the assumption that the pain has improved following treatment. This question may pressure the patient to respond with *'Well, perhaps a bit better'* although the patient may feel unchanged. The best way to phrase this question may be *'What has happened to your back pain since your last treatment?'* This lack of bias in the question should ensure that the therapist attains the most accurate information.

Leading questions may occasionally be used if the information sought concerns behaviour where the patient feels a positive response may be used to detrimentally judge or label them. For example, if a patient with chronic low back pain has been absent from work the physiotherapist, rather than enquiring whether the patient has had time off work, may ask how much time off work the patient has required. This may help to normalize the patient's behaviour and therefore result in a more accurate response (French, 1988).

Double-barrelled questions, or questions requiring two or more responses, should be avoided as they are often long, confusing and difficult to answer correctly. For example the following question *'Do you have any pain or pins and needles in your back, legs or feet?'* would be better posed as the following short, concise questions: *'Do you have any pain in your back?'*, *'Do you have any pain in your legs or feet?'*, *'Do you have any pins and needles in your legs or feet?'*.

Questions loaded with moral judgement should also be avoided as they may force the patient to respond in a specific way. An example of a loaded question may be *'I hope you haven't done anything to increase your neck pain since your last visit'*. This question suggests to the patient that if their neck pain is increased since their last visit then it is their fault.

Pain behaviours should be noted, and clarified with the patient if not understood. For example, if during a physical examination procedure the patient's facial expression indicates that they are in pain, although they are not verbally complaining of pain, this discrepancy should be clarified with the patient.

Conclusion

In summary, to ensure that reliable and valid information is obtained in the history it is necessary to recognize the factors that may threaten the quality of patient report data. These factors may include patient/therapist communication errors, poor questioning styles, poor memory or recall, the influence of motivational factors such as desire to please, and the difficulty in concentrating in the presence of severe pain. Several strategies to maximize reliability and validity are discussed. In order to obtain high-quality data that is useful in formulating a diagnosis and determining the best choice of treatment, the use of both an interview and a structured questionnaire is advocated.

The history

Procedure

Taking a good history requires good interpersonal skills as well as a good knowledge base. Much is known about how to use interpersonal skills to enhance the interview process and gain valuable information. It remains now to discuss what information is required, and how to use it. The kind of history now taken by musculoskeletal physiotherapists was first described by Maitland (1965), and it is a tribute to his thorough approach that it has changed little since that time.

The purpose of the history, as suggested above, is to formulate ideas or hypotheses about:

1. pathological diagnosis,
2. clinical diagnosis,
3. management strategies,
4. prognosis,
5. contraindications and precautions.

Judgements about each of the above categories of decision are made by comparing several different pieces of information. There is rarely a single piece of information that is definitive. However, rather than asking all questions relating to one *category*, such as prognosis, questions relating to one *aspect of the problem* are usually grouped together, so that, for example, information about the type and location of symptoms is gained before progressing to other aspects of the problem, such as when and how the injury occurred. This method increases both the efficiency and effectiveness of the interview process. Thus a somewhat routine set of questions has been developed to ensure that relevant information is gathered efficiently (Maitland, 1965). It is not intended that this routine should be strictly adhered to, but it serves as a guide for students just beginning, and even for experienced clinicians faced with solving new and challenging problems.

The order in which information is collected may affect its interpretation. It is suggested that our original hypotheses are made from the first information gained. With further information we then change or refine our early hypotheses. Often the order in which we collect information relates to the relative importance assigned to it, e.g. when a person presents with a knee problem, the mechanism of injury may be determined early in the history because this information is important diagnostically, whereas with low back pain, this information may have less diagnostic value.

Generally, the structure of the history consists of seven 'sections'. These are:

1. area of symptoms,
2. current history,
3. behaviour of symptoms over a 24 h period,
4. irritability of symptoms (how easily symptoms are aggravated),
5. past history,
6. questions to determine contraindications and precautions to examination and treatment ('special questions'),
7. 'social' history.

Some information about all categories of decisions (pathological and clinical diagnoses, treatment, precautions and contraindications and prognosis) will be obtained from each of the above sections. Thus ideas are formed on several categories of decision simultaneously, comparing new information with existing hypotheses. These categories of information and the use of information gained are presented in Table 5.1.

All information must be recorded. This means noting questions that were asked but were negative (e.g. the patient had no arm pain on the first visit). There are many occasions when records need to be consulted, such as on subsequent treatment occasions, or if the problem relapses in the future, as well as for research, audit or legal purposes. Records should therefore be complete, accurate and legally satisfactory.

Table 5.1   The history: Categories of questions asked, the information gathered and how this information is used by physiotherapists

Category	Information	Use of information
Area and type of symptoms	Spatial distribution, referral patterns	Diagnosis, prognosis, monitoring progress
	Type of symptoms: • pain • paraesthesia • anaesthesia	Diagnosis, monitoring progress
	Constant or intermittent	Diagnosis and prognosis
	Quality e.g. • dull ache • burning, sharp	Monitoring progress (? diagnosis)
	Intensity	Monitoring progress
	Depth	Diagnosis
	Relationship of symptoms	Diagnosis, treatment and prognosis
Current history	When injury occurred	Treatment and prognosis
	Mechanism of injury	Diagnosis and treatment
	Progress of symptoms	Treatment and prognosis
	Previous treatment and effect	Diagnosis, treatment and prognosis
Behaviour of symptoms (24 h behaviour)	Night pain • get to sleep? • wakens? • best/worst positions	Diagnosis, treatment
	Morning • pain • stiffness	Diagnosis
	Activities or position aggravating symptoms	Diagnosis and treatment
	Activities or positions easing symptoms	Diagnosis and treatment
	Symptom behaviour during the day	Diagnosis and treatment
Irritability of symptoms	What activity (and how much) aggravates symptoms?	Physical examination: • which tests? • vigour • treatment, strategy and dose
	Intensity of symptoms	
	Continuation of symptoms after cessation of activity	
Past history	First episode: • when did it occur? • how did it occur? • previous treatment and effect?	Diagnosis, treatment and prognosis
	Subsequent episodes: are they changing in • frequency? • intensity? • duration?	Treatment and prognosis

Category	Information	Use of information
Questions to determine precautions and contraindications to examination and treatment	General health Weight loss X-rays and other investigations Medications • steroids Presence of osteoporosis	These questions are aimed at excluding pathological diagnoses Certain pathologies may contraindicate all or selected treatment strategies and may require further medical investigation
(For spinal conditions)	Cord signs	
(For lumbar spine)	Cauda equina syndrome	
(For cervical spine)	Dizziness	
Social History	Age and gender	Diagnosis, treatment, prognosis
	Employment • status • type	Treatment
	Domestic role	Treatment
	Self-care	Other interventions
	Dependents	Treatment
	Leisure activities	Treatment

Area and type of symptoms (body chart)

The body chart is really a 'map' of the patient's symptoms outlined on a chart of the body, as shown in Figure 5.1. The purpose of completing such a 'map' is to identify possible sources of symptoms by:

1. identifying clearly all areas and types of symptoms;
2. initially determining the relationship of symptomatic areas.

Hypotheses raised from the body chart will be pursued throughout the remainder of the examination.

Information mapped on the body chart includes: the area, constancy, quality and severity of symptoms, and the relationship of symptoms if there is more than one area. The 'depth' of pain is sometimes also determined.

Area

The area of symptoms gives much information about the source of the problem, and perhaps about

prognosis. Knowledge of referral patterns (and receptive fields; see Schaible and Grubb, 1993) and of common patterns of presentation of particular pathologies is required to interpret the symptoms effectively. [Dermatomes and myotomes are illustrated in Williams and Warwick (1980)]. Pain radiating down the lateral aspect of the calf and foot, for example, may indicate involvement of the fifth lumbar segment (Williams and Warwick, 1980). Recently the pain referral patterns of the thoracic zygapophyseal joints have also been clearly documented (Dreyfuss, *et al.*, 1994) as have referral patterns for various lumbar spine somatic structures. Several studies have found that pain from the lumbar spine radiating below the knee is likely to be radicular in origin (McCulloch and Waddell, 1980; Austen, 1991).

The area and type of symptoms can also be used as a baseline measure to monitor treatment effects. For example, a decrease in area of pain or centralizing of pain towards the spine may indicate improvement in the condition (McKenzie, 1981), whereas a change from paraesthesia to anaesthesia would signify a worsening of the condition. For these reasons it is important to determine as accurately as possible all sites of symptoms. This

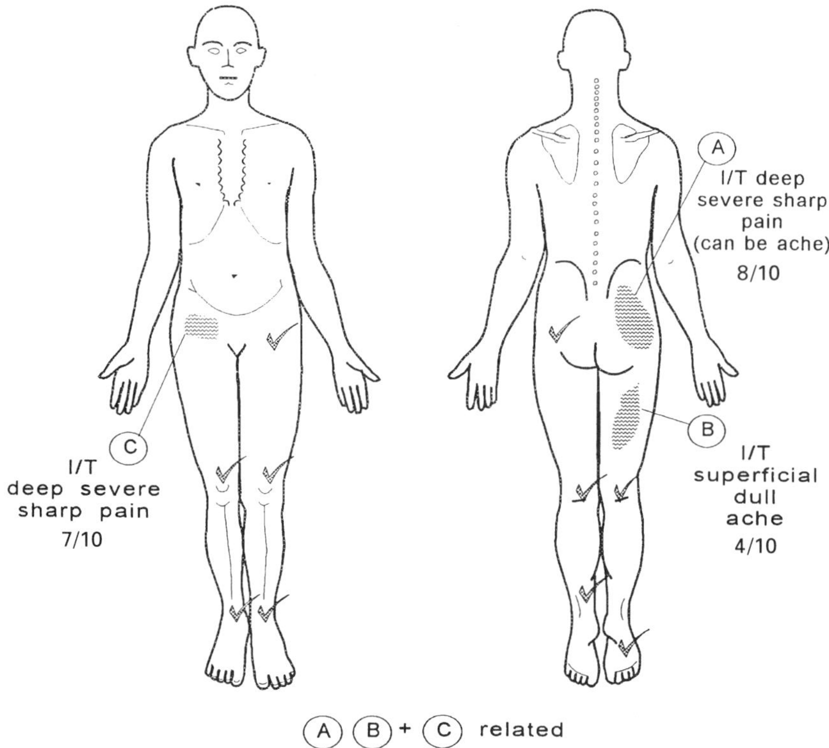

Figure 5.1 Body chart used to map spatial distribution and describe quality of patient's symptoms

often means asking specifically about the presence or absence of symptoms in the leg (in lumbar spine conditions) or arm (in disorders of the cervical spine). All possible sources of symptoms must be followed up throughout the examination.

Absence of symptoms should also be recorded. This indicates that the patient was asked about symptoms in these areas and they were not present.

The area of symptoms is also used to assist in determining prognosis. It is generally considered that a large area of pain with many associated symptoms such as pins and needles would take longer to fully recover than would a small localized area of pain with no other symptoms. For a thorough review of spinal pain see Schaible and Grubb (1993).

Anaesthesia or paraesthesia

Patients presenting with spinal musculoskeletal conditions are routinely asked whether they have any areas of paraesthesia (altered sensation such as pins and needles) or anaesthesia (absence of sensation, or numbness). The presence of any altered sensation is strongly suggestive of nerve compromise, particularly when the distribution of symptoms is dermatomal (Helfet and Gruebel, 1978; Sunderland, 1978; see Chapter 6 of this volume). Other conditions, including vascular compromise or perhaps altered afferent input from somatic structures, may also cause paraesthesia. However, the most common cause of altered sensation accompanying spinal disorders is compromise of the spinal nerve/nerve root (Bogduk, 1991).

Constancy

Constancy refers to whether the symptoms are continuously present and, more importantly, whether the intensity of the symptoms varies, particularly with movement or positioning. Generally, pain or paraesthesia that is made worse or better by certain movements or positions is likely to be musculoskeletal in origin or, as is often described, has a 'mechanical' component. This is because when the tissues involved are stressed they will transmit painful stimuli. Many pathologies will present with this pattern of signs and symptoms responding to movement such as some skeletal metastases or carcinoma, notably osteoid osteoma (Martire, 1987; O'Connor and Currier, 1992), but other information from the history and physical examination should warn the physiotherapist that the condition may be due to serious or identifiable pathology. Patients may have pain at rest, i.e. even when they are not moving, but if their pain does not vary (i.e. increase or decrease) with movement, the problem may not be a mechanical disorder of the musculoskeletal system. Rather, it may be systemic or organic, caused by pathologies such as arthritis or cancer or other diseases of the viscera. A patient may have constant pain (resting pain) because of accompanying inflammation or sensitization of receptors (Schaible and Grubb, 1993) but the pain will still vary with activity. Therefore, if symptoms are constant and unvarying, the physiotherapist should be suspicious about the nature of the problem. Such suspicions should be clarified throughout the remainder of the history.

Constancy of symptoms may also give some idea of prognosis. It is generally considered that the presence of resting pain indicates that the problem may take longer to improve than intermittent pain. Also, constant pain that becomes intermittent in nature may suggest that the patient's condition is improving.

Quality

The quality or description of pain (burning, throbbing, knife-like, dull ache etc.) has often been interpreted in terms of pathology and structures producing pain. For example, throbbing pain is thought to characterize inflammation, whereas burning or knife-like pain is thought to characterize neural involvement, and a dull ache to indicate joint involvement. Quality of pain, however, has been shown to have poor reliability and poor validity in detecting the structure or pathology involved, when investigating spinal problems with and without neural involvement (Dalton and Jull, 1989; Austen, 1991).

Quality of pain does have some uses, however. The quality of pain may be used to monitor a patient's progress with treatment. It is usually satisfying for the patient if the quality of the pain experience becomes less unpleasant. In addition, the quality of pain is used in disability questionnaires (e.g. the McGill pain questionnaire; Melzack, 1975). Combined with other information, then, the quality of the pain indicates the severity of the pain experience. In isolation, this information is probably of limited value.

Intensity

The usual way that physiotherapists determine the intensity of pain is to ask patients to rate the pain on a scale. The scale may be from 0 (no pain) to either 5 or 10 (the most severe pain). For research purposes and in disability questionnaires a visual analogue scale (AVAS) is used (Zusman, 1986). This is a line 10 cm long with pain descriptions at each end (e.g. no pain, and pain as bad as it could possibly be). This method of determining intensity has high intra-individual reliability (Kremer *et al.*, 1981).

Intensity of pain is used to indicate the severity of the symptoms as experienced by the patient and thus can be used as a reliable indicator of progress of the condition and effect of treatment. The intensity of symptoms possibly assists in determining prognosis, e.g. more severe pain may take longer to full recovery than mild pain. It is worthwhile to remember that intensity is not an objective measure of the pain experience. Different patients may nominate the same level on the scale for different pain experiences. However, it is a good indicator of change in pain. For example if pain were originally 8/10 and changed to 4/10 after intervention, the patient's pain has substantially reduced.

Depth

In the past it was thought that the depth of pain indicated the depth of the structure involved. However, this is not always a valid assumption (consider the superficial dermatomal symptoms caused by SN/NR compromise – a deep anatomical complex). Pain from musculoskeletal conditions is often described as a deep dull ache (Austen, 1991), although pain in superficial muscles may feel local. To make most sense of this information, knowledge of referral patterns for anatomical structures is essential. Muscles, for example, do not refer superficially (Mense, 1993), whereas viscera generally do have a cutaneous referral pattern, remembering that not all viscera are sensitive to noxious stimuli (Gebhart and Ness, 1991), and skin rarely (if ever) refers pain (Lewis, 1942). Joints, such as the zygapophyseal joints, appear to refer symptoms superficially (Mooney and Robertson, 1976). Autonomic symptoms, such as drop in blood pressure, sweating, and nausea may also be associated with visceral, and sometimes muscle, pain (Feinstein *et al.*, 1954). Since the source of spinal pain is not understood in most cases, but rarely seems to be muscles or skin, this information is probably less useful for diagnosis and treatment selection in disorders of the vertebral column than of the periphery.

Relationship of symptoms

A patient may have several symptomatic areas or several types of symptom. The physiotherapist must establish whether the various symptoms appear to originate from one source, or whether several sources are involved. This can be done by determining whether symptoms are provoked independently (unrelated symptoms) or they all worsen together (related symptoms). If symptoms are related, the physiotherapist will potentially treat one area and expect all symptoms to improve. On the other hand, if there are two or more separate sources of symptoms, several areas may require treatment. For example, it may be necessary to treat both the hip and lumbar spine to completely resolve a patient's leg pain. It is not always easy to establish a relationship by questioning in the history. If it is not possible, the relationship needs be clarified throughout the examination.

Current history

After clearly delineating the symptoms, physiotherapists often get information about the current history. The current history (history of the presenting condition) includes all relevant information about the onset of the disorder including; when the injury happened, how it happened (the mechanism of injury), the progress of symptoms, and what treatment has been used (if any) and its effect. This information assists in decisions about diagnosis, treatment and prognosis.

Onset of symptoms

When the injury occurred readily indicates whether the injury is acute, subacute or chronic. Acute injuries are defined as 0–7 days after the injury, subacute as 7 days to 7 weeks after the injury, and chronic as more than 7 weeks after the injury, although definitions vary (le Blanc *et al.*, 1987; see also Chapter 9 of this volume). This gives an idea of the stage of the pathology and the likelihood of the presence of inflammation, and thus indicates appropriate types of intervention. For example, a person with a severe whiplash injury that occurred 2 days ago would most likely require rest and perhaps gentle intervention, whereas a person with a 3-week-old ankle sprain would probably require exercise and mobilization. The length of time since injury may also give some idea of prognosis – the longer the patient has had the problem, the longer it may take to completely resolve.

Mechanism of injury

Mechanism of injury is used in formulating a diagnosis, especially in the periphery. The tissue damaged may be indicated by the direction and position of the injuring forces. It is also valuable to compare the magnitude of the injuring force with the severity of the injury sustained: a minor force causing a very severe injury may indicate abnormal tissue status, such as osteoporosis, before injury.

Progress of symptoms (whether the condition is better, worse or the same, and in what way)

Many musculoskeletal disorders will improve with the normal process of healing and repair, usually within 6 weeks e.g. for the spine (Evans, 1980; Sheldon, 1984). However, other disorders may worsen or require intervention. It is not uncommon, for example, for pain to start in a small area and radiate over time (e.g. 48 h) or increase in severity. The condition would also be considered to be worsening if paraesthesia commenced after the initial pain. Such progression of symptoms may indicate specific pathologies. For example, symptoms from fragments of intervertebral disc tissue impinging on a nerve root and aggravated by a lifting injury may radiate down the limb some hours or days after the insult; the symptoms of intermittent claudication from spinal canal stenosis may increase with time; but symptoms from a muscle strain with no complications should be improving within 1–2 weeks. Thus knowledge of progress of symptoms assists in diagnosis. It also probably assists in selecting the dose of treatment: a smaller dose may be applied if the problem is worsening, or a more vigorous dose may be selected if the problem is unchanged. Further, progress of symptoms may indicate prognosis. Generally, the prognosis is better if the condition is curently improving rather than worsening.

Previous treatment and effect

It is efficient to use all possible information to select a treatment, therefore, if the patient has previously been treated for a similar disorder, it is important to establish the treatment used and its effect. A treatment that has already been used successfully may again be an appropriate choice. On the other hand, if the condition worsened, or did not respond as quickly as predicted with treatment, this is an indication to alter the dose of the treatment or change the intervention strategy altogether. In addition, if the patient has already been treated well and responded poorly, the prognosis is poorer than if the condition had responded well. Knowing about previous treatments and their effects thus gives us ideas about treatment selection, dose and prognosis.

Behaviour of symptoms during the day and night (24 h behaviour)

Appreciation of the 24 h behaviour of symptoms includes knowing the status of symptoms at night and when the patient first wakes in the morning, how symptoms alter during the day, and specific activities that aggravate or alleviate symptoms. Understanding how symptoms behave during the day and at night assists in formulating a diagnosis, a treatment plan and to a lesser extent determining prognosis. Information about response of symptoms to various activities is also used to monitor progress of the condition.

Specific syndromes or diseases, such as spinal canal stenosis, vertebrobasilar insufficiency, the arthritides or other inflammatory diseases can frequently be recognized on the basis of the response of symptoms to various activities, since such conditions often have a characteristic presentation. Symptoms of spinal canal stenosis, for example, typically worsen when the patient walks, and are relieved on squatting or spinal flexion (Grieve, 1986). Commonly, however, spinal conditions seen by physiotherapists have a non-specific pathology; current knowledge is insufficient to identify the anatomic structure or pathology involved. Having determined that the condition originates in the musculoskeletal system, that there is apparently no specifically identifiable pathology, and that the condition is 'mechanical', further information about response of symptoms to various activities and positions becomes increasingly important because this may be used to formulate the clinical diagnosis and as the basis of the treatment plan.

Specific information gained

Night pain: does the patient get to sleep normally, and once asleep, do they stay asleep?

Establish whether the patient has more than usual difficulty getting to sleep, remembering that many people normally have trouble sleeping. Difficulty in getting to sleep may be caused by an inappropriate pillow or bed or particular sleeping positions. Before giving advice about pillows or beds, determine the status of the symptoms when the patient wakes in the morning (see below). If the bed or pillow is inappropriate (for example some thoracic spine conditions are more comfortable in a soft bed and some cervical spine conditions may prefer a slim feather pillow) advise your patient about changing them. Choice of bed and pillow, however, is related to individual comfort: there is no variable that will satisfy all painful conditions.

Sleeping positions or postures also often cause discomfort. Patients frequently report, for example, that lying on the symptomatic side is painful. Determine the worst and best sleeping positions. Information about sleeping positions is mainly used in determining a management plan. Intervention to enhance the patient's comfort and ability to sleep may be required, for example by using a pillow to avoid rolling on to the painful side. In addition, the provocative position may be used in treatment. If, for example, a patient cannot lie on their left side because it brings on their left leg pain, this position may be used as a treatment. On the other hand, if the condition is severe, this position may be avoided initially, and the most comfortable position used.

Does the pain wake the patient during the night? The answer to this question is extremely important because intractable night pain is generally indicative of serious pathology (O'Connor and Currier, 1992). This type of pain not only wakes the patient, but may force them to get out of bed, because nothing eases the pain. Unremitting pain may be caused by pathology such as the inflammation of rheumatoid arthritis or ankylosing spondylitis during exacerbation, or severe infections such as osteomyelitis, or advanced carcinomas. The reasons for the severity of the pain and its worsening during the night are largely unknown at this stage. Therefore, if patients tell you about pain at night that is very severe and unremitting, it is extremely important to follow up the possibilities of other more serious pathologies with further questioning and tests throughout the examination. Patients with musculoskeletal disorders often have night pain, but this can usually be relieved by a position of comfort. This pain needs to be differentiated from the unremitting night pain indicative of severe inflammation or other serious pathologies.

Morning pain and stiffness

The status of symptoms when the patient first wakes establishes whether the symptoms are better with rest. Generally, musculoskeletal conditions respond well to rest. Although there may be some stiffness in the morning it usually resolves quickly, often with a warm shower. Pain is also usually reduced in the morning. In contrast some arthritides, such as rheumatoid arthritis, respond poorly to rest. For example, when a patient with rheumatoid arthritis wakes, they often have marked stiffness lasting for more than 30 min (Kannangara and Shenstone, 1988; Schumacher, 1988). Therefore, the possibility of an inflammatory arthritis should be considered in patients who complain of morning stiffness lasting for more than 30 mins. If patients with a musculoskeletal disorder wake with increased pain in the morning, it is possible that the bed or pillow are inappropriate, or that the patient has slept in a provocative position. It seems wise not to recommend a change in bed or pillow unless you have determined that they are aggravating the condition.

Aggravating and easing activities

This involves identifying activities that make the condition better or worse. This information is particularly important, because the decision about whether or not the condition is 'mechanical' largely rests on this information. Therefore, the treatment approach to some extent also relies on this information. Musculoskeletal conditions generally respond well to appropriately prescribed rest in a position of comfort, and there is generally a particular movement(s) that will consistently cause pain or difficulty when attempted. For example, the pain from a sprained ankle often feels better after elevation for some time, and feels worse after walking for some distance. The ankle pain will respond in this same way consistently, until it has recovered. Systemic inflammation or arthritides such as ankylosing spondylitis, or osteoarthritis, will behave quite differently once the disease process is established. Such pathologies cause the patient to become stiffer and perhaps more painful after rest, and to become more mobile and less painful after appropriate exercise and movement (Kannangara and Shenstone, 1988; Schumacher, 1988). Too much exercise may exacerbate such conditions, all movements and positions probably becoming painful. Thus, the behaviour of the symptoms assists in diagnosis. When the condition is mechanical with non-specific pathology the movements aggravating the symptoms may also suggest the type of treatment that is appropriate. If activities involving spinal rotation aggravate the symptoms and the condition is not severe, then rotation may be a useful treatment option. If symptoms are severe, rotation may initially be avoided.

During the day symptoms may also behave in a manner typical of certain pathologies. Musculoskeletal mechanical conditions are generally better in the morning than in the evening, whereas inflammatory disorders and other pathologies may be worse in the morning, improve as the day progresses, and become worse again in the evening. This behaviour depends to some extent on the balance between exercise and rest.

It is often difficult to distinguish definitively between non-specific mechanical disorders and inflammatory joint pathology, since many musculoskeletal conditions may have an inflammatory component: lesions in the tissues of the musculoskeletal system heal with inflammation, and therefore musculoskeletal disorders would usually be accompanied by some symptoms of inflammation (Evans, 1980; Kannangara and Shenstone, 1988). Therefore, in many pathologies, features of inflammation may coexist with features of a non-specific mechanical musculoskeletal disorder. An important feature of inflammatory joint disease, however, is stiffness on first waking in the morning that lasts for more than 30 min (Kannangara and Shenstone, 1988; Schumacher, 1988).

Any functional activity that aggravates symptoms should be further examined in the physical examination. The patient may tell you, for example, that sitting causes immediate pain in the back, the buttock and the leg. Sitting and spinal flexion would therefore be examined in the physical examination, anticipating a painful response. In this patient, sitting can be used to monitor the patient's progress. After treatment, the patient may be able to sit for 10 min before any pain onset, and only pain in the back and the buttock is provoked. This represents a functional improvement, the most important improvement from the patient's point of view.

Irritability

Irritability is a theoretical concept proposed by Maitland (1986) to describe the ease with which a condition is exacerbated by movement. It provides a guide about how to approach the physical examination of a musculoskeletal condition. It is inappropriate to apply rigid rules to this concept since it is of undetermined reliability and validity.

There are three key questions which are asked to determine the irritability of a condition:

1. What activity (and how much) aggravates symptoms?
2. How severe is the pain?
3. After cessation of the activity, how long till the pain returns to resting level?

It is the combination of this information that determines irritability. Probably the most important information, however, is knowing the actual activity that aggravates symptoms. A condition that is considered irritable will prevent the patient from doing most activities. So, if a patient suggests that running, sporting activities or sitting for long periods aggravates symptoms, it is most unlikely that the condition is irritable. On the other hand, if pain in the neck and arm are provoked on the slightest movement, it is probable that the condition is very irritable. Severe pain alone does not indicate irritability of a condition. Severe pain may be provoked by a very stressful activity such as playing tennis, but the patient may be pain-free most of the time. The time the pain takes to settle

suggests the ease with which symptoms will settle if they are provoked during examination. The physiotherapist may be unwilling to provoke symptoms that will take a long time to settle.

The condition is then interpreted as irritable or non-irritable. Unfortunately most conditions are not so easily categorized and may be slightly irritable or moderately irritable, etc. It may be easier to think of irritability as a continuum, with two extremes; irritable conditions, and non-irritable conditions. Most disorders will fall between the two extremes.

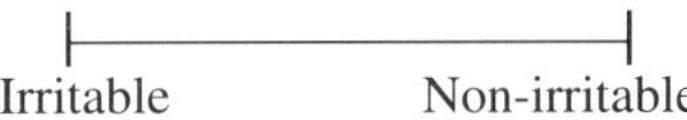

Irritable conditions require particular care when planning and executing the physical examination. For irritable conditions, only those examination procedures that give essential information, usually about diagnosis and treatment, will be performed. For non-irritable conditions on the other hand, a vigorous examination exploring extremes of range of movement and various combinations of activities would generally be required. By predicting the response of symptoms to movement, the concept of irritability is useful for determining the appropriate vigour of the physical examination of musculoskeletal conditions, ensuring that the examination is neither too gentle nor too vigorous for individual patients. With increasing clinical experience physiotherapists reach many of their examination and management decisions without rigidly adhering to these concepts.

Physical examination decisions affected by irritability

How many active movements to examine?

The number of active movements examined is guided by the time taken for symptoms to settle to the usual level, but it is frequently possible to examine all movements. It is important to recognize when the condition is being exacerbated, because this is the signal to stop performing movement testing. If it is not possible to examine all active movements, the physiotherapist would normally first examine those movements predicted to give the most useful information. Such movements have been identified on the basis of knowledge of the activities that aggravate the patient's symptoms.

How far through range to examine movements (active and passive)?

When dealing with irritable conditions, physiotherapists would usually examine several movements stopping each movement at the initial onset/increase in pain rather than examining one or two movements to end of range.

Which examination procedures to perform?

Physiotherapists usually prioritize examination procedures when assessing irritable conditions, ensuring that important procedures are performed early in the examination. Tests considered important for diagnosis or for treatment decisions, such as neurological testing, ligament tests or muscle tests, may be performed, even if symptoms may be exacerbated. Decisions to perform tests that will exacerbate an irritable condition are made on the basis of the certainty with which the test results can be interpreted (reliability and validity) and the importance of the test results to management decisions. If the results of tests are essential, then they will be performed, despite the probability of increasing symptoms. If the tests will have no impact on diagnostic or treatment decisions, they will probably not be performed until pain has settled at a subsequent visit. Consider the example of testing ligaments when your patient presents with an acute knee injury: ligament disruption may require surgical intervention, but the tests may be very painful for the patient. Some ligament tests are not reliable indicators of ligament disruption (such as the anterior drawer test; Feagin and Curl, 1976) although instrumented measuring devices provide reliable indicators of anterior cruciate ligament disruption (Daniel *et al.*, 1985). A physiotherapist experienced in treating knee injuries would probably choose to perform an instrumented ligament test, to decide the most appropriate method of management (which may require consultation with an orthopaedic surgeon), but may choose not to perform an anterior drawer test.

In patients presenting with an irritable disorder of the vertebral column, it is usually best to examine first the patient's worst active movement as identified from the aggravating activities. This will ensure that, should it be possible to examine only two or three active movements in these patients, information regarding the worst active movement, i.e. the active movement on which management and patient progress decisions are based, will have been examined.

The concept of irritability probably does not apply to all musculoskeletal conditions. In the presence of pathology such as rheumatoid arthritis, fractures, muscle rupture, joint replacements and other orthopaedic surgery, this concept is probably not very useful as treatment will be largely guided by the existing pathology, and the dose determined by the stage of healing and repair. Also, in patients with chronic low back pain the concept of irritability is not relevant.

Past history

Patients may never have experienced the presenting condition before or they may have had the same problem on one or several previous occasions. Previous episodes of the same problem may guide expectations for treatment and prognosis, and occasionally diagnosis. Sometimes patients may have had a different condition which may have an impact on the prognosis of the presenting condition, e.g. a patient may have had a fusion of the lumbar spine and now be presenting with thoracolumbar pain. The key features of the history of other relevant conditions should be understood, such as how and when the disorder started and the patient's normal health status. Some patients, for example, may 'normally' limp from a previous femoral fracture; the limp is not a feature of the presenting lumbar spine disorder and would not change with lumbar spine treatment, but may have implications for future recurrence of the presenting disorder and for prognosis.

For previous episodes of the same disorder, a detailed history of the first episode should be taken, including when and how the symptoms first started, and the type and effect of any previous treatment. In addition information should be sought about subsequent episodes: are they increasing or decreasing in frequency, intensity or duration?

This information provides guidelines for:

1. Prognosis; the duration of the current disorder will probably be similar to previous episodes if appropriate treatment had been administered, and other features are similar.
2. Treatment; based on knowledge about effective and/or ineffective treatments used in the past,
3. Diagnosis; there may be diagnostic information from previous episodes.

Recurrent problems may require further intervention to prevent future recurrence if factors contributing to onset can be identified.

Questions to determine precautions and contraindications (special questions)

Several questions are designed to identify pathology or a state of health that provides precautions or contraindications to various treatment strategies. These questions are routinely asked. The list is not exhaustive, and the physiotherapist may wish to ask further relevant questions. Information is routinely sought about the following:

1. state of general health;
2. recent unexplained weight loss;
3. X-rays or other investigations relevant to the presenting disorder;
4. medications the patient is currently taking;
5. presence of osteoporosis (use of oral steroids).

For all spinal conditions additional information is required about:

6. cord signs.

For lumbar spine disorders:

7. Cauda equina

For cervical spine disorders:

8. Dizziness (vertebrobasilar insufficiency).

General health

The health of a person is an indicator of many systemic diseases. A general question about the patient's health is therefore asked. Many diseases have extra-articular features, usually late in the disease process, for example, patients with rheumatoid arthritis may have eye or gastrointestinal involvement and may feel unwell, nauseated or lethargic (Schumacher, 1988), patients with cancer may feel unwell or fatigued (O'Connor and Currier, 1992), other diseases may manifest with fever or vomiting, etc. Since patients may present to the physiotherapist as the first health practitioner, the physiotherapist must know when to refer patients to other specialized care, and therefore to recognize early symptoms of pathology. If the physiotherapist suspects a particular pathology, further questions will be asked about symptoms relevant to that disease, such as swelling in other joints for no reason, which may accompany rheumatoid arthritis. In addition, certain illnesses, such as viral illnesses, may cause joint pain, but do not respond well to manual therapy. Other forms of physiotherapeutic intervention may be appropriate in many cases.

Weight loss

Weight loss occurring for no apparent reason can be a further indicator of systemic pathology. People may lose weight because they feel unwell or nauseated. However, loss of weight for no apparent reason generally suggests the presence of some pathology, such as with many cancers late in the disease process. Generally, by the time patients have started losing weight for no apparent reason, the disease is fairly advanced and has been diagnosed. Despite the fact that most people seem to want to lose weight, it is quite frightening when weight loss occurs for no apparent reason, and continues, perhaps because it signifies serious pathology. If a patient says they have lost weight, the physiotherapist should check whether they have been on a diet, or been particularly stressed. Weight loss should be investigated by the patient's medical practitioner.

X-rays and other medical investigations

X-rays will provide evidence of some diseases or abnormalities that may contraindicate certain procedures or advise caution in others. The identification of spondylolisthesis or spondylolysis on X-ray, for example, may indicate a poor response to posterior–anterior mobilizations at the level of the abnormality. Other medical tests, such as blood tests or liver function tests indicate the presence of pathology and the patient's general health status. If they have had such investigations, read the accompanying report, and view images (X-rays or CT scans, for example) in the light of the report. Any queries should be directed to the referring radiologist, remembering that physiotherapists are not professionally qualified to diagnose from such scans. Chapter 3 details common findings using various imaging techniques relevant to musculoskeletal physiotherapy.

Medications

Determine what medications the patient is taking, the dose and the effect. The patient may be taking medication to control blood pressure or diabetes, but may have omitted to tell you that they have these conditions. This is therefore a further check on their health status. In addition, patients with musculoskeletal disorders are often prescribed analgesics or non-steroidal anti-inflammatories. For a discussion of these pharmaceutical agents see Chapter 2. The physiotherapist needs to know the effect of these drugs on the presenting condition. A good response to anti-inflammatories suggests that there is an inflammatory component involved in the condition. If patients are taking analgesics, it may be wise in some cases to examine the patient before they take an effective medication so that signs and symptoms are not masked by the analgesic effect. In other cases, you may wish to treat after they have achieved some medication-induced analgesia, allowing a more vigorous intervention.

Presence of osteoporosis (including steroid use)

Oral and intra-articular steroids are fully discussed in Chapter 2. The main purpose of asking whether patients have taken oral steroids in the past is to determine the risk of osteoporosis. Osteoporosis is a precaution to vigorous manual treatments because the diminished bone density places the patient at greater risk of fracture (Pocock *et al.*, 1986). There are other factors contributing to reduced bone density, including hormonal status (particularly – postmenopausal women; Chow *et al.*, 1986), lack of calcium in the diet, smoking, slim build in early life and lack of exercise (Bailey *et al.*, 1986). In the presence of osteoporosis, manual treatments should be applied using small doses (with gentle forces).

Cord signs [questions to determine pathology in the central nervous system (CNS), particularly at spinal cord level]

The CNS is that part of the nervous system proximal to the anterior horn cell in the spinal cord (Williams and Warwick, 1980). Disorders of the CNS may therefore be the result of pathology anywhere in this part of the nervous system, including the brain and spinal cord. The location of the pathology must be established, because the cause of the CNS disorder may be pathology in the painful region of the spine. For example, cord compression secondary to rheumatoid arthritis in the upper cervical spine contraindicates management of upper cervical spine pain by manual therapy. CNS disorders will present with a variety of signs and symptoms, which include ataxia and diffuse (and therefore non-dermatomal) bilateral symptoms. When pathology affects the spinal cord at the level of the cervical spine, these symptoms will appear in both the arms and legs, whereas disturbances at the level of the lumbar spine will only affect the legs. The patient should therefore be asked about:

1. ataxia or unsteady gait,
2. bilateral non-dermatomal distribution of symptoms in the lower extremities for lumbar spine conditions, and in the upper and lower extremities for cervical spine conditions.

Further discussion of the CNS, testing and implications for treatment appears in Chapter 6.

Cauda equina syndrome

The spinal cord terminates at approximately the first lumbar segment. The long nerve roots continue, exiting at their appropriate intervertebral foramina and are collectively termed the cauda equina (Williams and Warwick, 1980). Cauda equina syndrome results from compromise of these nerve roots (Coscia *et al.*, 1994). Compromise of the cauda equina will therefore affect motor and sensory function in the whole lower extremity. Of particular importance is compromise of the S2 spinal segment, since S2 supplies the bladder and sphincters (Williams and Warwick, 1980; Coscia *et al.*, 1994). Compression of S2 will therefore result in loss of bladder and sphincter control, with a sensory loss in the genital region, commonly termed a 'saddle' distribution. Rarely, patients may present with urological dysfunction as the only sign or symptom (Coscia *et al.*, 1994). Since prolonged compromise of S2 may result in permanent dysfunction, acute cauda equina syndrome needs urgent recognition. Return of optimal neurological functioning requires surgical intervention, usually decompression (Coscia *et al.*, 1994). It is imperative that cauda equina syndrome be recognized immediately.

To determine the presence of acute cauda equina syndrome, questions are directed at ascertaining conduction in the S2 spinal segment. Patients are asked about:

1. alterations in voiding (frequency or absence of micturition, and perhaps bowel movements);

2. the presence of altered sensation (paraesthesia or anaesthesia) in the saddle area.

Cauda equina syndrome is further discussed in Chapter 6.

Dizziness (adequacy of cerebral blood flow)

The presence of vertebrobasilar insufficiency (VBI) causing inadequate blood supply to the brain is a contraindication or precaution to many physiotherapeutic procedures applied to the cervical spine. The most common presenting symptom is dizziness. Other disorders such as postural (orthostatic) hypotension, Meniere's disease, vestibular or labyrinthine disorders and cervical vertigo may also cause dizziness. The vertebrobasilar system supplies many intracranial structures. Ischaemia will result in symptoms from each of the affected structures and could include paralysis of gaze to the side of the lesion, diplopia (double vision), dysphagia, dysarthria, impaired trigeminal sensation (snout paraesthesia or anaesthesia) or transient ischaemic attacks. VBI is caused by reducing the volume of blood passing through the vertebrobasilar system. One cause of reduced blood flow may be a reduction in diameter of the vertebral arteries during cervical spine extension and/or rotation (Toole and Tucker, 1960; Refshauge, 1994). Therefore, if the cause of dizziness is VBI, patients will usually complain of dizziness, perhaps occurring with a slight delay, on assuming the provoking head position.

Postural hypotension (orthostatic hypotension), on the other hand, will occur with a sudden decrease in blood pressure resulting in a decrease in cerebral blood flow (Burton, 1965). The decreased blood pressure will usually result from changes in position, such as sitting up after lying down. Dizziness will not, therefore, be increased with cervical spine movements, but rather by positional changes. [For review see Rushmer (1976) or Rowell (1986).]

Meniere's disease is associated with other signs and symptoms such as fluctuating hearing loss, tinnitus and a feeling of pressure in the ears. Dizziness associated with Meniere's disease is unlikely to be associated with head movements, but will be associated with these other symptoms (Coman, 1986).

Vestibular/labyrinthine disorders also cause dizziness. Usually dizziness will be reproduced on specific head movement(s); the affected head movement(s) will be those causing movement of fluid to displace hairs in the affected canal (Kelly, 1991). The dizziness usually occurs immediately on head movement (unlike the slight delay associated with decreased blood flow). In addition, dizziness will not usually result from body movement that does not involve head movement (unlike VBI). However, it is sometimes difficult to distinguish vestibular or labyrinth disorders from VBI. The presence of pathological nystagmus (occurring even when the head is kept still) may assist in differentiation, since pathological nystagmus is a cardinal sign of disease of the labyrinth and its central connections (Goldberg *et al.*, 1991).

Cervical vertigo arises from abnormal afferent impulses from deep cervical spine structures such as muscles, zygapophyseal joints and the posterior longitudinal ligament (de Jong *et al.*, 1977). The disturbed afferent input can result in dizziness on head movement. It is therefore virtually impossible to differentiate between dizziness caused by VBI and that caused by cervical vertigo on the first treatment session. Differential diagnosis is usually confirmed after investigation, or after response to treatment is known.

Patients are questioned about the presence of dizziness. If they affirm that they experience periods of dizziness, further questioning will elicit the provocative manoeuvres. It is then important to follow up with questions about head movement, body movement and other signs and symptoms to determine the cause of the symptoms.

A full discussion of VBI appears in Chapter 6.

Social history

The social history provides useful information about management of the presenting disorder and occasionally cues regarding diagnosis or the presence of coexisting pathology. Pathology is sometimes exclusive to a particular age group or gender. For example, postmenopausal women are more likely to suffer osteoporosis than men in the same age group, and Scheuerman's disease most commonly affects young people.

Understanding the patient's social circumstances will ensure that overall management of the patient is appropriate and relevant. This requires learning about the patient's employment status (whether they work and the type of work engaged in), domestic role, requirements for assistance with self-care, existence of dependants and leisure pursuits. There may be other relevant aspects to the patient's life that need to be explored to ensure that home programmes and treatment goals are realistic, remembering that physiotherapists need to work within the constraints imposed upon their patients.

Details about employment status informs about the physical demands placed daily on the patient. This determines treatment goals to some degree. A patient may be unemployed and depressed, but have few other constraints in carrying out a home programme of exercises or rest. The goals of treatment will probably not be to return this patient to a particular work situation. For a patient who is currently employed, aspects of the work routine or postures adopted during the workday may require changing to benefit the patient in terms of avoiding re-injury or providing the optimal environment for tissue healing and repair. The demands placed on a patient at work may be identified during other sections of the history (e.g. aggravating activities in the Behaviour of symptoms over a 24-h period section). Other features of the patient's employment situation may need to be considered. For example, it is not always possible to make changes to a patient's work situation; employees might be frightened of losing their job, or a busy executive may be leading a company through organizational change. Although not ideal, physiotherapists sometimes need to work with patients within these constraints.

Leisure activities provide further information about desirable treatment outcomes. Type and level of activity, including specific requirements such as endurance of particular muscle groups, should be clearly ascertained. Retraining for these specific activities may form a necessary part of the management regimen.

When advising patients about home programmes and adequate rest, account must be taken of the patient's dependants. This may mean incorporating appropriate advice, e.g. mothers with small children may be unable to rest when physically it would be most desirable. They may also need advice about lifting and bathing small children, for example. Compliance with home programmes is impossible if consideration is not given to these factors.

Some patients may require domestic assistance. Sometimes this can be achieved by modifying the activity, but often means assistance from another person. If the patient lives alone, assistance may be required from other health personnel, e.g. occupational therapists or nurses.

It is important to be professional when discussing personal details with patients because it is easy to appear curious rather than proficient. In addition, a patient must trust you to give you honest personal details. It should also be remembered that it is unethical to discuss your patients publicly or disclose any information about a patient to unauthorized people or without consent.

A good knowledge of the patient's social history is particularly relevant when designing home programmes and setting treatment goals. Details about occupation and leisure activities are frequently a source of diagnostic information. Even when this is not the case, physiotherapists should understand the lifestyle the patient leads to enhance the possibility of successful treatment outcomes.

References

Patient report data

Chamberlain, G. and Johnstone, F. (1975). Reliability of the history. *Lancet*, **i**, 103.

Fairbank, J., Couper, J., Davies, J. and O'Brien, J. (1980). The Oswestry low back pain disability questionnaire. *Physiotherapy*, **66**, 271–3.

Fox, E. and Melzack, R. (1976). Transcutaneous electrical stimulation and acupuncture: comparison of treatment for low back pain. *Pain*, **2**, 141–8.

French, S. (1988). History taking in the physiotherapy assessment. *Physiotherapy*, **74**, 158–60.

Gerrard, B., Boniface, W. and Love, B. (1980). *Interpersonal Skills for Health Professionals*, pp. 31–7. Virginia: Reston Publishing Company.

Gilson, B., Gilson, J. and Bergner, M. (1985). The sickness impact profile. Development of an outcome measure of health care. *Am. J. Publi. Health*, **65**, 1304–10.

Kremer, E., Block, A. and Gaylor, M. (1981). Behavioral approaches to treatment of chronic pain: the inaccuracy of patient self-report measures. *Arch. Phys. Med. Rehabil.*, **62**, 188–91.

Linton, S. and Gotestam, K. (1983). A clinical comparison of 2 pain scales: correlation, remembering chronic pain, and a measure of compliance. *Pain*, **17**, 57–65.

Meade, T., Dyer, S., Browne, W. *et al.* (1990). Low back pain of mechanical origin: randomised comparison of chiropractic and hospital outpatient treatment. *Br. Med. J.*, **300**, 1431–7.

Melzack, R. (1975). The McGill pain questionnaire: major properties and scoring methods. *Pain*, **1**, 277–99.

Millard, R. (1989). The functional assessment screening questionnaire: application for evaluating pain related disability. *Arch. Phys. Med. Rehabil.*, **70**, 303–7.

Murphy, D., McDonald, A., Power, C. *et al.* (1988). Measurement of pain: a comparison of the visual analogue with a nonvisual analogue scale. *Clin. J. Pain*, **3**, 197–9.

Pollard, C. (1984). Preliminary validity study of Pain Disability Index. *Percept. Mot. Skills*, **59**, 974.

Roland, M. and Morris, R. (1983). A study of the natural history of back pain. Part 1: development of a reliable and sensitive measure of disability in low back pain. *Spine*, **8**, 141–4.

Scott, J. and Huskinson, E. (1976). Graphic representation of pain. *Pain*, **2**, 175–85.

Strong, J., Ashton, R., Cramond, T. and Chant, D. (1990). Pain intensity, attitude and function in back pain patients. *Austr. Occup. Ther. J.*, **37**, 179–83.

Tait, R., Pollard, A., Margolis, R. *et al.* (1987). The pain disability index: psychometric and validity data. *Arch. Phys. Med. Rehabil.*, **68**, 438–41.

Waddell, G., Main, C.J., Morris, E.W. *et al.* (1982). Normality and reliability in the clinical assessment of backache. *Br. Med. J.*, **284**, 1519–23.

The history

Austen, R. (1991). The distribution and characteristics of lumbar-lower limb symptoms in subjects with and without a neurological deficit. In *Proceedings of Manipulative Physiotherapists Association of Australia 7th Biennial Conference*, N.S.W, pp. 252–7.

Bailey, D.A., Martin, A.D., Houston, C.S. and Howie, L.J. (1986). Physical activity, nutrition, bone density and osteoporosis. *Austr. J. Sci. Med. Sports*, **18**, 3–7.

Bogduk, N. (1991). Innervation, pain patterns and mechanisms of pain production. In *Clinics in Physical Therapy. Physical Therapy of the Low Back* (L.T. Twomey and J.R. Taylor, eds), London: Churchill Livingstone.

Burton, A.C. (1965). Total fluid energy, gravitational potential energy, effects of posture. In *Physiology and Biophysics of the Circulation – An Introductory Text*, pp. 95–101. Chicago: Year Book Medical Publishers.

Chow, R.K., Harrison, J.E., Brown, C.F. and Hajek, V. (1986). Physical fitness effect on bone mass in post menopausal women. *Arch. Phys. Med. Rehabil.*, **67**, 231–4.

Coman, W.B. (1986). Dizziness related to ENT conditions. In *Modern Manual Therapy of the Vertebral Column* (Grieve, G., ed.), pp. 303–14. London: Churchill Livingstone.

Coscia, M., Leipzig, T. and Cooper, D. (1994). Acute cauda equina syndrome. *Spine*, **19**, 475–8.

Dalton, P.A. and Jull, G. (1989). The distribution and characteristics of neck–arm pain in patients with and without a neurological deficit. *Austr. J. Physiother.*, **35**, 3–8.

Daniel, D.M., Stone, M.L., Sachs, R. and Malcolm, L. (1985). Instrumented measurement of anterior knee laxity in patients with acute anterior cruciate ligament disruption. *Am. J. Sports Med.*, **13**, 401–7.

de Jong, P.T.V.M., de Jong, J.M.B.V., Cohen, B and. Jongkees, L.B.W. (1977). Ataxia and nystagmus induced by injection of local anesthetics in the neck. *Ann. Neurol.*, **1**, 240–6.

Dreyfuss, P., Tibiletti and C. Dreyer, S. (1994). Thoracic zygapophyseal joint pain patterns: a study in normal volunteers. *Spine*, **19**, 807–11.

Evans, P. (1980) The healing process at cellular level: a review. *Physiotherapy*, **66**, 256–9.

Feagin, J.A. and Curl, W.W. (1976) Isolated tear of the anterior cruciate ligament: 5 year follow-up study. *Am. J. Sports Med.*, **4**, 95–100.

Feinstein, B., Langton, J.N.K., Jameson, R.M. and Schiller, F. (1954). Experiments on pain referred from deep somatic tissues. *J. Bone Joint Surg.*, **36**, 981–97.

Gebhart, G.J. and Ness, T.J. (1991). Central mechanisms of visceral pain. *Can. J. Physiol. Pharmacol.*, **69**, 627–34.

Goldberg, M.E., Eggers, H.M., and Gouras, P. (1991). The ocular motor system. In *Principles of Neural Science*, (3rd edn) (E.R. Kandel, J.H. Schwartz and T.M. Jessell, eds), pp. 660–78, Connecticut: Prentice-Hall International.

Grieve, G.P. (1986). Bony and soft-tissue anomalies of the vertebral column. In *Modern Manual Therapy of the Vertebral Column*, pp. 3–20. London: Churchill Livingstone.

Helfet, A.J. and Gruebel, L. (1978). *Disorders of the Lumbar Spine*. Philadelphia: J.B. Lippincott Co.

Kannangara S. and Shenstone, B. (1988). Seronegative spondyloarthropathies. A distinct group of disorders. *Curr. Ther.*, April, 77–100.

Kelly, J.P. (1991). The sense of balance. In *Principles of Neural Science* (E.R. Kandell, J.H. Schwartz and T.M. Jessel, eds), pp. 500–11, Connecticut: Prentice-Hall International.

Kremer, E., Atkinson, J.H. and Ignelzi, R.J. (1981). Measurement of pain: Patient preference does not confound pain measurement. *Pain*, 24–248.

le Blanc, F., Cruess, R., Dupuis, M. *et al.* (1987). Scientific approach to the assessment and management of activity-related spinal disorders. *Spine*, **12**, (7 supplement) 20.

Lewis, T. (1942). *Pain*. London: Macmillan.

Maitland, G.D. (1965). *Vertebral Manipulation*. London: Butterworths.

Maitland, G.D. (1986). *Vertebral Manipulation*. (5th edn). London: Butterworths.

Martire, J.R. (1987). The role of nuclear medicine bone scans in evaluating pain in athletic injuries. In *Clinics in Sports Medicine*, pp. 713–38. Philadelphia: W.B. Saunders.

McKenzie, R.A. (1981). *The Lumbar Spine – Mechanical Diagnosis and Therapy*. Spinal Publications.

McCulloch, J.A. and Waddell, G. (1980). Variation of the lumbosacral myotomes with bony segmental anomalies. *J. Bone Joint Surg.*, **62B**, 475–80.

Melzack, R. (1975). The McGill pain questionnaire: major properties and scoring methods. *Pain*, **1**, 277–99.

Mense, S. (1993). Nociception from skeletal muscle in relation to clinical muscle pain. *Pain*, **54**, 241–89.

Mooney, V. and Robertson, J. (1976). The facet syndrome. *Clin. Orthop. Relat. Res.*, **115**, 149–56.

O'Connor, M.I. and Currier, B.L. (1992). Metastic bone disease: metastatic disease of the spine. *Orthopedics*, **15**, 611–20.

Pocock, N.A., Eisman, J.A., Yeates, M.G. *et al.* (1986). Physical fitness is a major determinant of femoral neck and lumbar spine bone mineral density. *J. Clin. Invest.*, **78**, 618–21.

Refshauge, K.M. (1994). Rotation: a valid premanipulative dizziness test? Does it predict safe manipulation? *J. Manip. and Physiol. Ther.*, **17**, 15–19.

Rowell, L.B. (1986) *Human Circulation Regulation During Physical Stress*. New York: Oxford University Press.

Rushmer, R.F. (1976). *Cardiovascular Dynamics* (4th edn.) pp. 217–45. Philadelphia: W.B. Saunders.

Schaible, H-G. and Grubb, B.D. (1993). Afferent and spinal mechanisms of joint pain. *Pain*, **55**, 5–54.

Sheldon, H. (1984) *Boyd's Introduction to the Study of Disease* (9th edn), pp. 131–57. Philadelphia: Lea and Febiger.

Schumacher, H.R. (1988). *Primer on the Rheumatic Diseases*, (9th edn). Atlanta: Arthritis Foundation.

Sunderland, S. (1978). *Nerve and Nerve Injuries* (2nd edn), London: Churchill Livingstone.

Toole, J.F. and Tucker, S.H. (1960). Influence of head position upon cerebral circulation. *Arch. Neurol.*, **2**, 616–23.

Williams, P.R. and Warwick, R. (eds) (1980). *Gray's Anatomy* (36th edn). London: Churchill Livingstone.

Zusman, M. (1986). The absolute visual analogue scale (AVAS) as a measure of pain intensity. *Austr. J. Physiother.*, **32**, 244–6.

Chapter 6

The physical examination

K.M. Refshauge and J. Latimer

Introduction

Our duty of care as physiotherapists is to offer appropriate care and advice to our patients. To be able to do this for each individual patient, physiotherapists must fully understand the nature, and the patient's experience of the presenting disorder. This is best achieved by performing a comprehensive examination, consisting of both a thorough history and physical examination. From the history, ideas are formed about the diagnosis, treatment, prognosis, factors contributing to the condition, contraindications and precautions to examination and treatment, as well as the patient's social circumstances. Many of these ideas are then tested in the physical examination. The extent and type of testing in the physical examination is therefore largely determined by information gained from the history.

The enormous growth in knowledge over the last few decades has led to new theories about diagnosis and treatment. New test procedures have been designed to examine many of these new theories. Most of these tests are comprehensively described in a wide variety of books (e.g. Grieve, 1984; Maitland, 1986; Magee, 1987). Only those tests commonly used by physiotherapists and considered important have been chosen for discussion here. It is not necessary (and, indeed, probably unwise) to perform all possible tests on a patient. Decisions about which tests to perform are mainly based on how the test results will be used. For example, many tests used by physiotherapists are also used by other health professionals such as doctors, chiropractors and osteopaths. However, some test procedures are predominantly used by physiotherapists because they are closely linked to physiotherapy diagnoses and treatments. Passive accessory motion is often assessed by physiotherapists, for example, because this information is used to predict whether the patient will benefit from treatment by mobilization, which specific region should be treated, and which treatment technique to apply. On the other hand, doctors rarely assess passive motion of the spine as this is not useful in forming a medical diagnosis or selecting medical intervention, such as medication or advice. Thus, testing is generally confined to those procedures relevant to ideas about diagnosis and overall management. When a patient complains of paraesthesia in the leg, neural conduction will be tested because impaired conduction from neural compromise is a possible cause of these symptoms, whereas a patient presenting with only local back pain will not undergo such testing because impaired conduction is not a likely source of symptoms.

Consent

Before any physical testing is performed valid consent should be obtained from the patient. A health professional should not, legally, touch or treat a patient without the patient's valid consent (irrespective of how foolish the patient's refusal may be), suggesting that paternalistic health care is no longer appropriate (Giesen, 1988). The ideals behind the obtaining of valid consent are that the decision about whether or not to accept intervention is the patient's decision and not the health professional's, and that every person has the right to decide what is done to his or her body (Giesen, 1988). In many countries the basic human right of self-determination is constitutionally protected. Valid consent consists of four parts (O'Sullivan, 1983).

1. Consent must be voluntarily given.
2. The consent should cover the act performed.
3. The person giving the consent must be legally competent to do so. If the patient is unable to give consent, as is the case with children, a relative can give consent on the patient's behalf.
4. The consent must be informed to some degree. This means that the patient should be given enough information to make a considered decision.

It is important that physiotherapists understand their legal responsibilities. Further information about aspects of law that affect health professionals can be found in, e.g. O'Sullivan (1983), Siegler *et al.* (1987), Buckley (1988) and Giesen (1988).

Diagnostic responsibility

As first contact practitioners, physiotherapists have specific legal and ethical responsibilities. These responsibilities include providing a high standard of care to all patients. To provide a high standard of care physiotherapists need to remain current in their knowledge and skills. This involves awareness of recent research findings, and incoroporation of these findings into clinical practice. Physiotherapists must also recognize the limitations both of their own practice, and of treatment options available to them. This means that physiotherapists need to recognize when to send patients for further investigation or management and who will be the most relevant practitioner for referral.

When assessing and treating patients, physiotherapists make judgements about:

1. The type of problem with which the patient presents (is physiotherapy appropriate?).
2. Whether the condition is progressing in the way expected (requiring knowledge of the natural history, or prognosis, of the disorder). This relates to the patient's status prior to treatment and after treatment has been instituted.

3. Any signs and symptoms in the clinical picture that might signal the possibility of pathology requiring further investigations (which may be urgent or non-urgent).

The reason for including this section on diagnostic responsibility is that we, as physiotherapists have some responsibility for recognizing signs and symptoms which indicate concern. This is not an academic or trivial consideration. Several real situations where important signs or symptoms were not recognized by the treating practitioner are presented in Table 6.1. All these patients were treated for at least 2 weeks with various procedures including mobilization, Feldenkrais techniques, relaxation, manipulation, and injection of local anaesthetic into trapezius muscle. In no case did the treating practitioners recognize cardinal signs of serious pathology that requires referral to an appropriate medical practitioner NOT treatment with manual techniques. Three patients suffered serious consequences from the inappropriate treatment. The other patients would have benefited enormously from early referral to the appropriate specialist for investigation and management. This point is further illustrated by a case study in Chapter 8 in which appropriate referral was the treatment of choice. Even if not working as a practitioner of first contact, physiotherapists are still responsible for deciding whether, indeed, any physiotherapy intervention is appropriate and also whether a specific intervention requires modification or progression. To do this requires the ability to determine the type of disorder, diagnose pathology not amenable to physiotherapy intervention, and monitor the effects of treatment. This, then, requires knowledge of the natural history of disorders.

It is difficult to be prescriptive and construct a list of signs and symptoms to watch for, particularly as in some cases the absolute presence of some signs is a signal, whereas in other cases, signs are important only in conjunction with other signs and symptoms, or the absence of a particular sign or symptom is vital in determining the pathology. In yet other cases the whole clinical picture is important. In all cases a judgement is required which is based upon sound up-to-date knowledge, skilful examination and thoughtful evaluation.

The following signs and symptoms are of particular importance in indicating concern. These signs and symptoms do not necessarily indicate a specific pathology, but whenever such signs or symptoms are encountered, it is particularly

Table 6.1   Illustrations where pathology requiring specific or urgent management was misdiagnosed

Physiotherapist's diagnosis and basis for treatment	*Treatment given*	*Actual cause of symptoms and consequences of lack of recognition*
1. Tension headache	Mobilization of upper cervical spine	Severe headache from cervical aneurysm, resulting in stroke
2. Stiffness of C2/3	Manipulation of C2/3 and mobilization of low cervical spine	Stenosis of C7/T1 intervertebral foramen and presence of disc/metaplastic tissue in canal at C5/6. Worsening of symptoms until unable to sleep or work. Surgery averted by complete bedrest
3. Non-specific mechanical low back pain	Mobilization of lumbar spine	Osteoid osteoma. Appropriate management eventually implemented, but after progression of disease
4. Non-specific mechanical low back pain with 'functional' overlay	SWD, interferential, traction, mobilization	Enormous disc bulge (or metaplastic tissue) causing cauda equina compromise
5. Tension headache with non-specific mechanical neck pain	Over 9 years, various procedures trialled: Feldenkrais approach, mobilization, acupuncture, massage, injection of anaesthetic into trapezius, relaxation techniques	Migraine headaches, co-existing with rheumatoid arthritis. Progress of disease unchecked for several years before controlled with medication

important that great care is taken to determine the underlying cause. Prompt referral to an appropriate medical practitioner may be required.

1. Any severe unremitting pain.
2. Severe unremitting pain that is staying the same or worsening despite rest, analgesia, appropriate intervention.
3. Severe pain with little disturbance of movement.
4. Severe night pain.
5. Worsening neurological deficit despite appropriate intervention and rest.
6. Non-mechanical behaviour, for example, excellent response to anti-inflammatory medication, little movement disturbance, lack of response to analgesia, unusual pain patterns, and inability to ease symptoms by positioning or postures, heat, movement or other modalities.
7. Severe pain without trauma (or severe undiagnosed pain following major trauma).
8. Severe spasm.

Many pathologies present as musculoskeletal pain. Such pathologies include vascular disorders, inflammatory diseases, tumours, arthritides, and compromise of nerve conduction particularly of the cauda equina. Since physiotherapists may be the first health professionals that the patient contacts, they must be alert to the possibility of

such pathology. Physiotherapists in many cases will not be able to make the actual diagnosis, but are able to recognize the necessity to refer to others with relevant expertise and access to appropriate testing procedures, who will make the diagnosis. Even if the patient has been referred to the physiotherapist by a medical practitioner, different information can be gathered by physiotherpaists, or signs and symptoms may develop that were not present when seen initially by the medical practitioner. To provide a high standard of care to patients, physiotherapists have a duty to ensure that they:

- recognize pathology outside their area of expertise and refer appropriately;
- maintain current practice (knowledge and skills);
- know natural history of common disorders so that they recognize when the disorder is not responding appropriately to treatment.

The general testing protocol: look, feel and move

In all fields of physical medicine, clinical diagnoses (diagnoses based on the patient's signs and symptoms), and pathological diagnoses, as well as appropriate treatment, are identified by the overall protocol of look, feel and move. This is particularly apt for the practice of physiotherapy, in which invasive procedures are rarely used. For all patients, therefore, at least some aspects of observation, palpation and movement testing will be performed. The assumptions underlying this practice appear to be that:

1. Visual cues aid recognition of patterns of signs and symptoms.
2. Painful structures are tender on palpation, and other clinical problems such as swelling or crepitus can be located by this procedure.
3. Testing the properties of structures involved in causing musculoskeletal pain will increase the pain or symptoms. Testing may include stretch, contraction or compression of the relevant tissues. In addition, functional impairment can be established.

This overall protocol appears to be effective and efficient. Additional procedures can be used to test for specific pathologies or dysfunction. However, the salient features of many musculoskeletal disorders and resultant functional deficits can be identified using the above protocol, resulting in accurate diagnosis and selection of appropriate management regimens.

The physical examination is therefore primarily aimed at confirming diagnoses suggested by the history and identifying the most appropriate treatment regimens. Some further information may also be gained about prognosis and factors contributing to the condition. Musculoskeletal conditions of the spine presenting to physiotherapists are often of non-specific pathology. In these cases, the clinical diagnosis is of great importance. Once the general functional deficit is established (e.g. ability to put on shoes and socks, walk or climb stairs) specific aspects of function are tested. Thus the nature of the presenting disorder guides the physical examination.

The physical examination

The physical examination generally involves observation, active movements with more stressful procedures applied when applicable, palpation, passive motion testing, and testing the adequacy of function of specific structures such as tension in neuromeningeal structures, neural conduction, vertebrobasilar sufficiency, and extensibility and strength of muscles. Various aspects of function or

movement control may also be tested, such as proprioception (for review see McCloskey, 1978), co-ordinated muscle activity or muscle activation levels, when relevant. Results of these tests are correlated with information previously gathered in the history and with results of preceding physical tests. The physiotherapist is looking for consistent patterns of signs and symptoms. If signs and symptoms are inconsistent, it is important to re-evaluate the data and the interpretations already made.

Hence the physical examination is performed systematically. This is because routines optimize efficiency. However, routines should not be performed thoughtlessly. If the purpose of each test is clearly understood, the results can be interpreted in light of results of other tests and ideas about diagnosis and treatment. By understanding this process, only appropriate information will be collected.

During testing all reasonable care must be taken to ensure comfort and safety of the patient. Comfort can be maximized by carrying out relevant tests in one position before moving on to the next position. This means, for example, that all relevant tests are performed in the standing position (or walking, etc.) before tests in the sitting position, and then tests in supine, side lying and finally prone positions. In each position, active movements are usually tested before passive movements, because this allows the patient to control the movement if there is any pain. When testing passive movements, the physiotherapist can then take into account the range of movement available and the amount of pain experienced by the patient during the movement. For example, active rotation of the lumbar spine would be tested before either passive rotation movements or rotation positioning of the lumbar spine.

The order of application of test procedures is important for some tests but not for others. Those tests with implications for further testing (such as the neurological examination) are usually performed early in the examination. Also, general tests are usually performed before specific tests therefore, for example, active cervical spine rotation would be assessed before rotation at individual intervertebral segments.

The vigour of the physical examination is determined by the irritability of the condition (how easily symptoms are provoked and their severity and persistence). If an examination is too gentle, the presenting problem may not be identified, as anatomical structures may not have been sufficiently stressed. On the other hand, an examination that is too vigorous may exacerbate the presenting symptoms to an extent where no more testing is possible, and insufficient information has been gained. If the condition is irritable, then the physiotherapist generally intends to modify the physical examination in some way, to prevent exacerbating the symptoms needlessly. Usually the number of tests performed under these circumstances is limited, so the most useful tests must be identified, i.e. those tests that give important information about the pathological or clinical diagnosis and about treatment, as well as investigating contraindications or precautions to treatment. In patients with irritable conditions it is still usually possible to perform most tests, including observation, all active movements (to initial onset or increase of pain), neurological tests (sensation and reflexes, and generally muscle power), tension tests, gentle palpation, and passive motion tests (again, performed gently, to first onset or increase in pain). Specific structures, such as muscles, are tested when the information is crucial to management decisions. If, however, management would not change with the results of a relevant test procedure, the physiotherapist may decide to perform these tests on subsequent treatment occasions when pain has settled.

Measurement

By performing various tests in the physical examination, physiotherapists are actually conducting a series of measurements on the patient. All test procedures included in the physical examination should therefore be performed not only appropriately for the individual patient, but also in a reproducible (standardized) manner. Since the results of our physical tests provide the basis for many diagnostic and management decisions, we must be confident that the results clearly reflect the patient's presenting status.

The variables that are measured depend on the test performed, but may include function, range of movement, pain response, muscle strength, sensory loss, degree of lordosis, kyphosis, etc. Some factors may be difficult to measure such as abnormalities found on observation or small changes perceived on passive motion testing, while other factors, such as general range of movement, may be easier to measure accurately. Rarely do we formally measure the outcome of all tests performed. In general the variables that should be accurately measured during the physical examination are:

1. Those related to the patient's main concern. For example, if a patient is attending physiotherapy because cervical spine pain and stiffness have reduced their ability to rotate when reversing the car, cervical rotation should be measured.
2. The variables that you expect to change with intervention. It would not appear logical to measure pain on performance of a certain movement before and after application of laser, when such an intervention has been repeatedly shown to have little effect on musculoskeletal pain (Gam *et al.*, 1993).

Thus appropriate variables should be measured, and they should be measured in a reliable and, where possible, valid way. This ensures that the measurement obtained is useful, with minimal measurement error (see Chapter 4). Measurement of specific test results is addressed further by the various authors who have contributed sections to this chapter.

The remainder of this chapter outlines test procedures used most frequently in the physical examination, describing the background to the tests, many of the test procedures themselves, the indications for testing, the interpretation of test results and the implications for treatment. Further reading for each section is located at the end of the chapter.

Observation

M. Goodsell and K.M. Refshauge

Using the protocol of look, feel and move, the first procedure in the physical examination is to look at, or observe, the patient. Physiotherapists 'informally' and 'formally' observe patients and the affected parts of the body before touching or moving them. The main purpose of observing the patient is to gain general information about functional deficits and about other abnormalities, particularly any abnormalities of alignment, either general or specifically of the spine, which might be manifestations of the presenting musculoskeletal disorder. It is often suggested that abnormalities of spinal curvature, such as the size of each regional curve, may contribute to the patient's presenting problem. The validity of associating these features of spinal alignment with the presence of symptoms is unclear. The relationship of the size of spinal curves to the onset or presence of pain has not been clearly demonstrated (Dieck *et al.*, 1985) except in the cervical spine where a more forward head position has been associated with the presence of headache (Griegel-Morris *et al.*, 1992; Watson and Trott, 1993).

Observation of posture in the clinic raises other questions, such as whether patients adopt their habitual sitting or standing posture while being formally observed by the physiotherapist, and also whether habitual standing or sitting posture reflects positions actually adopted during work or leisure activities. Therefore it is important to correlate the information gained from formal observation with the information gained informally when the patient was first greeted, was questioned during the history, during any functional testing and while undressing for the physical examination.

Whilst physiotherapists systematically observe patients as part of the physical examination, they have already informally noted the patient's demeanour, the ease of movement and the part of the body apparently affected when the patient enters the examination cubicle. When taking the history, they also note any positions of discomfort, for example, whether patients prefer to sit or stand, whether they hold their arm against their body, or whether they keep one leg extended while sitting. The physiotherapist then notices how the patient undresses in preparation for the examination. The difficulty experienced during undressing gives some information about the functional deficit as well as the movements that may provoke symptoms. It is imperative that it is explained to the patient that the reason for undressing is to expose the region for examination, as many people feel uncomfortable when scantily clad, particularly in the presence of a stranger, and with the possibility of other people entering the examination cubicle. The physical examination then commences with a formal observation of the patient and the affected part.

Test procedure

When the patient is undressed, formal observation are made. This consists of gaining a general impression of the overall posture of the patient before checking for any specific asymmetries or abnormalities. After this general check, it is usual to inspect the affected part more closely.

General postural overview

The patient is observed while standing (lumbar and thoracic spines) or sitting (cervical spine), undressed to expose the region to be examined. This means wearing underwear and no footwear for the lumbar and thoracic spines, but the lower body can remain clothed for cervical and upper thoracic spine observation.

For all regions of the spine, the physiotherapist notes:

1. muscle wasting (e.g. gastrocnemius, supraspinatus),
2. swelling,
3. scars,
4. skin changes,
5. bony alignment (e.g. spondylolisthesis may be evident by an anterior displacement at the level of the affected vertebra),
6. positional deformities (e.g. winged scapula).

For specific regions of the spine the physiotherapist also notes:

1. leg length discrepancies,
2. size of spinal curvature (thoracic kyphosis and lumbar lordosis),
3. scoliosis (rotational deformity),
4. sciatic scoliosis/list (antalgic position of lateral flexion without compensatory rotation).

For the cervical and upper thoracic spine, with the patient seated, the physiotherapist notes:

1. size of cervical lordosis,
2. size of cervicothoracic junction curvature,
3. lateral flexion or rotation deformities (e.g. wry neck),
4. shoulder height discrepancies.

Procedure

To gain this information efficiently, the physiotherapist usually observes posterior, anterior and lateral aspects.

From the posterior aspect, assessment consists of observing:

1. spinal alignment,
2. shoulder height,
3. scapular position,
4. level of posterior superior iliac spines (indicating level of pelvis),
5. height of iliac crests (level and rotation, indicating position of pelvis),
6. equality of gluteal folds,
7. height of knee creases,
8. calcaneal angle (equal, and not grossly pronated or supinated),
9. muscle bulk (e.g. gluteus maximus, gastrocnemius).

From the lateral aspect assessment consists of observing:

1. head position (poke neck/forward head position),
2. thoracic kyphosis (size and length – long thoracic curvature may indicate Scheuermann's disease),
3. rotation of rib cage (associated with scoliosis),
4. lumbar lordosis,
5. genu recurvatum.

From the anterior aspect assessment consists of observing:

1. head position (wry neck, asymmetry in rotation or lateral flexion),
2. shoulder height,
3. waist curves (increased asymmetry in structural and postural scoliosis),
4. height of anterior superior iliac spines (indicating level of pelvis),
5. patellar height and position,
6. forefoot position.

Relevant abnormalities or asymmetries should be measured if the physiotherapist intends to alter them. Some features are difficult to measure, e.g. skin changes or muscle wasting. Other features are easier to measure, such as leg length, which can be measured using a tape measure from the anterior superior iliac spine to the medial malleolus [see Grieve (1986) or Magee (1987) for further information]. Magnitude of spinal curves is also easily measured using a flexible ruler or photography, both of which have a demonstrated high reliability (Hart and Rose, 1986; Refshauge, *et al.*, 1994a). Other features are possible, although difficult, to measure, such as patellar position or calcaneal tilt, and results must therefore be interpreted cautiously.

Interpretation of information

Information about abnormalities and asymmetries derived from informal and formal observation of patients assists in making decisions about pathology, factors contributing to the presenting problem, which examination procedures to perform, and treatment selection. Some examples where observed abnormalities might indicate pathology in the affected area or suggest further examination procedures include:

1. Scars indicating either past trauma or surgery, both of which must be investigated for relevant past history (such as laminectomy, fusion) and for mobility of scar tissue during palpation.
2. Skin colour indicating state of the circulation (whether blood supply is adequate, such as in heart conditions or in thoracic outlet syndrome). A blueish tinge suggests anoxia, and redness indicates inflammation from any cause, although inflammation in deep tissues will not be obvious on visual inspection. Skin colour may also indicate the state of the patient's general health, sympathetic changes, bruising and presence of other diseases.
3. Substantial muscle wasting may indicate decreased conduction in a nerve at any point along its course before entry to the muscle. With musculoskeletal conditions arising in the spine, the nerve compromise may be at the level of the nerve root or spinal nerve (see under Neurological Examination in this chapter).
4. Winging of the scapula generally indicates reduced conduction in the long thoracic nerve. Serratus anterior, the affected muscle, is deep and therefore wasting will probably not be evident.
5. A 'step' in the low lumbar spine may indicate spondylolisthesis, where the affected vertebra has slipped forward, taking with it the attached superior vertebrae, giving the appearance of a step.

Asymmetries of posture may be directly related to the onset of symptoms. Such asymmetrical postures may be adopted as positions of pain relief, as in the case of an acute wry neck deformity in the cervical region, or a reduced lumbar lordosis or sciatic scoliosis in the lumbar region. In some cases such positions may suggest particular pathology, for example, sciatic scoliosis is thought to be associated with intervertebral disc pathology (McKenzie, 1981), although this clinical association has not been substantiated and intervertebral disc pathology is probably uncommon (Twomey, 1992). It seems that other postural features, for example size of spinal curvature, are observed because it is known that maintaining awkward or end of range positions for long periods causes pain (Harms-Ringdahl and Ekholm, 1986; Braun and Amundson, 1989). Extremes of spinal curvature are sometimes likened to end of range positions. Since tissues adapt to applied stress, it is speculated that adaptations such as muscle shortening occur in response to stresses applied in postures maintained for prolonged periods, such as an increased lumbar lordosis. It is possible that altered range of movement coinciding with postural abnormalities may alter function or movement patterns, resulting in increased strain in the tissues. The tissues may be unable to sustain the magnitude or type of this resultant stress. These hypotheses are tentative, however, because there is currently little evidence to support them.

Postural asymmetries are not clearly indicative of disorders. Evidence for a relationship between postural characteristics and presence of pain is equivocal, indicating that physiotherapists should be cautious in assuming a relationship. The size of lumbar lordosis has not been shown to be predictive of onset of pain or related to presence of pain (Dieck, *et al.*, 1985), even in pregnancy (Bullock *et al.*, 1987). The thoracic spine has not been investigated except in pregnancy. The cervical spine has been the subject of few studies, but preliminary work suggests that cervical spine posture may not be related to pain in the cervical spine or trapezius region (Refshauge *et al.*, 1995). On the other hand, people with frequent headaches have been shown to have a more forward head position than people with infrequent or no incidence of headache (Watson and Trott, 1993). There is also a wide range of normal postural variation, and asymmetries are common (During *et al.*, 1985; Raine and Twomey, 1994). Therefore the physiotherapist must decide whether observed asymmetries or other abnormalities are related to the patient's presenting symptoms. This cannot always be clearly established, but as a general rule, if the symptoms improve when the patient's posture is altered, then the asymmetry or alignment can be considered to be one of the factors related to the patient's symptoms. For example, using a lumbar roll to alter sitting posture by increasing the lumbar lordosis in sitting has been shown to reduce some patients' symptoms (Williams *et al.*, 1991). In this case some characteristic of the lordosis in sitting can be assumed to be associated with back and leg symptoms. However, it is not possible to demonstrate such an association when the patient has no symptoms at rest or when the symptoms are not easily provoked. In these circumstances the physiotherapist might choose to intervene to change posture and to evaluate the effect of intervention on symptoms over a period of time.

Other features of alignment of body segments such as that caused by inequality of leg length or magnitude of foot pronation have been raised as possible contributors to spinal pain. The association between mild leg length equality and pain is unclear, although it seems that a small discrepancy (up to 20 mm) is not associated with spinal pain (Pope *et al.*, 1985; Soukka *et al.*, 1991). This does not mean that unequal leg length is never related to spinal pain, but a relationship should be established in individual patients before intervening. This can be done, for example, by inserting a temporary orthotic into the patient's shoe, and noting any change in symptoms during functional activities, e.g. walking, or movement testing. If the pain decreases after equalizing leg length, it can be assumed that the symptoms were related to the inequality. The relevance of foot pronation to spinal or leg pain is also unclear. Although often described (McConnell, 1986), such a relationship has never been demonstrated when the magnitude of pronation is compared between symptomatic and asymptomatic states (see data in Gerrard, 1989).

Information about posture is still evolving. At present perceived postural abnormalities are difficult to interpret since normative data are not extensive: some postural characteristics may change with age (Milne and Lauder, 1974), although others may not alter with increasing age (Griegel-Morris *et al.*, 1992); there is a wide variation in normal (i.e. asymptomatic postures); slight asymmetries are common (e.g. few people appear to have equal shoulder height; Raine and Twomey, 1994); and as yet, 'ideal' posture has not been determined, nor conclusively established as desirable. In addition, surface contours do not appear to mirror bony vertebral alignment (Refshauge, *et al.*, 1994b) and therefore conclusions about magnitude of spinal curvature cannot easily be drawn from observation of surface contours. Thus the presence of any postural abnormalities must be interpreted with caution, and cannot be viewed in isolation. Rather, the information should be compared with the total clinical picture of signs and symptoms.

Implications for the physical examination and treatment

Few postural asymmetries or abnormalities are definitively associated with spinal pain. Nevertheless they may form part of a recognizable pattern of signs and symptoms, indicating specific pathology. Specific abnormalities, such as scars, signs of decreased nerve conduction (muscle wasting) or skin changes are usually further tested in the physical examination. Signs of reduced nerve conduction indicate that a neurological examination is required, scars should be palpated, and signs of circulatory disturbance (skin changes) tested by feeling strength of pulses and, when indicated, performing tests for thoracic outlet syndrome (see Magee, 1992).

Observed asymmetries or abnormalities in postural alignment might be further explored to determine whether they are associated with symptoms. This association may be investigated by facilitating a more 'ideal' alignment (e.g. correcting a sciatic scoliosis, facilitating chin retraction or altering pelvic tilt) and noting the effect on symptoms. For example, if chin retraction increases symptoms in a patient who has marked chin protraction, this suggests that the posture is antalgic, whereas if chin retraction decreases symptoms, this suggests that intervention to alter the position of chin protraction may be of benefit. A relationship between the patient's symptoms and any abnormal features should thus be established before intervening to change these features. When the physiotherapist chooses to intervene to change posture it is important to measure changes in the variable of interest, for example either pain or postural alignment. There has been surprisingly little investigation of the effect of intervention designed to alter posture either in terms of symptom relief or in changing the relevant postural characteristics. The few studies available suggest that the use of a lumbar support changed the intensity and area of back and leg pain (Williams *et al.*, 1991), but that exercises may not alter forward position of the head on the neck (Feldman *et al.*, 1994) in a healthy population.

Observation is useful for gaining an overall impression of the patient's alignment and general posture, as well as gaining some specific information about abnormalities that may be related to the presenting disorder. This information should be evaluated carefully, interpreted with caution and followed up with other tests during the physical examination.

Testing of active movements

K.M. Refshauge

After observation, the patient is asked to actively move the affected part(s) of the body. From active movement testing general information is gained about the clinical diagnosis and treatment. The clinical diagnosis is formulated in terms of movement dysfunction; the movements most affected, in what way these movements are altered, the effect of pain on movement and the range of movement available. From this information baseline measures are made for reassessment so that it can be clearly established whether the patient has improved following treatment. It is sometimes suggested, also, that an idea may be gained of the anatomical structures involved in the disorder because those structures stressed during a particular movement may be responsible for the symptoms reproduced during that movement. This seems possible in principle, but is probably more useful in the periphery than in the spine. The fact that the tissues involved in non-specific mechanical spinal pain have not been identified cautions against placing too much weight on such hypotheses, whereas, in the periphery, specific tissues may be readily identified as injured. For example a torn anterior talofibular ligament will usually cause pain when stressed in plantarflexion and inversion. The results of active movement testing also aid in treatment selection. For example, the most affected movement(s) may be used to increase the treatment dose for non-irritable conditions and the direction of movement that eases symptoms may be used for irritable conditions.

Procedure for testing active movements

This section is directed towards active movement testing in the spine, but the principles apply equally well to the periphery. Active movements are generally tested directly after the formal observation of the patient. All physiological active movements are usually examined systematically (flexion, extension, lateral flexion and rotation). The testing procedure should be standardized to enable accurate reassessment after treatment and before the next treatment session.

The movement causing the greatest functional disturbance is assessed whenever possible, because this is usually the movement that the patient most wants restored. This movement is often, but not always, the most symptomatic movement and may involve combinations of single plane movements. The most affected movement direction(s) will have been established in the history when discussing activities that provoke symptoms.

Although a sequence of active movement testing is normally implemented, the normal sequence may be altered when there is doubt about completion of testing in the case of an irritable condition. A patient may complain of difficulty in removing shoes and socks because of severe lumbar pain, for example. This may indicate that flexion is the main problem and therefore flexion may be among the first movements examined. More commonly, however, the patient's symptoms are closely monitored to identify immediately any exacerbation in symptoms, without necessarily requiring a change in the normal sequence of testing.

Clear and appropriate explanations to the patient are essential in achieving adequate testing of active movements. First, the patient is questioned about pain at rest. If pain is present before testing proceeds, it should be carefully monitored throughout the examination. Further instructions should reflect the irritability of the condition. If the condition is not easily exacerbated (is not irritable), the patient is asked to move as far as possible through a range of movement. The physiotherapist then identifies the limit of movement in terms of both what limits the movement (e.g. pain, stiffness), and the range of movement available. If the symptoms seem to be easily provoked, the patient is instructed only to move until the initial onset of pain, or in patients with resting pain, until the first increase in the resting pain.

Overall range of movement, or range to the first onset of pain in the case of irritable conditions, is measured. The intensity of pain provoked when performing the most symptomatic movement(s) is scaled, as this may be the variable that the physiotherapist aims to change. The shape of the spinal curves during movement is also observed as this may give information about areas of the spine where movement is either decreased or increased, although the reliability and validity of such observations is unknown. This information is further investigated during the physical examination using, for example, passive motion testing. Symmetry of movement is also noted in unilateral movements where comparisons with the contralateral side are possible. The quality of the movement may give information about ease of movement and antalgic deviations.

Active movement testing of the cervical and upper thoracic spine

Active movements are examined with the patient seated on a stool or on the end of a treatment plinth. Chairs with backs are generally avoided since the back support may encourage slumping. The lumbar lordosis should be maintained during active movement testing as the position of the lumbar and thoracic spines may affect the range of cervical movement observed.

Thus the starting (or neutral) position should be standardized with the patient looking ahead, and sitting comfortably upright. Unilateral movements, e.g. side flexion and rotation, are compared with movement to the contralateral side.

Active movement testing of the mid and low thoracic spine

Active movements of the thoracic spine can be assessed either in sitting or in standing positions. In the sitting position, however, movement in the thoracic spine rather than the lumbar spine seems to be better emphasized. In the seated position, the habitual lumbar lordosis should be maintained to prevent a starting position of thoracic and lumbar spine flexion. Patients cross their arms across the chest with hands on opposite shoulders, to standardize the starting position and to enable movement of the spine as a unit, thereby avoiding confounding movement of the shoulders and scapulae. Flexion, extension, lateral flexion and rotation can all be examined using this standardized starting position.

Active movement testing of the lumbar spine

Active movements of the lumbar spine are examined with the patient standing, with the possible exception of rotation. The region to be examined should be clearly exposed, to enable viewing movement of the intervertebral segments. The patient should not be wearing shoes because high heels or uneven wear of the heels or soles may alter the starting position of the spine and may not be comparable on repeat visits. For flexion, extension and lateral flexion patients slide their hands down their legs. Rotation is often examined with the patient seated to enhance stability, and, as for the thoracic spine, it is convenient for patients to cross their arms across the chest. The starting position should again be standardized, and unilateral movements compared with movement to the contralateral side.

As well as observing active movements, the physiotherapist may observe activities described by the patient in the history as provoking symptoms. Examples of activities that commonly aggravate symptoms and that can easily be assessed and measured in the clinical context include walking, stairclimbing, rising from sitting or putting on shoes. Variables of all these activities can be adequately measured (see under Motor performance: evaluation and intervention later in this chapter).

Measurement

The most affected movement(s) should be measured carefully. There are many methods that are simple to use, are widely available and provide reliable measurements. These include; tape measure for flexion, extension and lateral flexion of all spinal regions (Hsieh and Yeung, 1986; Beattie *et al.*, 1987), and for cervical spine rotation, the spondylometer for flexion and extension in the lumbar spine (Twomey and Taylor, 1979) and the cervical range of motion (CROM) measuring device for cervical spine movements (Youdas *et al.*, 1991; Garrett *et al.*, 1993). Rotation is difficult to measure in the lumbar spine, but infrequently appears to be the most affected movement. These measurement methods have a demonstrated high reliability, although only the spondylometer and the attraction–distraction use of the tape measure in the lumbar spine are likely to produce valid measurements of spinal motion. However, increase in overall range of movement (e.g. reaching the feet to put on trousers) is a more likely aim of treatment than increase in lumbar spine motion in isolation. Therefore, measuring overall movement such as finger tips to floor for lumbar spine flexion probably adequately reflects the aim of treatment. These measurement methods are illustrated in Figs. 6.1 and 6.2. The Lidcombe Template (Fig. 6.3) demonstrates a method of standardising the force applied to achieve the measured range of movement, particularly important in the periphery.

Applying further stress to active movements

If symptoms have not been provoked by active movement testing or have not been provoked to the desired extent (in the case of non-irritable conditions only), further stress may be applied to the movements. The reason for requiring symptom reproduction during active movement testing is that it is difficult to treat appropriately in the absence of an active reassessment baseline, because the physiotherapist cannot monitor the effect of treatment and dosage. The effect of an intervention is usually assessed during its application to identify changes in the condition as they occur, so that, for example, if the condition worsens, the dose can be altered immediately. The response to active movement testing is also used for treatment planning. Therefore, several methods of further stressing active movements have been suggested.

The most common procedure is to apply gentle pressure (*overpressure*) at the end of range. This is usually the first approach. The aim of applying overpressure is to observe the effect on symptoms of further stressing the movement. If no symptoms are reproduced on overpressure, it is generally considered that the movement is symptom-free and 'normal' (Maitland, 1986).

Combined movements are also commonly used to further stress active movements that are slightly

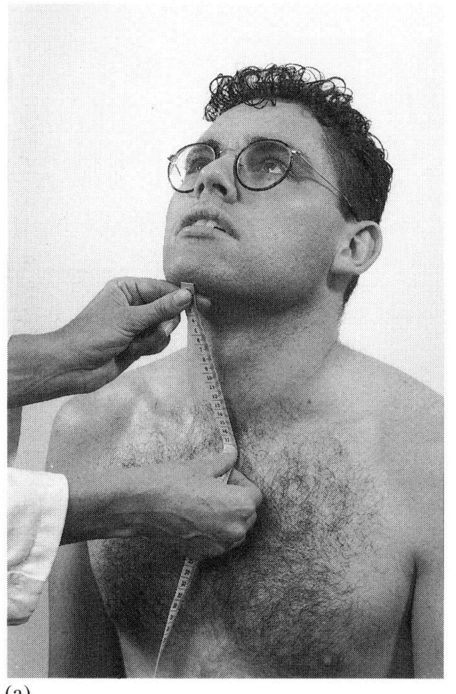
(a)

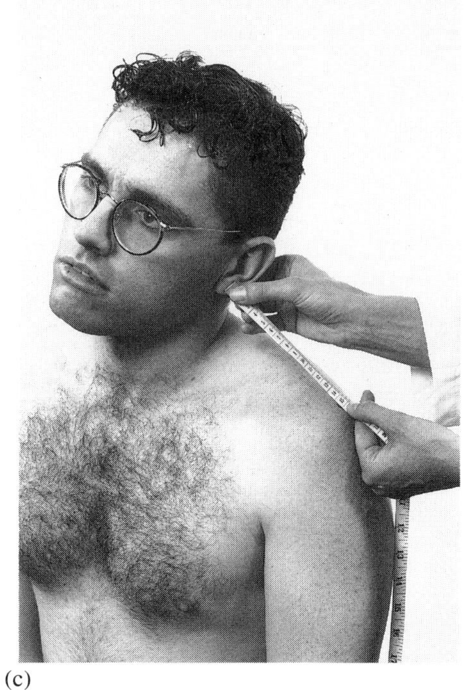
(c)

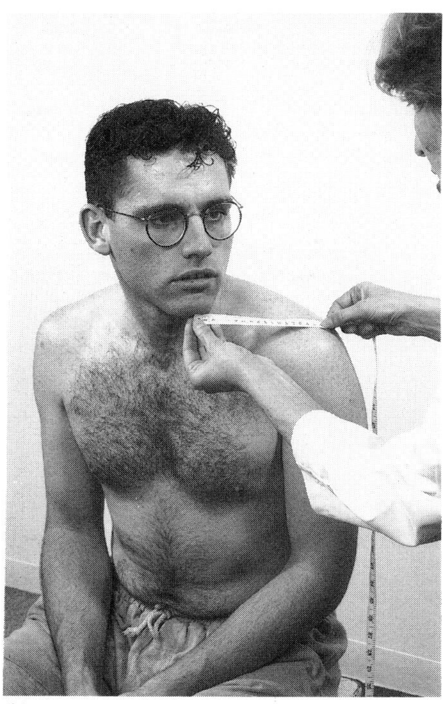
(b)

Figure 6.1 Measurement of active movements of the cervical spine using tape measure

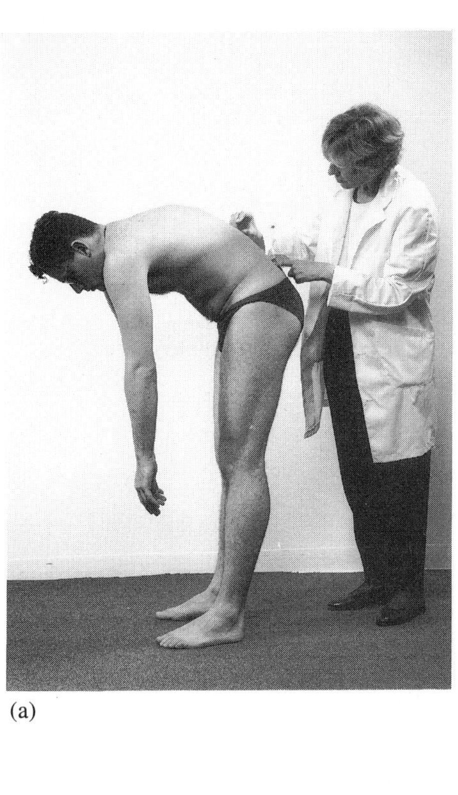

(a)

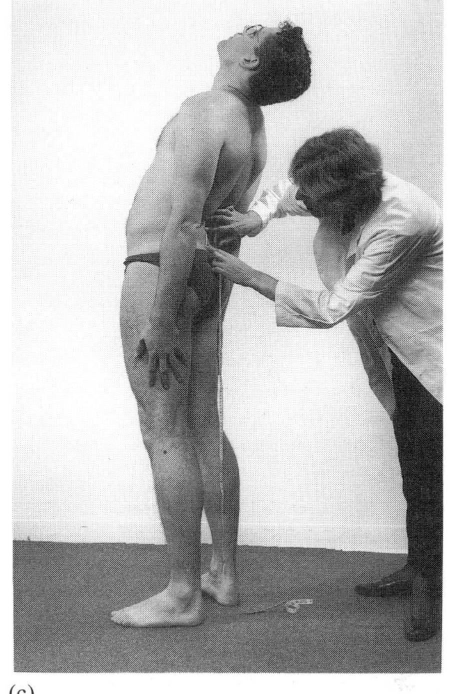

(c)

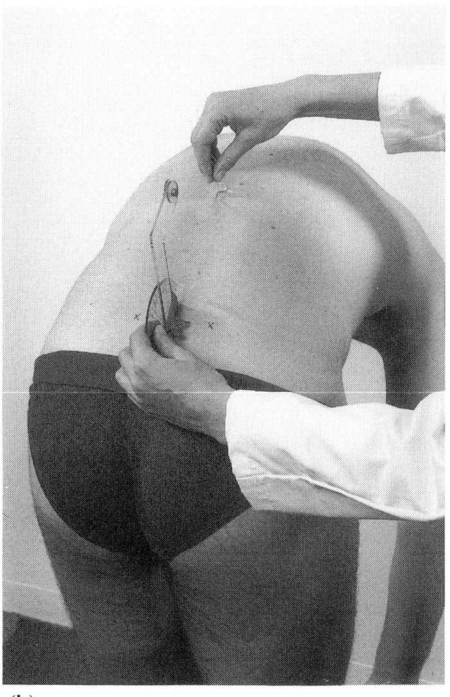

(b)

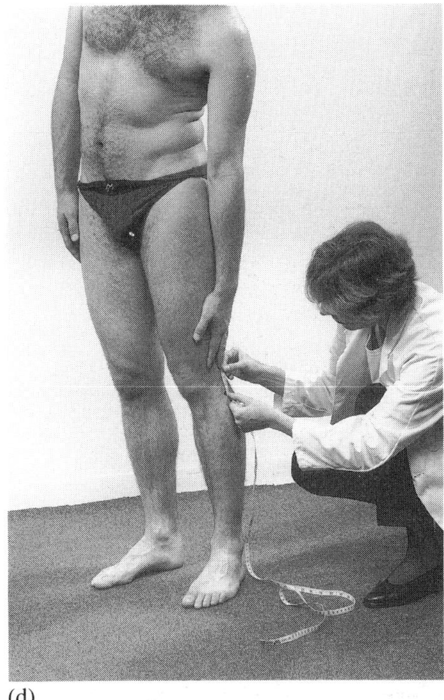

(d)

Figure 6.2 Measurement of active movements of the lumbar spine: using spondylometer in (a) and (b) to measure flexion; and using tape measure for extension (c) and lateral flexion (d)

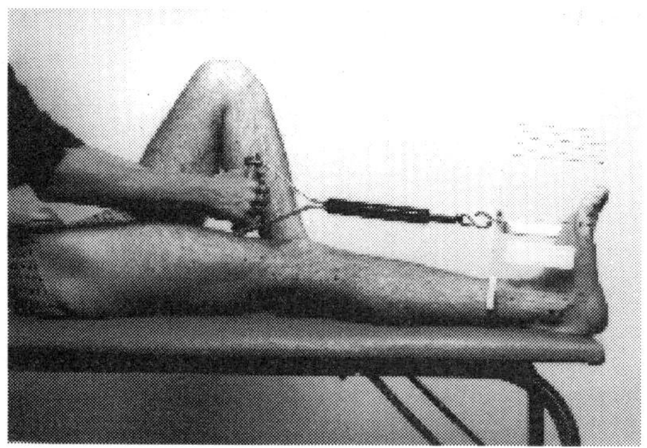

Figure 6.3 Measuring range of ankle dorsiflexion using Lidcombe Template, enabling standardization of force and starting position

symptomatic or have been reported as symptomatic in the history (Edwards, 1987). Although the concept of combining physiological movements in examination and treatment arose from knowledge of coupled movements (Edwards, 1987), combined movements do not simulate coupled movements (see Chapter 2 for further discussion).

When combining active movements, the most affected movement is usually performed first, and then the next most symptomatic movement is superimposed. If, for example, the patient complained of cervical spine pain when throwing the ball in the air in preparation for a tennis serve, and only slight pain was reproduced on cervical spine extension during active movement testing, the physiotherapist, might decide to stress extension further by superimposing movements in other planes (rotation or lateral flexion). It would be usual to ask the patient to extend the cervical spine, and then, while maintaining extension, to rotate the cervical spine. If this were pain-free, lateral flexion instead of rotation might be added to the extension. Combined movements are discussed fully in other musculoskeletal textbooks (Grieve, 1984; Maitland, 1986; Edwards, 1987, 1988).

Further stress may also be applied by *repeating movements*, that is several movements in the same direction are performed in quick succession. This is particularly relevant when repetitive activity has been reported as symptomatic, or when the physiotherapist anticipates that repeated active movements may be used as a treatment strategy. It has been suggested that repeated movements may decrease pain in some spinal conditions. The most common example of this is repeated extension in some instances of lumbar spine pain. McKenzie (1981) describes this approach in detail.

Movements or positions may be *sustained* if they are reported as provocative during the history. For example, lumbar spine flexion may be sustained if sitting is nominated as a problem, or cervical spine flexion sustained if reading, writing or watching television are provocative activities. It is more efficient (less time-consuming) to reassess dynamic activities, so movements are generally sustained only in the absence of provocative dynamic activities.

Implications for treatment

Information from active movement testing is used in several ways, but mainly for treatment decisions and as baseline measurements for reassessment. The ease of symptom provocation is elicited from the history. This information is then compared with the patient's actual ability to move during movement testing. Usually severe pain results in marked movement restriction, whereas mild pain results in minor movement restriction. Therefore, if a patient has very severe pain, but active movements are largely unaffected, this would arouse suspicion about the nature of the disorder. The results of active movement testing (which movement is affected, how it is affected, and the extent to which it is affected) assists in determining the vigour, or dose, of treatment.

Positions or movements to avoid or positions of comfort may also be identified for patients with irritable conditions. If a condition is irritable, the first goal of treatment is generally pain relief. It is therefore important to identify those movements that will exacerbate symptoms, and those movements or positions that may relieve symptoms. Movements or positions that relieve symptoms may be used as a treatment strategy, or may be used to position the patient during application of an alternative treatment strategy.

For non-irritable conditions, however, the most provocative direction of movement is often used for treatment or for positioning during treatment to increase the force or intensity of the treatment dose. Results of further testing, such as passive motion testing and tension tests, are also compared with the results of the active movement tests to monitor consistency of patterns of signs and symptoms.

Testing active movements in other joints that are potentially contributing to the symptoms

Patients presenting with pain of possible spinal origin often have pain radiating over several joints and other somatic structures. All potentially injured structures are tested during the physical examination. This includes structures located under the pain distribution or that could refer pain in the presenting distribution. It is mostly not possible or efficient to thoroughly examine all regions in a single visit, so screening tests are used to determine the potential contribution of anatomical structure(s) or regions to the patient's presenting problem. If a screening procedure is positive, then that structure(s) or region must be examined more specifically and thoroughly. If no symptoms are reproduced, then the structure or region is generally excluded from further consideration, depending on the sensitivity and specificity of the tests.

Joints potentially referring pain or lying beneath the pain pattern, are generally tested using active movements, with further stress applied as necessary (such as overpressure) to exclude the contribution of that joint to the pain pattern. Any joints can be implicated, as spinal pain can be referred to the most distal part of the extremity (Williams and Warwick, 1980). In all cases, the patient is asked to move the joint through its full active range, and if the movement is symptom-free, overpressure is applied.

It is important to test these joints in such a way that the spine or other potentially damaged structures are not also stressed, because these tests should differentiate one source of pain from another. When pain potentially originating in the lumbar spine crosses the sacroiliac (SIJ) and hip joints, and the history suggests that the hip and SIJ are possible sources of the symptoms, then the hip and SIJ must also be tested. If pain is reproduced during a test procedure, but the lumbar spine, the SIJ and the hip have been equally stressed, a judgement cannot be made about the most likely source of symptoms and where to direct further examination and treatment. It should be borne in mind also that since the physiotherapist believes that the joint being tested (in this case the hip or SIJ) could be contributing to the pain, it would be unwise to use the most stressful test as the initial test procedure. For these reasons, the hip is positioned in flexion (approximately 90° if this range is available with the knee flexed) and internal and external rotation are tested. This test is thought to stress the hip joint more than the lumbar spine or SIJ. Since there are no active movements specific to the SIJ, the SIJ is tested by palpation and passive motion testing. The initial screening procedure is to distract and compress the joint by pushing the iliac crests apart (compression of SIJ) and pushing them together (distraction of SIJ) in the frontal plane with the patient supine.

The shoulder is commonly suspected to be involved in cervical spine disorders. The shoulder is usually tested in flexion and abduction (different planes of movement) and more planes if required. Quadrant is not usually performed as the initial test procedure. If it is necessary to further examine the joint, then quadrant (described in Maitland, 1986) or any other procedures may be appropriate.

Usually, dorsiflexion and plantarflexion are tested in the ankle, and flexion and extension in the knee, elbow (in addition to supination/pronation if relevant) and the wrist (in addition to ulnar and radial deviation if relevant). These tests are preliminary examination tests to determine if the articular complex is contributing to symptoms. If these tests reproduce symptoms further examination should be directed at these structures.

Testing adequacy of cerebral blood flow (vertebral artery testing)

K. Refshauge

All patients who present with possible cervical spine disorders are routinely questioned in the history about whether they suffer from dizziness, because dizziness can be an early symptom of inadequate cerebral blood flow (see Chapter 5). Dizziness and vertigo have been described as different symptoms (Osol, 1972) indicative of different disorders. Dizziness is said to refer to the unpleasant sensation of giddiness or unsteadiness or of disturbed relationship to objects in space and is usually associated with a diminution in cerebral blood flow, while vertigo refers to the sensation that the outer world is revolving about the patient or that the patient is moving in space and is usually a symptom of vestibular disorders (Osol, 1972). However, it may be difficult to distinguish between the two, and the terms are often used synonymously.

Dizziness may be the first symptom of vertebrobasilar insufficiency (VBI) (Fisher *et al.*, 1965). It is also a symptom of other common clinical presentations such as disturbances of the vestibular/labyrinth system, postural hypotension, Meniere's disease and cervical vertigo. Of particular concern to physiotherapists is dizziness caused by VBI, because there is the potential for causing critical occlusion of cerebral blood flow when using some common therapeutic manoeuvres for the cervical spine. Such procedures include combining extension with rotation, and manipulation of the cervical spine, both of which can cause critical occlusion, with serious consequences, such as hemiplegia, 'locked-in' syndrome or, in extreme cases, death (Schellhas, *et al.*, 1980; Horn, 1983; Patjin, 1991). When examining the cervical spine, therefore, the presence of VBI must be identified as it will contraindicate certain examination and treatment procedures (e.g. cervical spine quadrant, manipulation), and will indicate caution when applying other procedures (e.g. end of range rotation manoeuvres, traction, forceful mobilizations). Differential diagnosis must be attempted through careful questioning and physical testing. Nevertheless, when dizziness is the only presenting symptom it may be impossible to make a definitive diagnosis (Lord, 1986; Grant, 1988).

Vertebrobasilar insufficiency

The vertebrobasilar system provides approximately 20% of intracranial blood supply, the carotid system providing the remainder (Lord, 1986; Zweibel, 1986). The cranial structures supplied by the vertebrobasilar system include the occipital cortex, the brain stem from the midbrain to the upper spinal cord, and the cerebellar hemispheres. This territory includes numerous motor and sensory tracts, the reticular formation, cranial nerves III–XII and their nuclei, including vestibular nuclei (Fisher *et al.*, 1965; Bogduk,

1986; Lord, 1986; Rowland, 1991). VBI occurs when either focal or overall blood volume is reduced to a level causing ischaemia (generally thought to require reduction by approximately 50%) (Stopford, 1916; Hardesty *et al.*, 1963; Lord, 1986). Symptoms are caused by ischaemia in the structures supplied by the vertebrobasilar system (Thiel, 1991). Thus, a great variety of symptoms are possible. Dizziness is the most common (in 45% of patients with transient ischaemic attacks of the vertebrobasilar system), and usually the first symptom (Fisher, *et al.*, 1965) and ataxia is the second most common symptom (Lord, 1986). Ataxia alone may be difficult to differentiate from that induced by vertigo or muscular weakness on the basis of the history. Other symptoms of VBI include diplopia (double vision), paralysis of gaze towards the side of the lesion, dysphagia, dysarthria, impaired trigeminal sensation (snout paraesthesia/anaesthesia) and drop attacks (in which the patient suddenly falls to the ground while remaining conscious). Drop attack is thought to be strongly indicative of VBI, but the ischaemic lesion responsible has not been clearly identified. However, evidence from autopsy examination suggests that drop attacks result from ischaemia of corticospinal tracts in the pons and medulla (Lord, 1986).

The vertebral arteries (VAs) are of concern to physiotherapists because their intimate relationship with the cervical spine (as they pass through the formina intertransversarii) makes them vulnerable to injury during certain therapeutic procedures such as sustained rotation or manipulation (see Fig. 6.4. Williams and Warwick, 1980; Lord, 1986). Blood flow through the VAs is normally reduced during cervical spine extension and/or rotation (Stevens, 1991; Refshauge, 1994). Symptoms probably occur when anomalies or pathology cause further compromise. Anomalies in the vertebrobasilar system are extremely common (Loeb and Meyer, 1965; Lord, 1986) and are normally overcome by adaptation of the vascular system, forming competent collateral circulation (Mishkin and Schreiber, 1974; Lord, 1986). It appears that symptoms arise when there is an acute change in the vertebrobasilar system, such as traumatic damage to the artery lumen, or compromised blood flow from sustained cervical spine rotation and/or extension (Okawarra and Nibbelink, 1974). The position of cervical spine rotation may result from either moving the head on a stable body or moving the body while the head remains stable, resulting in relative cervical rotation.

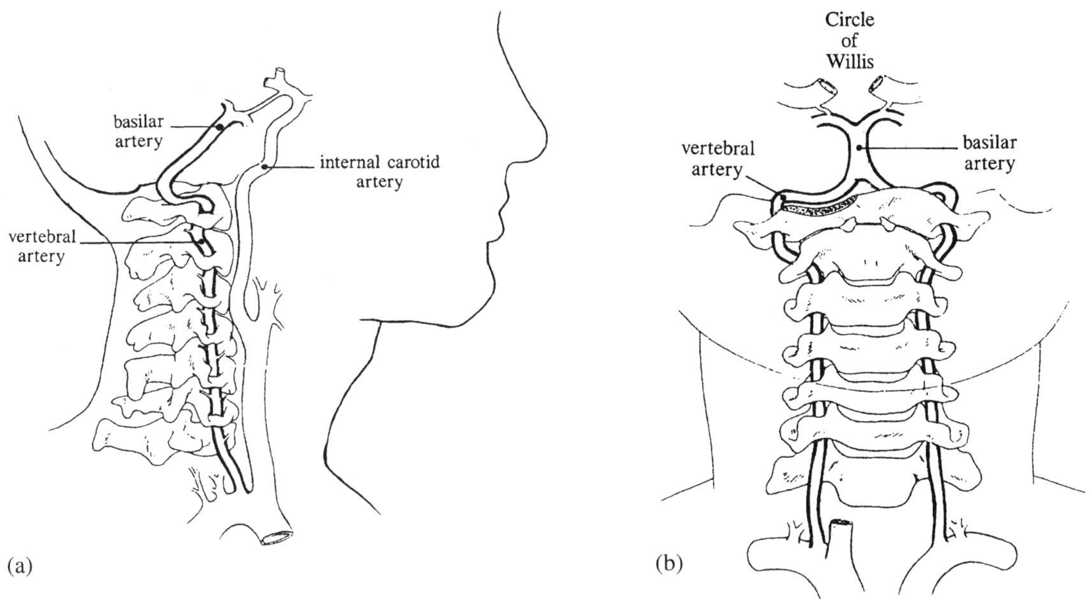

Figure 6.4 Intracranial arteries; lateral view (a) and anteroposterior view (b). The four parts of the vertebral arteries are shown, including the entry of the arteries into the cervical spine at approximately C6, the course through the transverse foramina of the cervical vertebrae, the 180° turn across C1 and the intracranial union with the basilar artery before joining the circle of Willis

The risk of injury to the VA during vigorous cervical spine procedures is thought to increase if there is an intrinsic disorder of the artery (such as atheroma and thrombosis) or in the presence of pathology that may impinge on the artery. Various extrinsic pathologies or anomalies have been shown to affect the VAs by impinging on the external wall and thereby narrowing the lumen. These extrinsic disorders and anomalies include:

1. osteophytes, especially of the uncovertebral joints and zygapophyseal joints, forcing the VA to deviate around them;
2. common anomalies in the vertebrobasilar system include the VA originating from the posterior aspect of the subclavian artery (a common phenomenon; Lord, 1986), the VA passing through the longus colli or the anterior scalene muscles, and the presence of a bony ring (normally present in 30% of cadavers) instead of the occipito atlantal membrane normally encircling the vertebral artery as it crosses the superior aspect of C1 – All of these anomalies may result in occlusion on contralateral rotation of the cervical spine.

3. The artery may pass beneath bands of cervical fascia, causing constriction on rotation (Bogduk, 1986; Lord, 1986).

There is no evidence that such disorders actually increase the risk of either critical reduction in cerebral blood flow or traumatic injury to the VA during vigorous procedures.

There is some evidence that other factors increase the potential hazard from manipulation, including asymmetry of the VAs (Lyness and Wagman, 1974), previous VA injury (Frumkin and Baloh, 1990), previous ischaemic symptoms (Kanshepolski *et al.*, 1972), excessive mobility in the cervical spine (Bogduk, 1986) and general vascular disease (Hart and Easton, 1986).

Differential diagnosis of VBI

Many conditions cause symptoms of dizziness. Those conditions most likely to present to physiotherapists, or to coexist with musculoskeletal disorders of the spine, are postural (orthostatic) hypotension, Meniere's disease, vestibular dysfunction and cervical vertigo. Some of these are also the most difficult to differentiate from VBI. In fact, if dizziness is the only presenting symptom, it may not be possible to differentiate Meniere's disease, vestibular disease or cervical vertigo from VBI. Features of these conditions that may assist in differential diagnosis include the following.

1. Orthostatic hypotension: symptoms of feeling faint or light-headed are caused by a sudden decrease in cerebral blood flow from altered blood pressure when changing posture. Therefore dizziness is experienced on moving from a low to high position, such as getting out of bed but is not caused by cervical spine movements (Burton, 1965; Rowell, 1986). Postural hypotension can usually be clearly differentiated from VBI.
2. Meniere's disease: this disease affects the endolymph in the labyrinth. Symptoms include fluctuating hearing loss associated with tinnitus, a feeling of pressure in the ears, episodic vertigo or dizziness, and nausea and vomiting. Although not usually difficult to distinguish from VBI, definitive diagnosis is made by audiometry (Coman, 1986).
3. Vestibular/labyrinth dysfunction: symptoms are caused by dysfunction in the labyrinth, such as in the semicircular canals. When fluid in the affected canal is disturbed, such as on movement of the head, hairs specific to that canal are moved (Kelly, 1991) and a rotating or turning sensation is experienced, commonly termed vertigo. The particular movements affected will depend on the canal affected, but may include flexion or lateral flexion (unlike dizziness caused by VBI, which may be worsened with extension and rotation) (Coman, 1986). The vestibular system can also be disordered as the result of ischaemia affecting the vestibular nuclei or altered afferent input from cervical spine structures (de Jong *et al.*, 1977). Since the vertebrobasilar system supplies both the brainstem and the vestibular nuclei, it is sometimes difficult to distinguish between vestibular or labyrinth disorders and VBI (brainstem) disorders (Coman, 1986). Pathological nystagmus is a cardinal feature of labyrinth disease, but may also be caused by VBI (causing ischaemia in the vestibular system) (Lord, 1986; Goldberg *et al.*, 1991).
4. Cervical vertigo: symptoms include ataxia and dizziness, and arise from abnormal afferent impulses from deep cervical spine structures, particularly muscles, zygapophyseal joints and the posterior longitudinal ligament (de Jong *et al.*, 1977; Abrahams, 1981). In laboratory-induced cervical vertigo, symptoms are thought to be mediated through the vestibular nuclei, occurring on movement of the head. It may therefore be difficult to distinguish cervical vertigo from lesions of the vestibular system or from VBI (de Jong *et al.*, 1977). Differential diagnosis is generally made retrospectively, after symptoms have responded to cervical spine treatment.

Differentiation of the cause of dizziness is generally based on the behaviour of dizziness, and therefore may often be established in the history. Frequency and duration of dizzy episodes may assist in determining the cause of symptoms: in cervical vertigo, the episode usually lasts for seconds only; in Meniere's disease, episodes last for hours; in acute vestibular failure episodes may last for weeks (Coman, 1986). In VBI, duration of episodes probably depends on magnitude of provocation, and therefore may result in transient episodes lasting from seconds to weeks, or may result in permanent impairment. If patients complain of dizziness, they should be tested in the physical examination to confirm the suspected diagnosis. Testing must be performed with extreme caution to avoid exacerbating potentially dangerous pathology.

Indications for VA testing

In 1988 the Australian Physiotherapy Association approved the test protocol outlined below [Australian Physiotherapy Association (APA), 1988] to enhance one aspect of safety during manipulation. The standard tests are performed whenever a patient complains of dizziness, but particularly when:

1. Patients present with cervical symptoms (pain including headache and/or stiffness) and dizziness, where the behaviour and history of the dizziness and other symptoms appear to be related.
2. Dizziness or symptoms of VBI are provoked during cervical spine treatment.
3. Symptoms of VBI are experienced following treatment.
4. The physiotherapist proposes using a technique that could compromise the VA (e.g. manipula-

tion), even in individuals who have not experienced symptoms of VBI. VA testing is *routinely* performed before every cervical spine manipulation.

VA tests should be performed after examination of active movements, but probably before examination of positions combining extension and rotation. Performing active movements before VA tests provides information about available range of movement and pain reproduction, allowing appropriate performance of extension and rotation during VA testing. VA tests are also performed before sustained positions (where applicable) as positive test results will contraindicate the use of these procedures.

Test procedures

Standard tests

Tests are performed in sitting and/or supine lying positions (as appropriate for each patient). Both positions are not usually necessary. The tests include:

- sustained extension;
- sustained rotation to the left and right;
- sustained rotation with extension, to left and right.

Each test position is maintained at end of range for a minimum of 10 s unless symptoms are provoked, in which case the head is immediately returned to the neutral position.

During each test and after each test position has been released, the patient should be questioned about the onset of dizziness. Patients should also keep their eyes open during testing to allow identification of nystagmus as a sign of vestibular disorder (Coman, 1986). Latent responses can occur after release of test positions (Grant, 1987). The tests are taken from the A.P.A. protocol (1988).

Additional tests performed when patients present with dizziness not provoked by standard testing

- testing the position or movement described by the patient which provokes dizziness;
- quick movement of the head through the available range of movement when the patient

relates dizziness to quick movements of the head rather than head postures or positions;
- where dizziness is provoked upon rotation, either during sustained postures or repetitive motion, these tests are further explored to differentiate dizziness arising from the vestibular apparatus of the inner ear from that caused by neck movement. These tests are commonly referred to as the labyrinthine tests.

The labyrinthine tests generally consist of:

- head held still, sustained trunk rotation to left and right, and could also include,
- head held still, repetitive trunk rotation to left and right.
- (A.P.A. protocol, 1988).

Positions are sustained for a minimum of 10 s, but released if symptoms are provoked. Positive results in these tests suggest that dizziness is not caused by inner ear labyrinth disturbance.

VA testing in the presence of an irritable condition

It may be difficult to perform all or any of the test procedures in a patient with an irritable condition. Irritable conditions are characterized by the range of movement being markedly restricted by pain. This may therefore preclude sustaining any cervical spine positions, particularly at the end of range. Since vigorous end of range procedures (provocative for VBI) would not normally be used to treat irritable conditions, it is generally safe to treat such conditions using gentle manoeuvres in the absence of knowledge of VA test results. Testing must be performed, however, when range of movement has increased, and the physiotherapist intends to use more vigorous procedures. It would therefore also be considered unwise to manipulate an irritable condition, such as an acute wry neck, since full VA testing is impossible, and these tests are considered mandatory before manipulation.

Manipulation

Manipulation of the cervical spine has resulted in many severe accidents, reports appearing in the literature primarily recording incidence of Wallenberg's syndrome, 'locked in' syndrome and death (Terrett, 1987; Patjin, 1991). Since the consequences can be grave, all precautions must be taken to ensure the procedure is made as safe as possible. Generally, the reported deaths seem to have been due to multiple large-range generalized rotation manipulations of the cervical spine. In other words, responsible and careful use of manipulation and procedures to monitor cerebral blood flow may assist in avoiding the occurrence of such accidents.

VA testing is therefore *routinely* performed before every cervical spine manipulation, even in the *absence* of reports of dizziness. This does not ensure safety of the manipulation since the ability of the arteries to withstand externally applied forces has not been tested, but it does ensure adequate vertebrobasilar or collateral circulation in provocative positions, important in the event of occlusion of the VA occurring. When manipulation of the cervical spine is intended, therefore, patients are placed in the position of manipulation in addition to the standard test positions. Testing before every cervical spine manipulation therefore consists of positioning the patient in either sitting or supine lying, and investigating:

- sustained extension;
- sustained rotation to left and right;
- sustained rotation with extension, to left and right;
- simulated manipulation position. The patient's head and neck are held in the manipulation position as a sustained premanipulative procedure.

Each test position is sustained for 10 s, but immediately released if symptoms are reproduced. Latent responses may occur following release of a test position.

When using manipulative procedures, consideration should be given to issues of informed consent [see Introduction to this chapter, and the Australian Physiotherapy Association protocol (1988) for further explanation, and for suggested information given to patients]. Informed consent should be gained before any procedure, but the potential risks associated with cervical spine manipulation demand particular stringency in gaining and recording clear consent. Results of all tests undertaken should also be accurately recorded.

investigated, there is information to suggest that the VA test procedures will frequently identify position-induced VBI. Several cadaver studies demonstrated reduced fluid flow (sometimes becoming absent) through contralateral vertebral and internal carotid arteries in combined extension and rotation, (Tissington-Tatlow and Bammer, 1957; Toole and Tucker, 1960) and flow was further reduced by the addition of cervical spine traction (Tissington-Tatlow and Bammer, 1957). *In vivo* studies have demonstrated decreased blood flow in extension and rotation (Schmitt, 1991; Refshauge, 1994), altered flow occurring as early as 45° range of rotation (Stevens, 1991; Refshauge, 1994). Therefore, current information suggests that the tests may be valid in terms of compromising blood flow, but that the high number of false positive and false negative test results suggest low sensitivity and specificity of the test (Bolton *et al.*, 1989).

Sensitivity of the tests has also been investigated by Hutchinson (1989), who determined that:

1. The most sensitive tests were combined extension and rotation in the sitting position and rotation in the supine position. The use of the sustained manipulation position was relatively insensitive.
2. The patient's haemodynamic status changes with increasing range of motion, a negative test result sometimes becoming positive; therefore repeat testing is essential before each provocative treatment occasion.

Current understanding of the tests suggests that they are probably valid for detecting position-induced dizziness, the most sensitive tests being combined rotation and extension in sitting, and rotation in supine, but false positive and negative results can occur. Results must therefore be interpreted with caution, the severity of consequences dictating that it is prudent to err conservatively. On the basis of current knowledge, these tests appear to be the most reasonable available for testing adequate cerebral blood flow, but they give no information about the safety of the actual manipulation.

Interpretation of test results

If any of the test results are positive, it is initially assumed that VBI is the cause. Although reliability and validity of the tests have not been extensively

Implications for treatment

Positive results during or after any of the test or other examination procedures contraindicate examining the quadrant position (Maitland, 1986), any procedure that provokes dizziness, and treating with cervical manipulation. When patients complain of dizziness which is not reproduced during testing, it is generally considered wise to avoid potentially provocative treatments initially such as manipulation or any procedure that provokes dizziness, until symptoms respond and the nature of the dizziness is clarified. Precautions and constant questioning about dizziness and associated symptoms must accompany forceful application of mobilization, rotation and traction procedures. Traction combined with rotation is best avoided. Patients with suspected VBI who have not reported their symptoms to their medical practitioner should be referred for confirmation and further investigation if appropriate.

Tension tests

R. Boland

In the last few decades intervertebral disc pathology (disc protrusion in particular) was considered to be the main cause of low back pain, and the straight leg raise (SLR) tension test was strongly associated with identifying disc protrusions (Charnley, 1951). The SLR therefore became an important test procedure and was generally carried out routinely in patients with low back pain. This convention has persevered, despite the current view that disc pathology is not the only major cause of low back pain. Many tension tests have now been described, some of them being routinely performed in patients presenting with spinal pain. This suggests that interpretation of the results of tension tests has broadened considerably from the original purpose of detecting disc pathology.

Tension tests are widely used by physiotherapists and medical practitioners to examine the response of the nerve, its surrounding connective tissue and associated vessels to applied tension. The tension tests most frequently used are SLR, prone knee bend (PKB) and passive neck flexion (PNF). While not unknown in orthopaedic medicine, the upper limb tension test (ULTT; Elvey, 1983) and slump test (Maitland, 1978, 1985) are predominantly used by physiotherapists. The combination of joint movements applied during the slump and ULTT tests is thought to stress neuromeningeal structures to a greater extent than non-neural structures.

Nociceptive responses do not usually occur when normal spinal nerves and nerve roots are stretched or compressed (Howe, *et al.*, 1977). Ectopic and nociceptive impulses are only generated if the nerves have been structurally damaged causing an increase in sensitivity to stimulation. Much of the work investigating the response of damaged nerve to mechanical stimuli has used pressure as the deforming stimulus. Some authors have demonstrated that minor compression of damaged nerve roots and spinal nerves will generate painful or nociceptive discharge (Smyth and Wright, 1958; Howe, *et al.*, 1977). Brieg (1978) argues that within the spinal canal, tension is the pathologically significant force and describes the close relationship between pressure and tension, and the way in which application of a compressive force may increase axial tension over a small area. It should also be noted that after trauma to a nerve (such as a compression injury) neural tissues become stiffer during the repair phase (Beel, *et al.*, 1984). Thus, not only may pain be reproduced during tension testing, but increased stiffness of neural tissue may limit movement.

Information gained from tension tests differs from that gained from the neurological examination (see under Neurological Examination section in this chapter). In the neurological examination, the conduction properties of a nerve are tested, whereas tension tests examine the ability of neural connective tissue to move relative to the surrounding tissues and to resist tension. Although tension tests are widely used to determine the contribution of neuromeningeal structures to a patient's symptoms, physiotherapists also use them as treatment procedures and to monitor a patient's progress.

Indications for testing

On the basis of knowledge of the structures stressed by each test procedure and expected patterns of symptom reproduction, it would appear logical that:

1. In the lumbar spine:
   (a) PNF and SLR be performed routinely in patients with low back pain (Maitland, 1986; Butler, 1991);
   (b) PKB be performed only in patients with low back pain and anterior thigh pain;
   (c) Slump be performed when a patient has lumbar spine and posterior leg pain, the condition is not irritable, and:
      (i) it is thought that neuromeningeal structures are a source of symptoms, but symptoms have not been sufficiently reproduced with SLR and PNF; or
      (ii) the patient complains of symptoms reproduced in positions similar to slump, such as on long sitting (with the straight leg outstretched), e.g. when reading in bed, or getting into or out of a car.
2. In the cervical spine and upper limb: ULTT be performed when a patient has cervical spine and arm pain, and:
   (a) it is thought that neuromeningeal structures could be the cause of the patient's upper limb symptoms, for example the patient describes symptom provocation during activities similar to the ULTT position;
   (b) the physical examination of the cervical spine and shoulder has not sufficiently reproduced the upper limb and cervical spine pain.

Test procedures

Tension tests routinely examined

Only two tension tests are routinely examined, both applicable to lumbar spine conditions.

Straight Leg Raise (SLR)

The SLR produces tension and movement in the sciatic nerve and the spinal nerves and nerve roots (SN/NR) which contribute to it (L4–S3) (Goddard and Reid, 1965).

Standard test procedure

For examination of SLR the patient lies supine and completely relaxed. The physiotherapist supports the ankle posteriorly and the anterior aspect of the knee superior to the patella to lift the leg passively into hip flexion, while maintaining knee extension. The test should initially be standardized, with the hip in neutral abduction/adduction and neutral rotation, the head unsupported (no pillow is necessary unless pain demands one) and the ankle relaxed (usually in some plantarflexion; Brieg and Troup, 1979). This standard procedure can be reliably reproduced (Matyas and Bach, 1985) and range of hip flexion measured using a tape measure or goniometer (Hsieh *et al.*, 1983). This is illustrated in Figure 6.5 (a).

Sensitizing procedures

Neuromeningeal structures may be further stressed by using 'sensitizing' manoeuvres. Sensitizing manoeuvres aim to further stress neural connective tissue whilst only minimally stressing other tissues that could produce the patient's symptoms (Brieg and Troup, 1979).

The commonest sensitizing procedure for SLR is ankle dorsiflexion. Hip flexion is reduced a little (usually approximately 5°) from the point in range where pain first increases. Dorsiflexion of the ankle is then added while the position of hip flexion remains unchanged (Brieg and Troup, 1979). Current opinion holds that the addition of ankle dorsiflexion to SLR increases tension in the sciatic nerve and its contributing SN/NR while not significantly increasing tension in other lumbar spine structures or in the hamstrings muscle group. An increase in pain with the addition of dorsiflexion is therefore thought to indicate an abnormal response to tension in the neuromeningeal structures. When relevant, PNF, hip adduction or hip internal rotation can be added to SLR in the same way, with the intention of further increasing tension (Brieg and Troup, 1979).

Passive neck flexion (PNF)

PNF is thought to apply tension to the spinal cord and associated dura and the lumbar nerve roots (Brieg and Marions, 1963; Maitland, 1986).

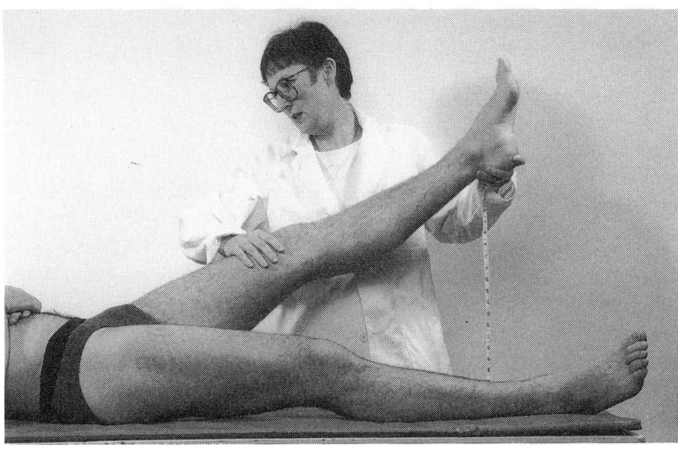

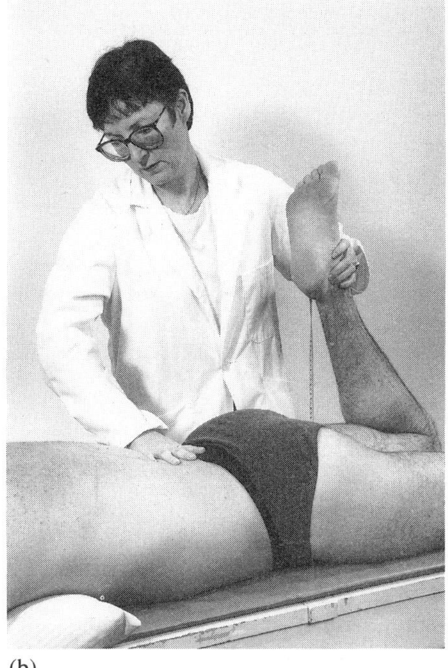

Figure 6.5 Standardized tension testing: (a) straight leg raise, and (b) prone knee bend. In both cases range of movement is measured using tape measure

Standard test procedure

PNF is tested with the patient lying comfortably in supine. The physiotherapist carefully flexes the patient's cervical spine, ensuring control during the movement to avoid rotation and side flexion. The cervical spine must be fully flexed rather than causing an anterior shearing movement in the lower part.

Sensitizing procedure

SLR can be combined with PNF in the same way as described during SLR above.

Other tension tests performed when relevant to the patient's signs and symptoms

For lumbar spine conditions the following tests can be carried out.

Prone knee bend (PKB)

PKB produces tension in the femoral nerve and the SN/NR which contribute to it (L2–L4; Dyck,

1976). It is therefore tested when the patient has pain in the lumbar spine and anterior thigh (the dermatomes corresponding to L2–L4 spinal segments).

Standard test procedure

PKB is tested with the patient lying comfortably relaxed in the prone position. The physiotherapist carefully flexes the knee while the hip remains in neutral on the plinth (Figure 6.5(b)). Initially the test is standardized, with the hip in neutral. Knee flexion can be measured with a goniometer or using a tape measure to record the distance from the heal to gluteal crease.

Sensitizing procedure

Hip extension can be added as a sensitizing manoeuvre to further increase tension in the femoral nerve and its contributing SN/NR (Dyck, 1976). Care should be taken to avoid lumbar spine rotation and extension, confining movement as much as possible to the hip and knee. Interpretation of results from the addition of cervical flexion/extension to PKB is equivocal, being unsubstantiated by appropriate investigation (Davidson, 1987), hence their value as additions to PKB is unclear.

Slump

The slump test is thought to apply more tension to neuromeningeal structures than SLR, PNF or a combination of the two tests (Maitland, 1978, 1985). Slump is therefore applied when lumbar spine and leg symptoms have not been reproduced to the extent required by these tests, and further examination of tension in neuromeningeal structures is indicated.

Slump is tested with the patient seated comfortably on the end of a plinth. The standard protocol for examining slump consists of (Maitland, 1985):

1. Active flexion of thoracic spine by the patient, while the head remains erect and the sacrum remains vertical. Overpressure is applied to thoracic flexion, and maintained throughout the remainder of the procedure.
2. Active flexion of cervical spine. Overpressure is applied and maintained.
3. The knee on asymptomatic side is actively extended and dorsiflexion applied.
4. The patient is asked to extend the cervical spine, and the effect on symptoms is noted.
5. The patient is asked to attempt further knee extension while the cervical spine is in the neutral or extended position, and changes in symptoms are noted.
6. The patient flexes the cervical spine again, and knee extension, ankle dorsiflexion, cervical spine extension are repeated on the symptomatic side.

Results from testing the symptomatic side are compared with those of the asymptomatic side. At each step symptoms are noted before adding the next step of the protocol. An abnormal response to tension testing in the lumbar neuromeningeal structures is indicated by:

1. reproduction of symptoms when the spine is fully flexed and the leg fully extended, followed by a decrease in symptoms with cervical extension;
2. an increase in knee extension and/or ankle dorsiflexion with cervical extension;
3. a difference in range of knee extension/ankle dorsiflexion between sides.

Upper limb tension test (ULTT)

The ULTT is performed when cervical spine and arm symptoms have not been adequately reproduced with other examination procedures. It is thought to increase stress in the cervical spine neuromeningeal structures including mid-low cervical SN/NR (C5–T1), the brachial plexus and peripheral nerves (Selvaratnam, *et al.*, 1989, 1994).

The standard test is performed, with the patient lying comfortably in the supine position, the use of a small pillow under the head being standardized, and consists of the following steps (Elvey, 1983; Kenneally, 1985).

- shoulder depression,
- glenohumeral abduction behind the coronal plane (i.e. slight extension),
- glenohumeral external rotation,
- forearm supination,
- elbow extension,
- wrist and finger extension,
- contralateral cervical lateral flexion,
- ipsilateral cervical lateral flexion is also added to determine change in symptoms.

Results of testing the symptomatic arm are compared with those of the asymptomatic arm. At each step symptoms are noted before adding the next step of the protocol. An abnormal response to testing cervical neuromeningeal structures is indicated by (Elvey, 1983):

1. reproduction of symptoms when the arm is fully extended which are increased with cervical contralateral lateral flexion followed by a decrease in symptoms with ipsilateral cervical spine lateral flexion;
2. an increase in elbow and finger extension with ipsilateral cervical spine lateral flexion;
3. a difference in range of movement between sides in any of the components.

Many variations of the ULTT have been described (see Butler, 1991). The rationale underlying these variations is that tension can be altered in the cervical neuromeningeal tissues by changing the position of limb segments. It is therefore speculated that some variations are specific to different peripheral nerves. It has been demonstrated that variations to the test alter the test response (Elvey, 1979; 1981; Yaxley and Jull, 1991); however, explanations for these observations are yet to be validated. For a full exploration of these issues see Butler (1991).

Interpretation of test results

The degree to which results of tests are used to formulate decisions about diagnosis and treatment depends on the validity and reliability of the tests. Since most information about reliability and validity relates to the standard tension test procedures (Kenneally, 1985; Pullos, 1986), results can be best interpreted when tests are performed in a standardized way. It is therefore suggested that the standard procedures be performed before adding sensitizing manoeuvres or varying the procedure.

A positive response

The term 'positive' is generally used in orthopaedic medicine to denote a response that suggests the presence of pathology. Although the term has been broadened by physiotherapists to encompass any symptom-producing manoeuvre, when interpreting tension tests, identification of a positive response should be consistent with that understood in orthopaedic medicine. The situation is somewhat confusing, however, because a 'positive' tension test of the lumbar spine neuromeningeal structures, until recently, was interpreted as indicating a disc protrusion. This is no longer the only interpretation. Nevertheless, the term 'positive' should be reserved for specific test results, as described below.

Physiotherapists, however, are interested in any response during performance of tension tests. Tension tests are often a useful method of monitoring the patient's immediate response to treatment, progress of the condition, and may also be used as treatment procedures. Therefore, all responses and the point in range in which they occur are noted.

SLR

A positive response is considered to be reproduction of leg symptoms early in range of hip movement ($< 30°-45°$ hip flexion). This response may be caused by various pathologies, but the most frequently cited is that of a space-occupying lesion (usually a fragment of intervertebral disc) (Charnley, 1951; Smyth and Wright, 1958; McNab, 1971). This may produce changes in the nerve causing an abnormal response to tension. It should be noted, however, that the intervertebral disc is not the sole cause of decreased SLR (see diagnostic validity).

PNF

A positive response is reproduction of any lumbar spine, perhaps thoracic spine, or leg pain (Butler, 1991). This is thought to result from tensioning the dura mater or lumbar nerve roots.

PKB

A positive response is reproduction of lumbar spine and anterior leg pain early in range of knee flexion ($< 60°-90°$ knee flexion). It is thought that pathology such as a space-occupying lesion affecting the SN/NR associated with the femoral nerve is responsible for a positive PKB (Dyck, 1976; Estridge *et al.*, 1982).

Slump and ULTT

Slump and ULTT procedures have not been investigated as thoroughly as SLR. Since they are vigorous procedures, it is unlikely that they would be used to identify serious pathology in the presence of marked pain. These tests therefore probably do not have the same diagnostic significance as SLR, PNF and PKB.

Diagnostic validity

SLR

The SLR was originally described to differentiate hip from sciatic symptoms, a purpose it is still used for today. Over the years the diagnostic utility of the SLR has been frequently debated. Charnley's (1951) widely held view that a severely restricted SLR indicates the presence of a protruding disc has been challenged by several authors (Fahrni, 1966; Lerman and Drasnin, 1975). It has been subsequently demonstrated that some patients with SLR restricted to 35° or less do not have disc pathology at surgery, but rather a nerve root adherent to the disc or intradural adhesions of specific nerve roots (Fahrni, 1966; McNab, 1971). Hence a severely restricted SLR should not be used in isolation to implicate the disc as the source of the patient's symptoms. Similarly the test is not diagnostically useful in deciding whether the symptoms are due to intra- or extra-thecal dural adhesions, intraneural pathology or venous congestion within the intervertebral foramen.

A crossed SLR has also been identified as a possible diagnostic indicator of disc pathology. A crossed SLR occurs when SLR performed on the asymptomatic leg reproduces symptoms in the symptomatic leg. In some patient groups this has been demonstrated to be a better diagnostic indicator of a space-occupying lesion than the standard SLR (Hudgins, 1975).

The standard SLR does appear to increase tension in neuromeningeal structures and cause pain in sensitized neural tissues. It is therefore valid, but does not appear to have high specificity.

PNF

PNF was originally advocated as a test for meningitis [Brudzinski (1909), cited in O'Connell (1946)] before Brieg and Marions (1963) described the cephalad movement of the lumbar nerve roots and dura during the manoeuvre. PNF has not been further investigated, therefore little is known of its diagnostic validity.

PKB

PKB, first described by Wasserman (1918, cited in Dyck, 1982), is probably the least useful of the tension tests and, like PNF, has not been rigorously investigated. The test was devised as an aid in diagnosing upper lumbar disc lesions. Most authors agree that symptom reproduction may be from increased tension in nerve roots (Estridge *et al.*, 1982; Dyck, 1984). Since the upper lumbar nerve roots are thought to be subjected to the most tension during PKB, it is expected that anterior thigh pain will be reproduced. Christodoulis (1989), however, argues that the L4 nerve root is most affected, and therefore that posterolateral thigh pain should be reproduced, although there is no further supporting evidence for this view. The usual assumption is that PKB is performed to reproduce anterior thigh and lumbar spine pain, although the test gives little information about cause of the symptoms.

Slump

The slump test was devised to identify sources of leg symptoms other than pathology of the intervertebral disc or intervertebral foramina (Maitland, 1978). There is some evidence to show that the slump test fulfils this purpose.

ULTT

The ULTT as originally described was thought to stress the ulnar nerve more than other peripheral nerves, as well as more proximal neuromeningeal tissue (Elvey, 1979). The current standard test procedure is thought to stress the median nerve more than other peripheral nerves (Elvey, 1983; Kenneally, 1985; Butler, 1991). Butler (1991) has further described tests that he believes impose stress on radial, musculocutaneous, axillary and other nerves of the brachial plexus.

Normative responses have been reported for the standard ULTT procedure (Kenneally, 1985; Rubenach, 1985; Bell, 1987; Landers, 1987), and for a variation hypothesized to affect the radial nerve (Yaxley and Jull, 1991). From this information, and from comparison with the response when testing the patient's asymptomatic arm, it is possible to identify an abnormal response. Until further investigations are completed, it is not possible either to establish clearly the location or type of pathology. It is possible, however, to distinguish pain caused by tension in upper limb neuromeningeal tissues from pain caused by other somatic structures (Selveratnam *et al.*, 1987, 1994; Simionato *et al.*, 1988; Quinter, 1989; Yaxley and Jull, 1991).

Discriminative validity

During the performance of each of the tension tests many structures are moved and stressed. For example, during SLR, other lumbar spine structures, the SIJ, hip and hamstrings are also stressed. In fact, SLR is also a test of hamstrings' length, and putting hamstrings on maximal tension as during SLR would be expected to reproduce pain from a hamstrings' lesion. The PNF maximally stresses the cervical and upper thoracic spines in flexion. The slump test stresses all the above structures as well as the low thoracic spine and ankle. PKB affects the knee and the quadriceps muscle group in addition to the femoral nerve. The ULTT stresses cervical spine and shoulder structures and the elbow, wrist and finger joints. This suggests relatively poor discriminative validity for most of the tension tests. Discriminative validity has only been investigated for SLR and ULTT, and it has been found that SLR, without the addition of sensitizing manœuvres, has high sensitivity and low specificity (Fahrni, 1966; McNab, 1971; Hudgins, 1975). ULTT appears to be able to discriminate between radicular and other somatic sources of symptoms (Selveratnam *et al.*, 1987; Quinter, 1989). It is clearly difficult to interpret results of tension tests in isolation without other information from the history and physical tests.

The response to sensitizing manœuvres probably enhances the diagnostic capacity of the tests. If a sensitizing manœuvre increases symptoms, it is generally believed that neuromeningeal tissue is responsible for the symptoms, as other structures may not be further stressed. Since this belief is still being investigated, it is again advised that results of the tension tests should be correlated with the full clinical presentation.

Implications for treatment

If a positive response is found on SLR or PKB, i.e. severe pain causes a marked restriction during the test movement, and this does not appear to be consistent with the history and other findings in the physical examination, it is probably wise to confer with the patient's medical practitioner. Of itself, a positive response does not necessarily indicate specific pathology, nor constitute a contraindication or precaution to any management strategy. However, serious pathology should be excluded.

Each of the tension tests described in this section can also be used as a treatment technique. Usually one element of the test is selected, e.g. elbow extension in the ULTT position or ankle dorsiflexion in the slump position, and is either mobilized using a rhythmic oscillatory physiological procedure, or is sustained in a gentle stretch.

It is appropriate to use a tension test procedure as a treatment when it is the most provocative physical test (i.e. reproduces symptoms maximally during the physical examination), the condition is not irritable, and especially when there is no other physical finding. Tension test procedures are infrequently used as the technique of choice at the first treatment session. Responses to treatment using these techniques can vary, occasionally markedly increasing symptoms. It is therefore recommended, particularly for the novice, that the patient's signs and symptoms are clearly understood before using a tension test procedure as a treatment technique.

Proposed mode of action

Given our knowledge of tissue mechanics including hysteresis and creep (Fung, 1981; Bogduk and Twomey, 1991; Herbert, 1988) and the fact that neural tissue behaves in a similar manner to other biological tissues (Sunderland and Bradley, 1961a, b) it is difficult to see how stretching neural tissue could have other than short-term reversible mechanical effects. Butler (1991) has provided several possible explanations for the prolonged effects observed after treatment with stretches of neural tissues. He hypothesized that the effects could be mediated by dispersion of intraneural œdema, lengthening of neural tissue, improved intraneural blood supply or improved axonal transport. Although each of these proposed mechanisms is sustainable from a theoretical viewpoint, there is little evidence that any of them actually occurs.

Dose

In pharmacological practice therapeutic doses of pharmaceutical agents can be clearly established; however, in the area of neural treatment techniques, physiotherapists rely on personal experience, anecdotal evidence and recommendations from experienced clinicians when deciding treatment dose (Grieve, 1984; Maitland, 1986; Butler, 1991). There are no data that clarify the relationship between symptoms and dose, and since the mode of action is unclear, it is difficult to propose appropriate dosages. The usual dose on the first treatment occasion may be to sustain the treatment position (e.g. ankle dorsiflexion in the slump position) for approximately 30 s. If the patient's signs and symptoms improve this dose may be repeated a further two times or until reassessment indicates that signs and symptoms have ceased improving. It is recommended that the patient's signs and symptoms are closely monitored during the first treatment session. Reassessment after treatment and before the second treatment occasion will clarify the response and enable modification of dosage as required.

Conclusion

Tension tests are a useful adjunct to other examination and treatment procedures. Since they have high sensitivity but low specificity, they cannot be interpreted in isolation to formulate pathological diagnoses. Physiotherapists, however, compare results of tension tests with findings from the history and the physical examination to refine clinical diagnoses and treatment options. To be most useful, the tests must be performed in a reproducible manner.

The tension tests themselves can be used as treatment procedures. It is likely that the novice will have difficulty interpreting findings from tension tests, because of their low specificity and high sensitivity. Many anatomical structures are exposed to various biomechanical stresses during testing, and many varied pathologies may exhibit a painful response. It is therefore recommended that novices use tension tests as treatment procedures only in the absence of other treatment possibilities, until they are clear about the nature of the patient's disorder, and can predict the likely response to treatment.

Tension tests have enjoyed an increased interest in recent years, particularly with the development of the ULTT and its several variations. These tests are useful in clinical practice, but it should be remembered that test development has outpaced rigorous investigation into reliability, validity and clinical effectiveness of the tests.

The neurological examination

K. Refshauge and E. Gass

Many patients with spinal conditions have pain or other symptoms referred into the limb in addition to local spinal pain. In such cases neurological tests are performed by physiotherapists to determine whether conduction properties in the relevant parts of the nervous system are normal. The results of these tests are often considered diagnostically important and have implications for both assessment and treatment (Rydevick *et al.*, 1989). These tests are also used to monitor progress of the patient's condition. The parts of the nervous system of particular interest when dealing with spinal musculoskeletal conditions are the spinal nerve, nerve root, spinal cord and the cauda equina (see Figures 6.6–6.8).

Spinal nerve/nerve root (SN/NR)

Conduction in the SN/NR is tested when symptoms could originate from compromise of these structures. Compromise of the SN/NR can result from:

1. mechanical compromise of the nerve resulting in intraneural œdema which would in turn cause pressure on axons (Hayland *et al.*, 1989);
2. compromise of the blood vessels associated with the SN/NR, causing ischaemia;
3. traction injuries;
4. friction fibrosis (Sunderland, 1978).

It is difficult, if not impossible, to distinguish clinically between compromise of a spinal nerve and nerve root. Many authors refer only to compromise of nerve roots (Helfet and Gruebel, 1978), but others include the spinal nerve, as symptoms are often the same, and pathology in the intervertebral foramen is frequently postulated as a potential site of nerve compromise (Hayland *et al.*, 1989; MacNab, 1972). Therefore, the complex is referred to as SN/NR in this text, and is tested as an anatomical complex. Integrity of SN/NR is tested by determining the presence of a dermatomal distribution of altered sensation and myotomal pattern of motor weakness and decreased reflex response. A dermatome is the area of skin supplied by a single spinal nerve, and a myotome is the muscle supplied by (or largely supplied by) a single spinal nerve (Osol, 1972).

Indications for testing

Testing of the SN/NR complex should be undertaken when symptoms are present that could originate from compromise of this complex, including:

1. pain in a dermatomal distribution (for dermatomal maps see Williams and Warwick, 1980);
2. pain referred from the lumbar spine past the buttock, or from the cervical spine referred beyond the point of the shoulder;

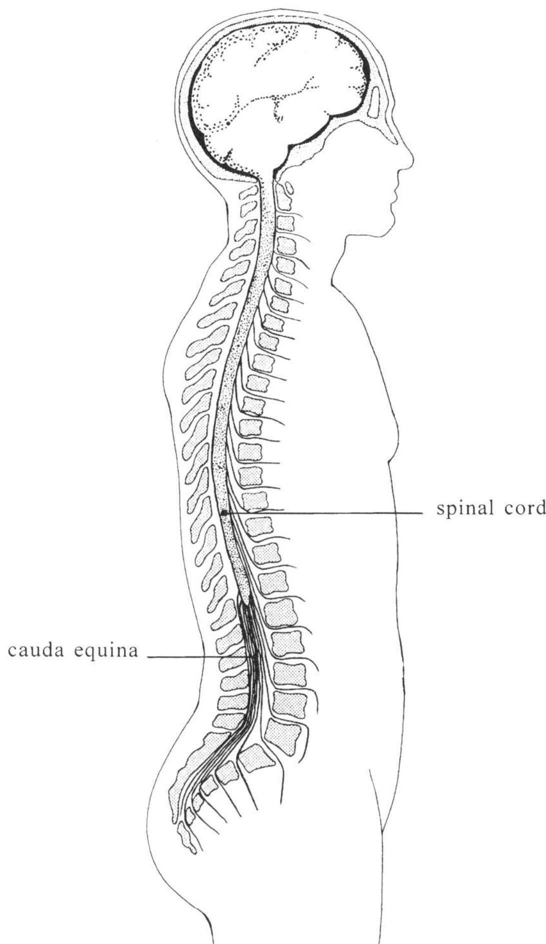

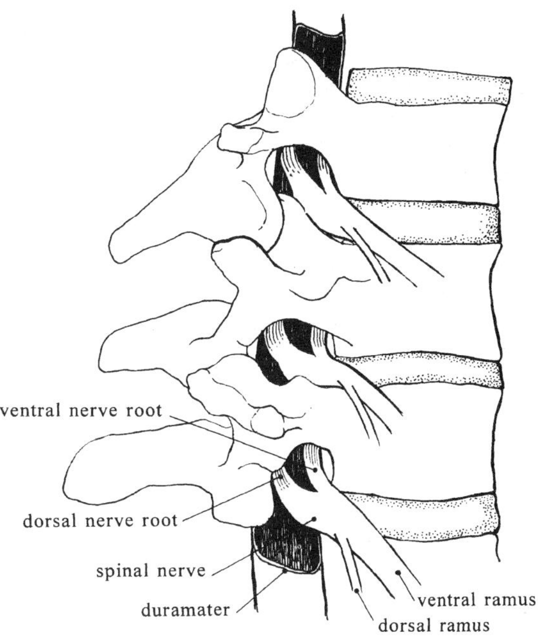

Figure 6.7 Dorsal and ventral roots exiting the spinal canal, uniting in the intervertebral foramen to form the spinal nerve, and dividing into ventral and dorsal rami after exit from the foramen

Figure 6.6 Location of spinal cord and cauda equina in spinal canal

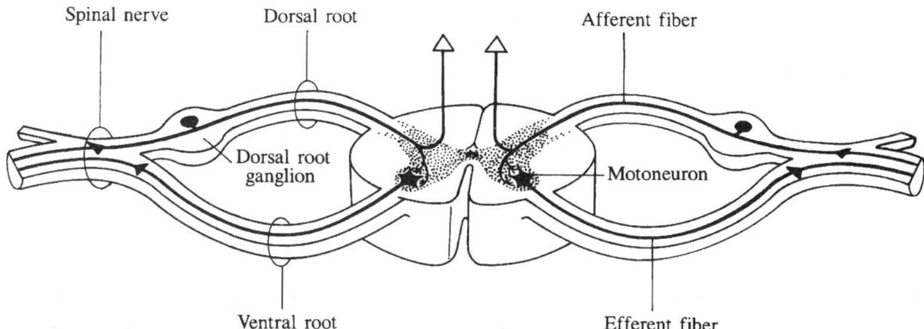

Figure 6.8 Diagrammatic representation of a section of the spinal cord, with afferents entering posteriorly and ascending through tracts to various intracranial centres, and efferent information exiting the spinal cord anteriorly

3. altered sensation (e.g. paraesthesia, anaesthesia) in the limb (lower extremity for the lumbar spine, upper extremity for the cervical spine);
4. pain in the lower extremity that may be related to a lumbar spine condition, or in the upper extremity that may be related to a cervical spine condition.

Test procedures

Compromise of SN/NR can affect neural conduction, and therefore result in reduction in one or more of the following: sensation, reflexes, muscle power. These modalities are therefore tested by the physiotherapist to determine the presence of a neurological deficit.

Testing of sensation

Physiotherapists commonly test response to light touch and pin prick as these sensations are carried by the large-diameter Group II afferent fibres to the dorsal column. These large diameter fibres are particularly vulnerable to compression (because they are located at the periphery of the nerve) and to ischaemia (because they require a greater supply of oxygen and nutrients to function normally than do small diameter fibres). Therefore, altered conduction in Group II afferents may be one of the first indicators of SN/NR compromise.

Testing consists of running cotton wool lightly around either both lower or both upper limbs simultaneously (i.e. across several dermatomes with each sweep), asking the patient to report any differences in sensation in one part of the limb or from one limb to the other. If areas of altered sensation are identified they are delineated using gentle pin prick. This pin prick should be sharp not painful, ensuring that the large Group II fibres carrying non-noxious information are tested rather than the smaller Group III or Group IV carrying noxious stimuli (Kandell *et al.*, 1991). Areas of sensory change are recorded (generally on a body chart) and compared with dermatomal areas of innervation (Bickerstaff, 1980) to determine firstly, whether there is SN/NR compromise, and secondly, the affected level, i.e. the segmental level corresponding to the dermatome.

Several other aspects of sensation could be tested, for example:

1. Two-point discrimination, testing the integrity of the dorsal column and lemniscal systems (Foreman and Croft, 1988), although it has been suggested that this test is not sensitive to SN/NR compromise (Gelberman *et al.*, 1983).
2. Vibration, testing integrity of Group II fibres, dorsal column and medial lemniscal systems (Kandell *et al.*, 1991). This test appears to be sensitive to compression (Gelberman *et al.*, 1983).
3. Temperature sensibility, testing the integrity of the lateral spinothalamic tract of the spinal cord (Kandell, *et al.*, 1991) and the Group III fibres (Barr, 1974). Extremes of temperature, however, are perceived as painful stimuli.
4. Proprioception, testing skin and joint receptors, muscle spindles, Group I and Group II fibres, and dorsal column and medial lemniscus systems (Foreman and Croft, 1988).

These other sensory modalities are not routinely tested. The purpose of sensibility testing is to use efficient testing procedures to detect SN/NR compromise and the affected level, rather than differential diagnosis of affected spinal tract. Light touch and pin prick, testing large-diameter fibres, are currently the most appropriate to achieve this purpose.

Testing of reflexes

There are four types of reflex that can be tested in the peripheral nervous system; deep tendon reflexes, superficial, visceral and pathological (Foreman and Croft, 1988). Deep tendon reflexes are tested by physiotherapists to determine the presence and segmental level of SN/NR compromise. An intact deep tendon reflex requires integrity of the stretch reflex arc (Lance and McLeod, 1975).

The stretch reflex is elicited by briskly striking the tendon with a tendon hammer while the muscle is on slight stretch and the patient is relaxed. The number of times the reflex is elicited is arbitrary, the test being repeated until the examiner is satisfied that the response can be interpreted. The response is compared with the other side and with the known range of normal (Skre, 1972). A decreased or absent reflex may indicate a compromise of the corresponding SN/NR or peripheral nerve, and an increased response may indicate a lesion in the central nervous system (see under central nervous system, later in this chapter).

Testing of muscle strength

Muscles are tested for isometric strength to determine whether nerve conduction is affected. The muscles tested are innervated or largely innervated by a single SN/NR and therefore represent myotomes. Myotomes C5–T1 are tested in the cervical spine and L2–S2 for the lumbar spine.

There are no clearly defined myotomes in the upper cervical spine (above C4), most muscles in this region being innervated by multiple segments (Williams and Warwick, 1980). Occasionally muscle power is tested in the upper cervical spine. The results, however, must be interpreted with caution since weakness will not indicate involvement of a single SN/NR. Note that when testing the mid-low cervical spine SN/NR, C4 is not tested. Although trapezius is often recommended as a myotome for C4 (Maitland, 1986; Magee, 1987), trapezius receives its motor supply from cranial nerve XI (spinal accessory nerve), although the C4 dermatome overlies the upper trapezius region (Williams and Warwick, 1980). Muscle strength is not tested in the thoracic spine since segmentally innervated muscles (intercostal muscles) are not accessible for this type of testing. In the lumbar spine, L1 is not tested, as there is no corresponding myotome; again, muscles in this region are supplied by several segmental levels.

Myotomes are generally tested using maximum voluntary isometric contraction. This practice is supported by some authors who suggest that decreases in strength may only be detected on maximum sustained or repeated contractions (Lieberman *et al.*, 1983), while others claim that resisted contraction through a range of motion may be more sensitive (Bickerstaff, 1980). The presence of pain may reduce the strength of contraction. If weakness appears to be caused by pain on contraction, results must be interpreted in the light of the other neurological tests, and not weighted heavily, in isolation. The most valid and sensitive method of testing myotomes therefore remains somewhat controversial. The current practice of testing maximum voluntary isometric contraction will probably continue in use until another clinically viable method is demonstrated to be more appropriate. Muscle power can be measured using a hand-held dynamometer, weights or numerous mechanical devices, such as the Cybex of Kincom.

Interpretation of test results

Our interpretation of neurological findings will be influenced by the reliability and validity of the tests, as well as by the rest of the clinical presentation.

Testing of sensation

Standardization of the test procedure will enhance reliability. During testing a stimulus of constant intensity should be applied (Sunderland, 1978). This pressure must also be appropriate: if intensity is too gentle, only the exquisitely sensitive hair follicles may be stimulated rather than all light touch receptors, perhaps reducing the response.

Identification of the spinal segmental level inolved from the area of sensory loss probably does not have high discriminative validity. Dermatomal maps of segmental sensation vary between individuals (Skre, 1972) and between the right and left limb of the same individual, this difference not being related to limb dominance (Weiss, *et al.*, 1985; De Palma and Rothman, 1970). Some of this variation may be attributed to bony and neural anomalies (Young, *et al.*, 1983; McCulloch and Waddell, 1980; Neidre and McNab, 1983). Dermatomes are also known to overlap. However, dermatomes vary in a minor way, overlapping rather than varying in a completely random manner. Therefore, although a single affected level may be difficult to identify with certainty, it is probable that the SN/NR compromised can be isolated to two possible levels. It may be important, however, to identify the anatomical location of the compromise, which may not be at the level of exit of the SN/NR, particularly in the lumbar spine (Kortelainen *et al.*, 1985).

Reflexes

Reflexes like sensation are subject to large normal variation. It is not uncommon for normal hyper- or hypo-reflexia to occur and there may be some normal difference between right and left (Luhan, 1968). There is also an apparent reduction in magnitude of response with increasing age (Skre, 1972), indicating that hyporeflexia in the elderly, either unilateral or bilateral, may be an insignificant finding.

The reflex arc is influenced by converging input. The CNS can directly influence the alpha and gamma motor neurons, and it is thought that skin and joint receptors could also have an effect (Appelberg *et al.*, 1983), suggesting that both the CNS and other somatic structures could affect the reflex response. The effects of this may be demonstrated when using reinforcement (Jendrassic's manoeuvre), when contraction of a muscle distant from the site of the reflex can increase the response (Lance and McLeod, 1975). Hagbath *et al.*, (1975) suggest that slight muscle contraction gives a more reliably enhanced response than does Jendrassic's manoeuvre. To enhance reliability of response, testing should be standardized considering particularly the amount and direction of applied force.

When interpreting reflex response it is therefore prudent to note only large discrepancies or asymmetry of the stretch reflex and compare these findings with the overall clinical picture (Lance and McLeod, 1975).

Muscle strength

Interpretation of muscle testing is complicated by several factors. Myotomes overlap with variations between individuals, perhaps due to anomalies in the bony or neural system. This reduces specificity of myotomal identification. Overlap of myotomes also maintains innervation to a muscle when conduction from one spinal segment is interrupted, if other contributing segments are uninterrupted. In addition, there appears to be a compensatory mechanism that may occur in patients with chronic SN/NR compromise, whereby the motor units still conducting nerve impulses increase their firing frequency and collateral axon sprouting reinnervates denervated muscles, resulting in little or no apparent strength deficit (Bohannon and Gajdosik, 1987). The muscle could therefore have approximately normal strength.

Testing muscles manually is known to have low sensitivity (Gelberman *et al.*, 1983) demonstrating that altered strength is not detected until there is a substantial reduction (approximately 30%) in motor action potentials. This indicates that a large asymmetry may be present, yet not evident on muscle testing (Bohannon and Gajdosik, 1987).

Muscles also exhibit a length–tension relationship, generating different forces at different lengths, therefore joint position must be standardized for testing. To enhance the probability of detecting abnormalities, it is important to standardize the test procedure, including position of both patient and tester, hand position, external cues, and dominance of the physiotherapist's resisting arm. Manual muscle testing appears to be reliable when using a dynamometer (Bohannon, 1986). Use of mechanical devices may allow detection of small changes; however, small changes need to be interpreted with caution, being aware of normal limb differences.

Conclusion

These neurological tests considered independently do not have high reliability or high specificity and sensitivity. The tests are rarely considered in isolation, however. All three tests (or two in the absence of a relevant reflex) are performed and the results considered in the context of the total clinical picture, e.g. the patient's age, the area and quality of symptoms, mode of onset, provocative movements, and comparison with the other side and known normal ranges. It appears, therefore, that a decreased response in only one neurological test may not be as diagnostically significant as a decreased response in two or three tests. This is particularly true when the finding is indicative of a segmental level different from that suggested by the area of pain.

Neurological deficit and other somatic structures

There is no doubt that altered sensation, loss of motor power and reflex changes can be caused by SN/NR compromise (Helfet and Gruebel, 1978). However, it may be possible that neurological changes could be caused by a disturbance of somatic structures other than nerve, particularly where there is an isolated neurological deficit with no other supportive clinical findings. To date this has not been clearly demonstrated and remains hypothetical based on theory and clinical observation.

Compromise of normal SN/NR does not cause pain (Loeser, 1985; MacNab, 1972), therefore, a neurological deficit can occur without pain. Under certain conditions, however, compromise of the nerve root may cause pain. Such conditions include previous damage to the nerve root, intra-neural oedema causing axon compression and ischaemia from radicular artery compression (McNab, 1972; Olmarker *et al.*, 1989; Rydevick *et al.*, 1989). This pain should be accompanied by neurological deficit (Bogduk, 1987) since the function of large-diameter sensory and motor afferents is affected by compromise before the small-diameter nociceptive afferents (groups III and IV) within the SN/NR complex (Sunderland, 1978). Therefore, the absence of a neurological deficit, even when pain appears to be dermato-mally distributed, may indicate that SN/NR is unlikely to be involved in symptom production.

The diagnostic decision is less clear when a dermatomal area of pain is accompanied by an isolated neurological deficit, such as a small area of sensory change, or a slightly altered reflex, or equivocal alteration in muscle power. It is poss-ible that such a deficit is due to altered afferent input from somatic structures converging at spinal cord level, from altered facilitation in C3–4 propriospinal neurons (Burke, *et al.*, 1992a,b) or from descending control from higher centres. Such neurophysiological phenomena occur, but evidence of their clinical manifestation is still only hypothesized.

There is scant, but consistent, clinical evidence that somatic structures other than nerve may cause neurological deficit. Resolution of neuro-logical deficit (normalized reflex) has been observed after injection of xylocaine into the zygapophyseal joints (Mooney and Robertson, 1976). This study has often been criticized for the volume of injection material (2–5 cc) used which would not only fill the zygapophyseal joint cap-sule but also disseminate into surrounding tissues (McCall *et al.*, 1979). Nevertheless if SN/NR compression had been the cause of the decreased reflex due to direct compression or intraneural oedema, it seems unlikely that introducing more fluid to the region (further increasing pressure) would restore the reflex. The xylocaine may have affected the joint receptors which could affect the alpha and gamma motor neurons (Appleberg *et al.*, 1983) and thus the reflex arc. It is perhaps possible, therefore, that somatic structures may cause changes in deep tendon reflexes. Normal-ized muscle strength has also been observed immediately after traction (Knutsson *et al.*, 1988).

Somatic structures other than nerves are some-times thought to cause isolated changes in sensa-tion. However, there are no substantiating reports, perhaps because most studies involving intra-capsular zygapophyseal joint injections have been primarily concerned with pain relief rather than normalizing neurological signs.

In general, a decrease in response to neuro-logical testing indicates the possibility of SN/NR compromise. In fact, if there is a decrease in at least two tests, it should be assumed that SN/NR compromise is the cause. This situation is less clear where pain is accompanied by a small decrease in response to one neurological test, with no other clinical evidence suggestive of SN/NR compromise. It seems possible that in this case, the isolated neurological deficit in the presence of an inconsistent clinical picture is caused by somatic structures other than neural structures.

Implications for further testing and treatment

In the presence of a clinical picture indicative of definitive or possible SN/NR compromise, phys-ical tests that are thought to reduce the size of the intervertebral foramen, increase the com-promise of the nerve or increase intraneural inflammation are avoided. These tests include passive accessory movements and possibly oscil-latory passive physiological movements. Treat-ments aimed at increasing the size of the inter-vertebral foramen are generally recommended (Maitland, 1986). Such treatments are thought to include sustained traction, rotation and perhaps lateral flexion away from the affected side. Other treatments may be used when the neurological deficit is chronic and/or stable (i.e. response has not changed to testing over approximately 1–2 weeks), when the deficit is unrelated to the presenting problem (and would not be affected by treatment of the presenting problem) and when the therapist is certain that the deficit is not caused by relevant neural structures (usually not on the first day presenting for treatment). In these latter instances, the treatment most appro-priate to the presenting problem (e.g. oscillatory techniques) may be implemented, but the neuro-logical deficit must be constantly monitored to ensure no further decrement. It is recommended that performance of manipulation for patients with neurological deficit be restricted to those physiotherapists who have completed further study in manipulative procedures.

Central nervous system (spinal cord)

The CNS is comprised of all parts of the nervous system proximal to the anterior horn cell in the spinal cord. Disorders of the central nervous system, termed upper motor neuron lesions (UMNL), can therefore arise from lesions anywhere in this part of the nervous system, for example in the brain (e.g. hemiplegia, brain trauma) or in the spinal cord (e.g. rheumatoid arthritis in the cervical spine, causing displacement of C1 on C2, compressing the spinal cord at this level), or both the brain and the spinal cord (e.g. multiple sclerosis). It is important for physiotherapists to determine whether pathology exists locally in the painful region of the spine, because sometimes this pathology can be serious and contraindicate manual treatments in this region. On the other hand, an UMNL affecting the brain, such as stroke, does not have implications for local treatment of musculoskeletal disorders of the spine. Physiotherapists therefore need to determine whether there is upper motor neuron involvement in the disorder, the cause of the UMNL, and the location of the pathology.

Indications for testing

Testing of the central nervous system (CNS) is not routine, being performed only as indicated. Tests to identify UMNL will be incorporated into the neurological examination in the presence of:

1. ataxia (sometimes people describe vertigo or dizziness as unsteadiness of gait, but this is not ataxia);
2. bilateral non-dermatomal distribution of symptoms in the lower extremities for the lumbar spine, and in the upper as well as lower extremities for the cervical spine (symptoms may initially manifest unilaterally, and as the condition worsens, become bilateral, therefore, an early presentation may not appear typical);
3. findings on SN/NR testing suggestive of UMNL, such as exaggerated tendon reflexes or bilateral non-dermatomal distribution of sensory changes.

Test procedures

Procedures to identify UMNL would usually be performed in addition to the tests for sensation, reflexes and muscle strength described in the SN/NR section. The procedures below performed by physiotherapists identify a general UMNL only, and are:

- testing for the presence of clonus,
- testing the Babinski reflex,
- sensation, reflex and muscle strength testing as part of the SN/NR test.

Other tests can be performed, but do not appear to give additional information useful for management of the musculoskeletal condition. Additional tests include: Chaddock sign, Gordon reflex, Schoffer's reflex, Hoffmann's sign, as well as many others (described in Kandell, *et al.*, 1991).

Testing for the presence of clonus

Rationale

Clonus is the term used to describe the abnormal, rhythmic, repetitive reflex twitches elicited when tension is suddenly applied to a muscle or muscle group and maintained (Zimmerman, 1978). The phenomenon is observed when pathological changes in the CNS, probably affecting the corticospinal tract, lead to a facilitation of the spinal stretch reflexes (Bannister, 1992).

The stretch reflex can be thought of as a dynamic closed loop functioning to regulate muscle length, particularly in the presence of perturbations (Zimmerman, 1978). Pathological CNS changes can increase the gain of the dynamic closed loop leading to situations of instability and overcompensation, manifested as undesirable oscillations of muscle contraction/relaxation following the sudden change in muscle length.

Clonus may therefore be observed in many muscles and may not need a specific test procedure as, in some patients, it may be demonstrated during reflex testing, or even while sitting with their feet on the floor. More commonly, however, a specific test to elicit clonus is performed.

Test procedure

Clonus can be tested in many muscle groups, but the ankle plantarflexors are usually tested. With the patient relaxed and well supported the physiotherapist applies a sudden dorsiflexion movement to the patient's ankle, thus applying a stretch to the plantarflexors. Dorsiflexion is maintained for a short time and the presence of clonus is detected by observation and palpation. The test is generally considered positive (abnormal) if clonus is present (more than five reflex twitches).

Testing for the presence of Babinski reflex (extensor plantar reflex)

Rationale

After the first year of life, a normal response to a firm scratch along the lateral aspect of the foot is plantarflexion of the toes with dorsiflexion of the foot and possibly some contraction of other leg muscles such as tensor fascia latae (Bannister, 1992). In 1896 Babinski suggested that in the presence of any UMNL, commonly a corticospinal tract lesion, the normal plantar reflex is replaced by an abnormal upward extensor movement of the great toe. With an UMNL the local plantar reflexes (extensor reflex) to the toes are lost and the flexion reflex dominates so that blunt scratch stimulation to the sole of the foot not only evokes flexion of the ankle and leg but dorsiflexion of the toes (Bouchier and Morris, 1982). The abnormal extensor plantar reflex is part of widespread nociceptive reflex activity of the whole lower limb. When fully demonstrated the reflex includes flexion of hip, knee and ankle joints, dorsiflexion of the great toe and abduction or fanning of the other toes with dorsiflexion. This abnormal response is not normally present and therefore indicates the presence of an UMNL.

Test procedure

The patient should be relaxed and well supported. The physiotherapist gently keeps the patient's foot stable while firmly scratching the outer surface of the sole with a blunt object (such as the end of the percussion hammer). The manoeuvre should start at the heel, continue along the lateral aspect of the sole, and curve medially at the forefoot terminating beneath the first metatarsophalangeal joint. Care should be taken to provide neither a painful nor a light and ticklish stimulus as strong withdrawal of the foot and leg will make test interpretation difficult. The physiotherapist should observe the big toe carefully, because the decision about a positive test response predominantly rests upon accurate observation of movement of the big toe and, to a lesser extent, the other four toes.

The test is positive or abnormal if the big toe dorsiflexes. The other toes may also fan outwards in abduction and dorsiflex. Response of the big toe is the most important, and if no response is elicited (no movement of the big toe into either dorsiflexion or plantarflexion) the test should be repeated more firmly.

Positive Babinski test is often described as an 'upgoing toe' and gives a general indication of the presence of an UMNL. 'Upgoing toe' is preferable to terms involving flexion and extension which can be confusing.

Testing reflex response

Rationale

In the presence of compromise of SN/NR conduction, reflex response is decreased. An increased response, however, may indicate an UMNL, as the gamma efferent system supplying the ends of the muscle spindles is regulated by inhibitory descending motor pathways (Lance and McLeod, 1975). Thus, any block to this inhibitory regulation may cause hyper-reflexic responses.

Test procedure

Reflexes are tested during the SN/NR examination described earlier. If an increased response is identified during this examination, reflexes in the untested extremities are investigated. For example, a person with spinal cord compromise due to local pathology in the lumbar spine may have an increased response in L3/4 and S1/2 reflexes, while the upper extremity reflexes may remain normal. On the other hand, if the spinal cord compromise is due to cervical spine pathology, both upper and lower extremity reflex responses would be increased. In other words, reflexes below the level of the lesion will be increased.

Interpretation of test results

The tests used to identify an UMNL have not been subjected to rigorous investigation of their reliability or validity. Nevertheless, they are in widespread use amongst all health personnel managing patients with neurological disorders. Information is available about reflex testing, indicating that reflexes vary within and between individuals and may decrease in size of response with increasing age (Skre, 1972). It is also known that some clonus may be present normally in the elderly, although the response is usually less than three beats (Skre, 1972). A clonus response can also be elicited in normal asymptomatic young people, if the plantar-flexors are stretched at a particular point in range of movement. It seems, however, that a positive Babinski response is rarely present in a normal population. Therefore, in the presence of equivocal findings, such as the presence of clonus in the absence of positive results in the other two tests, a diagnosis of UMNL is not clearly established. As with other examination procedures, the presence of a positive response in all three tests is required for definitive diagnosis of an UMNL, although hyper-reflexia is probably most heavily weighted.

Implications for treatment

The clinical significance of the presence of an UMNL must be determined in conjunction with the patient's medical practitioner. Since the purpose of the tests is to identify contraindications or precautions to manual therapy treatment for spinal pain, it is the cause of the UMNL and location of any pathology that is of concern. Manual therapy can be used safely to treat spinal pain in the presence of an UMNL if the cause of the UMNL is distant from, and unrelated to, the cause of the spinal pain (e.g. hemiplegia or brain injury). Manual therapy would be contraindicated, however, for treating cervical spine pain in the presence of severe rheumatoid arthritis causing compression of the spinal cord. It is recommended, therefore, that when a physiotherapist recognizes the possibility of an UMNL, contact is made with the relevant medical practitioner to definitively establish the cause. The suitability of manual therapy can then be determined.

Cauda equina (lumbosacrococcygeal SN/NR)

The cauda equina is anatomically composed of the ventral and dorsal nerve roots from lumbar, sacral and coccygeal spinal cord segments (Williams and Warwick, 1980). In adults, the lumbar, sacral and coccygeal segments of the spinal cord lie in the region between the tenth thoracic vertebra and the first lumbar vertebra. The nerve roots descend

from the spinal segment of origin to their point of exit from the vertebral canal as segmental spinal nerves. Since this arrangement of obliquely descending nerve roots within the spinal canal resembles a horses tail, it is termed the cauda equina. A lesion of the cauda equina may therefore interrupt conduction in several nerve roots resulting in diffuse leg pain and signs and symptoms consistent with every level affected (Coscia *et al.*, 1994). In musculoskeletal physiotherapy clinical practice, the principal concern is compromise of S2 SN/NR because this segmental level supplies the bladder, rectum and male sexual organs. Persistent compromise of S2 SN/NR may lead to necrosis, causing permanent loss of function of bladder and bowel, resulting in permanent disturbances in micturition and defaecation (Coscia, *et al.*, 1994). It is therefore imperative that such a disorder is immediately recognized.

Micturition

The main structures involved in micturition are the urinary bladder and internal sphincter, composed of smooth muscle, and the external sphincter composed of skeletal muscle. The smooth muscle of the bladder and internal sphincter are usually innervated by T11–L2 sympathetic nerves and S1–S2 parasympathetic nerves (Ganong, 1975). The sympathetic preganglionic fibres synapse in the coeliac and mesenteric ganglia, becoming postganglionic hypogastric nerves, while the para-sympathetic preganglionic nerves reach the bladder. The skeletal muscle of the external sphincter is supplied by the pudendal nerve composed of spinal segments S2–S4.

Micturition is a spinal reflex under voluntary control. It occurs when mechanoreceptors in the bladder wall are stimulated, causing excitation of the micturition centre in the anterior pons (Ganong, 1975; Thorn, 1977). Descending output excites parasympathetic S1 and S2 neurons, causing contraction of the smooth muscle (expansion of the internal sphincter). Concurrently, skeletal muscle of the external sphincter is relaxed, allowing micturition.

It appears that the major role of the sympathetic nervous system in micturition is maintenance of smooth muscle tone at the neck of the bladder to provide continence. In addition, sympathetic stimulation in males causes closure of the neck of the bladder during ejaculation (Ganong. 1975; Janig, 1978).

Defaecation

The main structures involved in defaecation are the internal sphincter (smooth muscle) and the external sphincter (skeletal muscle). Sympathetic preganglionic efferent fibres to the rectum originate in the lateral grey matter of lower thoracic and possibly upper lumbar spinal cord and synapse in the inferior mesenteric plexus before reaching the rectum. Parasympathetic efferent fibres are distributed via pelvic splanchnic nerves probably originating from S1–S2. The skeletal muscle of the anal sphincter is supplied by the pudendal nerve (S2–S4).

Defaecation, like micturition, is a spinal reflex under voluntary control. Sympathetic nerve supply to the internal sphincter is excitatory whereas parasympathetic and somatic are inhibitory. Reflex evacuation of the distended rectum occurs when there is a transected cord if sacral segments of the cord remain intact.

Bladder and bowel dysfunction can result from neural lesions such as:

1. interruption to afferent nerves from bladder and rectum (e.g. tabes dorsalis);
2. interruption to both afferent and efferent nerves (e.g. diabetic neuropathy, tumours of cauda equina, sacral SN/NR compromise, traumatic cauda equina lesions);
3. disturbance to facilitatory and inhibitory pathways between sacral spinal cord and brain (e.g. tumours, spinal cord transection, multiple sclerosis)

Indications for testing cauda equina (S2 SN/NR)

Testing for conduction in S2 SN/NR is performed when the patient complains of recent onset of:

1. frequency of micturition (uncontrolled and urgent) or urinary retention. There may also be complaints of disturbances to defaecation;
2. paraesthesia and/or anaesthesia in the 'saddle' area, i.e. the genital area and around the natal cleft.

Test procedures and interpretation of tests

The test procedure is the same as that described in the neurological examination for the SN/NR complex in the preceding section of this chapter, but should include sensibility testing (light touch) of the saddle area. There are no further specific tests to identify a cauda equina lesion, or specifically, S2 SN/NR compromise, but neurological testing would determine the segmental level affected (in this case S2 dermatome and myotome).

Interpretation of test results

It is extremely important that the physiotherapist recognizes compromise of conduction in S2 SN/NR immediately (Coscia *et al.*, 1994). Recognition of S2 SN/NR compromise is made from;

1. history – reports of frequency of micturition and symptoms of saddle paraesthesia/anaesthesia;
2. decreased muscle power in S2 myotome (toe flexors) (with possible involvement of multiple segments);
3. decreased sensibility in S2 dermatome (with possible involvement of multiple segments).

Where cauda equina compromise is suspected, i.e. in the presence of history findings, with or without decreased muscle power or sensibility in S2 distribution, the patient should immediately be referred back to the medical practitioner. These patients should not be treated, especially with manual therapy. Clinical judgement must be used to decide what information to provide to the patient at this stage. An explanation of the findings and possible implications should be conveyed but in a manner mindful of the fact that a definitive diagnosis has not yet been made.

Palpation and passive motion tests

J. Latimer and C. Maher

During the physical examination physiotherapists frequently perform assessment procedures that involve the manual application of forces to selected regions of the spine or periphery. These assessment procedures are commonly referred to as 'passive motion tests' and in the spine include tests of both passive accessory intervertebral movement (PAIVM) and passive physiological intervertebral movement (PPIVM). During the performance of these tests the physiotherapist notes any report of symptoms by the patient and also makes a judgement about the quality of the movement produced, e.g. whether the movement feels stiffer than normal. This information is used to select patients suitable for manual therapy, to assist in establishing a clinical diagnosis, to select the region to be treated, and the most appropriate treatment technique.

Before performing passive motion tests in patients with spinal pain, the physiotherapist will have observed the patient, performed active movement tests, tension tests and a neurological examination in those patients whose symptoms are thought to be due to spinal nerve or nerve root compromise. In patients with acute neurological signs the therapist may decide not to perform passive movement testing as the information gained from these tests will not help further in isolating the symptomatic level, nor in selecting the best treatment. The neurological signs have already indicated the SN/NR involved, and traction or sustained rotation are often the treatment of choice. Rarely are passive accessory mobilizations used to treat patients with acute nerve root compromise.

Indications (and contraindications) for testing

Soft tissue palpation may be performed on all patients with spinal pain. Passive motion testing, however, is only performed on patients with spinal pain when there is no known contraindication to the application of forces to the spine. Disease processes that affect the structural integrity of the vertebral column or conditions that may be exacerbated by movement of the spine are the two main concerns regarding contra-indications of the physiotherapist. Such contraindications may include malignancy involving the vertebral column, cauda equina compromise, recent fracture, active inflammatory or infective bone disease and acute spinal cord compromise. Special care should be taken when performing passive motion tests on patients with acute neurological signs, osteoporosis, spondylolisthesis and, when assessing the cervical spine, rheumatoid arthritis and vertebral artery signs or symptoms.

Test procedures

Soft tissue palpation

Before passive motion tests to the affected spinal region are performed, the soft tissues are gently palpated to help gain the confidence of the patient, and to provide information regarding:

- temperature, sweating,
- muscle spasm,
- bony anomalies,
- soft tissue thickening, tightness, swelling (either paravertebrally or involving the interspinous space),
- pain.

Temperature and the presence of sweating are usually assessed using the backs of the fingers. In patients with mechanical non-specific spinal pain the presence of sweating may only provide information about the room temperature or the state of anxiety of the patient. This information is probably more useful in detecting patients presenting with inflammatory diseases affecting peripheral joints, or assessing the extent and timing of trauma to a peripheral joint or involvement of the autonomic nervous system.

In the spine, muscle spasm and thickening or tightness of the paravertebral tissues are detected using the tips of the middle three fingers to palpate the area. Bony prominences and interspinous spaces are also palpated. During this examination the patient is also questioned about the reproduction of any symptoms. Because of the morphology of the spine it is generally not possible to directly palpate the structures that may be the cause of symptoms and so the test cannot be used to identify the symptomatic structure.

Judgements made regarding the presence of muscle spasm or bony anomalies have been found to be relatively unreliable (Keating *et al.*, 1990) and so some physiotherapists do not collect this information. However, the test yields reliable information regarding pain and symptom reproduction (Keating *et al.*, 1990). It is this aspect of the test that best helps indicate the vertebral levels to be tested using passive accessory and physiological tests. (It needs to be remembered, however, that a patient may present with referred tenderness and hence the site of dysfunction may be well removed from the tender or painful area.)

In the periphery, palpation of the symptomatic area is also performed before testing of passive accessory movements. Unlike the spine this palpation may help identify the symptomatic structure especially where the structure is readily accessible, for example, the medial collateral ligament of the knee or the supraspinatus tendon of the shoulder. Hence palpation in the periphery provides more diagnostically useful information than palpation in the spine.

Testing passive motion

After soft tissue palpation the physiotherapist proceeds to test the passive motion of the symptomatic spinal region or peripheral joint. Detailed descriptions of how to perform these assessment procedures are available in many of the manual therapy texts (see Kaltenborn, 1980; Grieve, 1984; Maitland, 1986) and therefore will not be described in detail here.

Passive accessory motion tests

There are two different types of information collected from passive accessory motion tests. The first is the patient's report of symptom behaviour in response to the test, and the second is the physiotherapist's perception of the quality of the movement that results from the forces applied during the test. The physiotherapist makes a judgement regarding stiffness based on the amount of force applied and the amount of displacement that results. This stiffness is then compared with adjacent levels and the physiotherapist's expectation of normal stiffness for that level, to determine whether abnormal stiffness is present. The patient is then reassessed to establish whether there has been any change in signs and symptoms. Because PAIVM testing and PAIVM treatment procedures are quite similar, improvement in the patient's condition following PAIVM testing is regarded by many physiotherapists as a good sign that PAIVM treatment will be successful.

Passive physiological intervertebral movement tests

To gain more specific information about the range of physiological movement available at various intervertebral segments, PPIVM techniques can be performed. Information gained from accessory movement testing of the spine is used to establish which levels to examine using PPIVM testing,

although PPIVMs are also performed a few levels above and below the symptomatic spinal region. The results of active movement testing help select the physiological movements to be examined. For example, if a patient with low back pain is restricted in flexion and lateral flexion, these are the PPIVMs that are assessed. PPIVM techniques are primarily performed to identify intervertebral segments with restricted range of movement by comparison with the contralateral side and adjacent levels. It needs to be remembered, however, that different spinal levels will demonstrate varying ranges of motion, and that a unilateral movement restriction will affect movement of the contralateral side. Little information is gained from PPIVM testing in relation to symptoms. After PPIVM testing the patient's signs and symptoms are reassessed and, if the patient appears improved, passive physiological mobilization techniques, such as rotation, flexion or lateral flexion, may be selected as a treatment.

Current use of passive motion tests

In the spine

Passive motion tests are used by physiotherapists for a number of purposes in addition to establishing a clinical diagnosis and selecting treatment. They are also used to predict prognosis and to document patient recovery. Although these tests have been used for all of these purposes, current evidence suggests that not all of these uses are in fact valid.

It is probably important to state first of all that passive motion tests are not useful in establishing a structural diagnosis to explain the patient's spinal pain. In fact, current opinion is that it is not possible to make a structural diagnosis for the majority of patients with spinal pain even after a full clinical examination and the use of imaging and laboratory tests (Spitzer, 1987; Nachemson, 1992). In the common case where a structural diagnosis cannot be made, the patient is usually described as having non-specific spinal pain.

Caution needs to be employed when using the test results to document patient recovery. Considerable evidence has shown that the patient's report of symptom provocation with the test is more reliable than the physiotherapist's perception of movement. It is probably more useful therefore to use information regarding the degree of symptoms reproduced on a passive motion test when deciding whether a patient has improved or not.

Similarly the symptom response may be more helpful when selecting the region to be treated and the technique to apply. This point is taken up further when discussing reliability and validity in this section.

To date there is little experimental evidence to suggest that the presence of pain and/or movement abnormalities on passive motion tests are a prerequisite for a patient to benefit from manual therapy. DiFabio in 1992 reviewed the large number of clinical trials that have evaluated spinal manipulation to provide a profile of the type of patient that would respond to manipulation. Interestingly subjects with pain or reduced range on passive motion testing were not a feature of this group of patients, whereas factors related to the area and duration of pain and the presence of pending litigation were more indicative of whether a patient would improve after manipulation. Koes *et al.* (1993) came to a similar conclusion in a subgroup analysis of their manipulation clinical trial. These results suggest that passive motion tests may not help select patients likely to benefit from manipulation. Information from the history such as central or bilateral low back pain of less than one month's duration and no pending litigation best describes the patient likely to benefit from manipulation.

The few clinical trials that have demonstrated a positive effect after vertebral mobilization have been poorly designed and therefore provide little information about the group most likely to benefit from this treatment. It is probable that, similarly to manipulation, the history findings may be more useful in selecting the patient most likely to respond to mobilization. These history findings are likely to be very similar to those documented for manipulation.

Passive motion tests are probably of most value in helping to select a region to be treated and the technique to apply. The reproduction of symptoms or the recognition of movement abnormalities such as abnormal stiffness during the performance of the test is usually regarded as an indication that treatment should be directed to that spinal segment. The direction of application of the force may be inclined medially or laterally, and in a cephalad or caudad direction depending on which is most provocative in patients with non-irritable conditions, and least provocative in patients with irritable conditions. Frequently the manual test that reveals these findings is used as the actual treatment technique. Improvement in the patient's signs and symptoms after a passive motion test is also regarded as a strong indication that the testing procedure should be used as a treatment at that level.

All this information must be considered in relation to the history findings. In this regard a useful guide is the concept of 'comparability' advocated by Maitland (1986). This concept suggests that positive passive motion test results are only of clinical significance if they can logically be related to the patient's symptoms. For example, increased stiffness noted at T4 is not anatomically linked to a patient's buttock pain whereas tenderness and stiffness at L5 are anatomically related.

In summary the decision to perform passive motion testing in patients with spinal disorders is based upon a proposed relationship between symptoms and abnormal passive movement or stiffness, and the hypothesized mechanism of action of mobilization and manipulation. The usefulness of passive motion testing in helping to isolate symptomatic structures, assisting in determining patient prognosis and predicting whether a patient is improving or not has still to be investigated. It is unlikely that passive motion tests alone will provide this information, but they may prove useful when combined with information from other tests. These issues will be discussed further below when the validity and reliability of passive motion testing is examined.

In the periphery

Passive motion testing is frequently performed on patients presenting with disorders of peripheral joints. In contrast to the spine, passive motion testing in the periphery can be used to help establish which structure is the source of symptoms. For example, in patients with knee pain and instability following an injury, there are a range of passive motion tests such as the Lachman test and the valgus stress test (Magee, 1987) that can be used to help establish which anatomical structure has been damaged. It is important to note that in isolation the results of a single test may not accurately determine the diagnosis but will need to be considered along with the results of other physical tests and relevant history findings.

Similarly to the situation with spinal pain, when a structural diagnosis cannot be made for a peripheral disorder and serious pathology such as cancer has been excluded as a source of symptoms, passive motion tests can be used as treatment procedures to decrease pain and increase range of movement. Where the pathology of the disorder has been clearly established these passive mobilization procedures may still be useful; however, they need to be applied with respect to the nature of the pathology present. For example if the patient has an acute partial disruption of the medial collateral ligament, mobilization procedures have the potential to adversely affect the underlying pathology and should probably be avoided. In contrast, these procedures are unlikely to affect the pathology of an osteoarthritic knee and can be safely used to address any associated pain or loss of range.

Kaltenborn (1980) has suggested an indirect method for determining the most appropriate direction in which to assess and treat peripheral joints. This method is mainly based on the work of MacConnaill and Basmajian (1969) who theorized that the type of movement occurring between joint surfaces is primarily determined by the shape of the joint surfaces. MacConnaill and Basmajian described joint surface movement as a combination of spin, slide and roll – a slide occurring when the same point on one surface contacts a new point on the opposing surface, and a roll occuring when equidistant points on two surfaces contact each other. He suggested that when a convex surface moves on a concave one the direction of the slide that accompanies the roll is in the opposite direction to that of the roll. Thus when the arm is moved into abduction Kaltenborn suggests that the convex humeral head not only rolls upwards but also slides downwards on the concave glenoid cavity. Therefore caudal gliding mobilization of the humeral head may be performed to improve abduction. Kaltenborn states that this indirect method of determining the direction of mobilization should be used when the patient has severe pain, the joint is very hypomobile, or the examiner has insufficient expertise to feel the joint gliding movement (Kaltenborn, 1980).

More recently several studies (Poppen and Walker, 1976; Harryman *et al.*, 1990; McClure and Flowers, 1992) have challenged this convex/concave rule of joint surface motion. It has been demonstrated that during physiological movement, accessory movement occurs in the direction opposite to that predicted by the convex/concave rule. It is most likely that the degree and direction of accessory motion is dependent on many factors other than the joint surface shape, including the external forces generated by the muscles and periarticular structures. It would appear sensible therefore, that after a decision to include passive motion testing in the physical examination, all directions of passive motion be assessed.

Interpretation of test results

Reliability of passive motion tests

The degree to which we rely on the results of passive motion tests in helping to select the treatment is dependent upon the amount of error involved in these clinical measurements. Measurements with large errors should not be used as the basis for important clinical decisions. This section will consider the error associated with these tests by reviewing the reliability and validity of these tests.

The reliability of manual assessment procedures is typically affected by the type of judgement made with the test. When the tests are used to make a judgement on factors such as joint range of motion, end-feel, compliance, the presence of muscle spasm, trigger points or bony anomalies, the tests yield results of poor to fair reliability. In contrast when the test is used to make judgements related to pain, the test yields results of good reliability. This result has been observed in the assessment of the cervical, thoracic and lumbar spine and the SIJ by physiotherapists, doctors, chiropractors and osteopaths (Maher and Latimer, 1992). Interestingly while clinical experience does seem to result in higher intra-tester reliability, the more important inter-rater reliability is not affected. While these results in isolation may not strongly support the use of manual assessment procedures, they must be viewed in context.

It is important to note that few tests have perfect reliability and in fact some important judgements made by health workers have surprisingly low reliability. For example, recent studies (Sidor *et al.*, 1993; Siebenrock and Gerber, 1993) have shown that shoulder fracture classification by orthopaedic surgeons and radiologists similarly has reliability as poor as that of manual posteroanterior (PA) stiffness assessment (e.g. I.C.C. < 0.4: Maher and Adams, 1994). None of the physical assessment procedures used to examine the spine have perfect reliability but rather range from very good to poor reliability. Where instruments such as an inclinometer or flexible rule are used to measure the range of movement of the spine, very good reliability can be attained by trained testers; however, inexperienced raters can produce results of only fair reliability. Visual estimation of spinal range and posture can yield measurements of poor reliability as can reflex and sensation testing and manual muscle testing. The reality is that all the information collected in the physical assessment contains some error and so is fallible and this should be reflected in how information is used to make clinical decisions. Against this background it seems sensible that measurements with a large error should not be used as the sole basis for important clinical decisions.

The results of the studies on the reliability of manual assessment procedures suggest that, if a clinical decision is to be made based upon a single test, the more reliable pain provocation tests should be used in preference to other manual tests. However, a clinical decision is rarely made using the results of one test. Usually an overall impression is made based upon the results of a pool of tests. Unfortunately there have been few studies that have examined the reliability of judgements based upon the results of several tests.

One study, that of Cibulka *et al.* (1988), found that judgements on the presence or absence of SIJ dysfunction were highly reliable ($K = 0.88$) when the physiotherapists based their judgement upon a number of SIJ mobility and alignment tests adopting a decision rule that required that at least three of the four tests be positive. This strategy of basing clinical decisions upon the results of a number of manual tests has a firm basis. One principle of statistics is that the mean of several measurements is a more accurate measure than a single measure (Fleiss, 1986). This strategy may also be applied to other regions of the spine. For example, if passive motion tests are positive at both L4 and L5, but more of the passive motion tests are positive at L5, then treatment should be directed to L5. Further, tests that reproduce the patient's symptoms (which are more reliable and so contain less error) are probably an even stronger suggestion that treatment should be directed to that level.

Validity of passive motion tests

Several studies have examined the validity of manual assessment procedures. For the purposes of this text, however, only the validity of PAIVM testing will be considered. Although Maitland (1986) describes the test as one of accessory intervertebral movement, the true nature of the movement produced by the test is somewhat different. Although the tests do produce movement of the contact vertebra relative to its starting position, not all of this movement could be invertebral movement. Lee and Moseley (1991) have measured PA movement of the contact vertebra of 15 mm when a PA force of 150 N is applied to L3. If this movement is purely inter-vertebral movement, i.e. movement of the tested level on its neighbour, then significant encroachment of the cauda equina would result, because the diameter of the lumber dural sac is of the same magnitude, being approximately 15 mm (Penning, 1992).

The spine is in fact a series of linked segments and so it is to be expected that when a PA force is applied to one lumbar vertebra, movement of the whole lumbar region would occur (Figure 6.9). Lee and Moseley (1991) have modelled the response of the spine to a PA central pressure and predicted

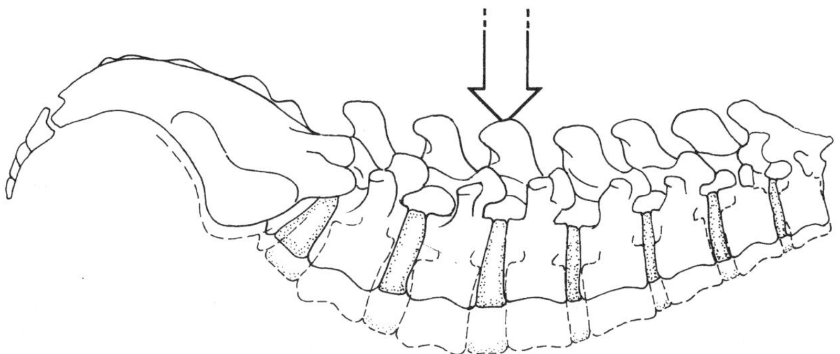

Figure 6.9 Posteroanterior pressure applied to the spinous process results in movement of the whole spine, even at levels quite distant to the site at which pressure is applied, although movement is emphasized at the level sustaining the force

that, with a 100 N PA force applied to the L4 spinous process, only 5–7% of the movement perceived by the therapist would be true intervertebral joint movement. This prediction is consistent with an earlier radiographic study by Ward (1988). This study showed that 50% of the perceived displacement seems to be taken up in compression of the soft tissues overlying the spinous process, with some lumbar spine extension occurring. The study did not note any substantial intervertebral shear displacement.

It therefore seems clear that PAIVM tests cannot be validly used to make inferences about intervertebral motion. However, this does not preclude the tests from being used to make a judgement of the stiffness of the complex movement that results from the PA pressure. Because of the complex movement that results from a PA central pressure it may be more useful to talk of tests of PA stiffness rather than passive accessory intervertebral movement tests.

It is also important to consider whether the passive accessory motion tests are useful in discriminating asymptomatic subjects from symptomatic subjects. Sturesson *et al.* in 1989 investigated the range of motion of the SIJ in subjects with and without SIJ pain. The study used tantalum markers implanted in the sacrum and ilium and stereophotogrammetric analysis and found that the range of motion was in fact quite small with sagittal rotation ranging from 0.8 to 3.9° and movement between joint surfaces ranging from 0.1 to 1.6 mm. The study found that there was no difference in range of motion in SIJ between the symptomatic subjects presumed to have low back pain arising from SIJ, and so raises questions about the value of performing clinical SIJ mobility tests to screen patients for SIJ dysfunction.

Finally it is useful to consider whether these 'PAIVM tests', when compared with other tests used to identify which vertebral levels are symptomatic, give the same results. Jull *et al.* (1988) found that a manipulative physiotherapist using PAIVM testing was able to correctly identify all symptomatic zygapophyseal joints that had previously been identified using a radiologically controlled diagnostic block. The physiotherapist also used these manual tests to reproduce the patient's pain and it may have been this more reliable pain information, rather than information about spinal compliance, that contributed to the high success in identification. This suggestion is supported by the study of Phillips and Twomey (1993) which compared a manipulative physio-

therapist's diagnosis of the symptomatic level with the level established by a unilevel lumbar spinal block procedure. This study found that when the physiotherapist used the verbal patient response during PAIVM testing to identify the symptomatic level there was 100% sensitivity in diagnosing the symptomatic level. In contrast when the physiotherapist did not attend to the verbal patient response but only to what they could feel during the performance of the test, sensitivity fell to 60%. Considered together these studies provide strong support for the suggestion that the verbal patient response is probably the most valuable piece of information to collect during PAIVM testing.

Sensitivity of passive motion tests

For a test to be useful it must be sufficiently sensitive to detect clinically relevant differences with at least the ability to discriminate asymptomatic subjects from symptomatic subjects. Jull and Bullock (1987) suggest that the PA central pressure is sensitive; however all the physiotherapy studies that have evaluated the sensitivity of the test to detect differences in stiffness have shown a poor ability to discriminate stiffness (Trott *et al.*, 1989; Viner *et al.*, 1991). This relatively poor ability of physiotherapists to discriminate stiffness is intriguing because studies outside the physiotherapy literature have shown that subjects have a good ability to discriminate stiffness, e.g. Scott-Blair and Coppen (1939) showed that subjects could discriminate differences in stiffness as small as 9%. In contrast, the study of Trott, *et al.* (1989) found that physiotherapists could only reliably detect differences in PA stiffness when the difference was of the order of 200%. Given this background it is not possible to provide a meaningful estimate of the sensitivity of tests of stiffness save to say that it is an area that needs further investigation.

Implications for treatment

Consideration of the reliability, validity and sensitivity of passive motion tests suggests that at present treatment decisions should be guided more by symptom reproduction than by the perceived quality of movement. The first treatment option should be to direct treatment to the most painful spinal level (unless of course that level is not anatomically capable of producing the patient's symptoms). If this treatment strategy is unsuccessful, then the less reliable stiffness findings can be used to select the level to treat but the physiotherapist needs to acknowledge that the stiffness information is less reliable, i.e. error prone, and so they may waste time directing treatment to the wrong level.

Because the most effective treatment dose is yet to be determined for manual treatments the appropriateness of dose can only be established through close monitoring of the patient's condition. After each repetition of the mobilization, the patient should be reassessed and the dosage altered accordingly. The duration of each repetition is best determined by the patient's pain response and the spinal compliance perceived by the therapist while performing the mobilization. If in a patient with an irritable condition, the patient complains that the symptoms are worsening or the therapist perceives an increase in tissue compliance, then the mobilization should be halted and the patient reassessed. If during the mobilization there is an improvement or no change in the patient's status then the mobilization is usually continued for 30–45 s.

In patients with non-irritable conditions, pain is often provoked during the mobilization. The mobilization is generally continued until the therapist perceives a change in stiffness, the patient reports that the symptoms have significantly changed, or, in the absence of these factors, 45–60 s has elapsed. The number of repetitions to be performed is usually based on reassessment of signs and symptoms after one repetition of mobilization.

Generally if the patient is continuing to improve, the repetition should be repeated. However, when treating a patient on the first occasion, it is safest to adhere to the guidelines suggested by Maitland (1986): two repetitions are given to patients with irritable conditions, whereas patients with non-irritable conditions may be treated with three to four repetitions.

One parameter of treatment dose, the grade of movement, can be quantified reliably if defined in relation to range (Matyas and Bach, 1985) and the pain response rather than a perceived resistance curve. If this approach is adopted, then the dose of treatment can be recorded and allows meaningful communication between therapists.

Conclusion

Passive motion tests are widely used by physiotherapists to select patients likely to benefit from mobilization, to formulate a clinical diagnosis and to help select the region and the most appropriate form of treatment for patients with both spinal and peripheral musculoskeletal disorders. Many studies have examined the reliability of these tests, but the more difficult task of establishing validity has been largely avoided. Physiotherapists need to consider that decisions based on the patient's pain response to passive motion testing are likely to provide a more accurate guide to patient management.

Muscle testing

R. Herbert

This section will examine some principles underlying clinical testing of muscle strength and muscle length.

Testing of muscle strength

Clinicians test muscle strength both to provide information for diagnosis and to assess the effectiveness of intervention aimed at increasing muscle strength.

Diagnosis

People develop weakness for many different reasons. Sometimes the cause of the weakness may not be obvious from the person's history. Then a careful physical examination can provide clues, especially about the distribution of weakness, which can aid diagnosis.

Manual muscle testing is widely used for diagnostic purposes, probably because the simplicity of the test procedures means that many muscle groups can be tested in a short period of time. A number of different manual muscle testing protocols are in wide clinical use (Lamb, 1985), but all use similar criteria to assign grades based on the ability of the muscles to contract through range and against gravity or manual resistance. Some protocols are designed to test individual muscles (Daniels and Worthingham, 1986), whereas others test muscle groups (Kendall *et al.*, 1993). Although tests of individual muscles are desirable for diagnostic purposes, the validity of assumptions underlying procedures which profess to test individual muscles is dubious; in reality it is often difficult to differentiate the weakness of one muscle from weakness of other muscles from the same muscle group. For this reason, it would seem more appropriate to test muscle groups, rather than individual muscles.

Studies of the reliability of manual muscle testing suggest that test–retest and inter-therapist reliability is moderate [see Lamb (1985) for a brief review]. Typically, when several therapists use manual muscle testing to measure the strength of the same patients they agree on 50 or 60% of their measures, and they agree to within one grade on more than 90% of their measures. Given this finding, and that some of the manual muscle test grades (especially grades III and IV) encompass an enormous range of strengths (Munsat, 1990), it would appear that manual muscle testing is likely to be useful for detecting gross muscle weakness or for detecting large changes in muscle strength over time, but it is not sufficiently sensitive or reliable to detect subtle weakness or small changes in strength.

Muscle testing is used for another purpose which arguably also falls under the heading of diagnosis. Tests of muscle can help localize pain-causing lesions. In particular, muscle testing is often used to determine if a muscle is the source of a person's pain (Corrigan and Maitland, 1983). For example, if a person's history is indicative of a hamstring muscle tear, a therapist may choose to see if pain is elicited with a strong isometric knee flexor contraction. The rationale is that if the muscle or its tendon is a source of pain, muscle contraction will stress the injured tissues and reproduce the person's pain. Other pain-sensitive structures will experience relatively little stress, and therefore this strategy should not elicit pain if tissues other than the muscle are responsible for the pain. Clinicians (and even some academics) know, however, that there is a tendency for isometric tests of muscle to produce false positives, because muscle contraction may stress other (non-muscle) structures. In particular, strong muscle contractions compress joint surfaces and stress ligaments. Therefore, positive findings should be taken with a grain of salt, but negative findings can be considered quite strong evidence that the tested muscles are not the source of pain.

Quantifying the effect of intervention

It can be useful to measure muscle strength to determine if training has been aimed at appropriate muscle groups and is appropriate in terms of intensity, achieving clients' goals etc. Also, measurements of muscle strength can be useful for motivating people to 'comply' with training protocols in cases of prolonged rehabilitation.

Three criteria should be applied to determine the suitability of any strength test.

1. Reliability – the test must be sufficiently reliable to distinguish 'signal' from 'noise', i.e. it must be possible to be confident that observed changes that are of a clinically significant magnitude are not simply measurement error. Typically, with training, people can be expected to experience strength gains of 0.5–3% per day (McDonagh and Davies, 1984). This means that, if measurements of strength are to be made weekly, they must be able to reliably detect changes in strength of between about 4% and 20%. The reliability of many clinical strength measurement procedures has been reviewed by Mayhew and Rothstein (1985) and Bohannon (1990).

2. Validity – refers to the degree to which useful inferences can be drawn from test measures. When physiotherapists test strength to monitor progress, their concern usually is to make inferences about the ability of muscles to produce tension for the performance of motor tasks. For example, measurements of knee extensor strength after knee reconstruction are really only of interest in so far as they tell us something about how well the person is able to use their knee extensor muscles for tasks such as running, jumping and kicking.

There have been very few studies which directly tackle the issue of the degree to which measures of muscle strength provide information about the ability of muscles to generate tension during the performance of motor tasks. One study that provides some insights into this issue simply looked at the relationship between a number of different measures (e.g. isokinetic, hydraulic and free-weight measures) of bench-press strength (Hortobagyi, *et al.*, 1989). This study found that, after measurement errors were accounted for, there was a moderate correlation between different measures of strength, i.e. people who performed well on one measure often, but not always, performed well on other measures of strength. To the extent that the different tests agreed they could be said to be measuring the same thing, but there was not perfect agreement between tests. This means that proficiency in one test may partly reflect a specific proficiency at the type of muscle contraction required for that test, rather than in some generalizable strength parameter.

There are still not enough data to be certain about the degree of generality that can be attached to most currently used measures of strength. However, it is probably reasonable to conclude provisionally that any reliable meas-ure of muscle strength will provide some measure of 'functional' strength (i.e. people with muscle weakness will tend to perform poorly on most measures of the strength of their weak muscles). However, the more closely the testing conditions resemble the task of interest the more valid the test is likely to be (i.e. the more inferences can be made about the ability of the muscles to generate tension during the performance of those tasks). Clearly more research should be directed to investigating the validity of clinical measures of muscle strength.

3. Practicalities – some measuring tools are quick and easy to use, whereas others are time-consuming and useful for testing only a few muscle groups. The former are obviously pre-ferred.

There are many procedures used by clinical therapists for measuring muscle strength. The next section briefly discusses the reliability, validity and practicalities of four of the most widely used procedures for measuring muscle strength.

Hand-held dynamometers

The available literature suggests that hand-held dynamometers provide a highly reliable way of measuring isometric strength (for review see Bohannon, 1990). The exception is when the subject being tested is capable of producing such large forces that the tester has difficulty keeping the dynamometer still (Bohannon, 1990). Hand-held dynamometers are suitable for measuring the strength of most large peripheral muscle groups, and some specialized versions are available for testing smaller peripheral muscle groups, such as the muscles of the hand.

The appeal of these devices is that they can provide a highly reliable measure of isometric muscle strength with little more difficulty than manual muscle testing. The major drawback is that they can only be used to measure isometric strength, and (as discussed above under Validity) it is not clear how well inferences can be made from tests of this type to the ability of muscle to generate tension for task performance.

In the author's opinion, the reliability and ease of use of hand-held dynamometers make them the tool of choice for a wide range of clinical situations in which it is necessary to measure muscle strength.

Isokinetics

Isokinetic testing machines enable the measure-ment of torque produced by muscles as they perform constant-velocity contractions. These devices have increased in popularity over the past decade to the extent that many clinics now have one or several of them. Perhaps the most useful feature of isokinetic machines is their high reliabil-ity – typically test–retest reliability is sufficiently high that measured changes of as little as 10% can be confidently considered to be real changes in strength, rather than measurement error (for review see Mayhew and Rothstein, 1985).

Despite their popularity, however, isokinetic machines have some distinct disadvantages. At a technical level, isokinetic torque measures are prone to a number of artifacts [particularly inertial artifacts caused by unwanted accelerations of the limb during testing (Winter *et al.*, 1981; Sapega, *et al.*, 1982; Herzog, 1988)], although these can now be dealt with reasonably satisfactorily with features such as 'preloading' (e.g. Gravel *et al.*, 1988; for a fuller discussion of these issues the reader is referred to Mayhew and Rothstein, 1985). More significantly, it can be argued that isokinetic testing conditions are far removed from the way in which muscles are required to contract for the performance of everyday tasks, and that therefore isokinetic tests may provide a less valid test of the ability to generate muscle tension during the performance of meaningful motor tasks. Equally problematic is the inflexibility of isokinetic devices – they do not lend themselves easily to testing of many different muscle groups, and few clinics can afford to have a suite of isokinetic machines specifically configured for every key muscle group.

Manual muscle testing

The reliability of manual muscle testing was discussed above, where it was noted that it provides an insensitive and only moderately reliable test of muscle strength. Although convenient, manual muscle testing is unlikely to be sufficiently sensitive and reliable to provide a satisfactory measure of the changes in strength of a magnitude that are often of interest clinically.

Functional tests

Functional measures of muscle strength are probably widely used in practice, but they have not often been described in the literature, and they have rarely been subjected to experimental investigation. With a little bit of imagination, simple functional tasks such as stepping on to a block or standing up from a chair can easily be turned into a measure of strength. For example, to obtain a measure of the strength of lower limb muscle groups a person could be asked to step up on blocks of increasing height (see Figure 6.10). The highest block on to which the person could step provides an indirect measure of the torque-generating capacity of muscles of the lower limb.

The types of muscle contraction utilized in these tests explicitly resemble those required for motor task performance, so they have a face validity – it is likely that these functional tests provide the best possible validity for this sort of inference. On the negative side, the reliability of these tests is not known. Reliability of functional tests probably varies with the functional task being tested. Also, functional tests demand that therapists are able to ensure that subjects do not utilize compensatory movement strategies which might enable successful task performance without generating large forces with weak muscle groups. For example, when testing lower limb strength in the manner described above, it is necessary to prevent subjects throwing their arms forward and pushing-off with the contralateral leg (this can be done by asking subjects to hold their hands behind their backs,

keeping the contralateral knee extended, and standing on the heel of the contralateral leg, Fig. 6.10). Only then can the therapist be sure that the lower limb muscles of the test leg are being tested. Lastly, because these tests often examine a number of muscle groups simultaneously they provide relatively little information about which muscle groups are weak, and sometimes this information is useful when structuring training.

Measuring the length of muscles

Measurement of 'muscle length' really involves testing whether muscle–tendon units are short or inextensible. A number of clinical observations may be suggestive of muscle shortening, but it is often not possible to be certain that adaptive shortening of muscle (as distinct from other tissues that cross the joint) is responsible for a loss of passive joint range of motion. For example, it would be reasonable to suspect that soleus muscle

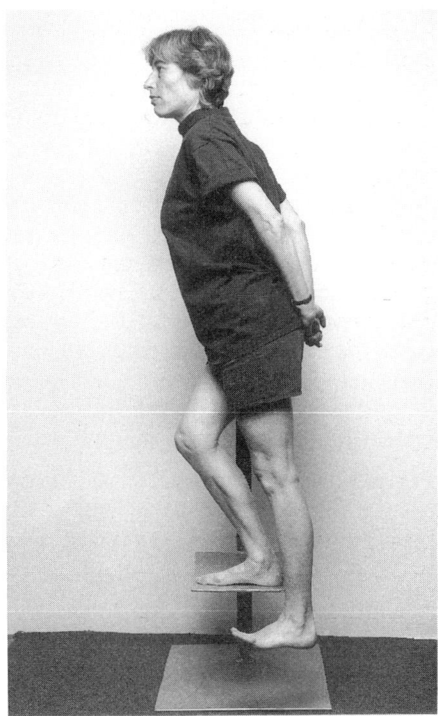

Figure 6.10 Functional exercises such as climbing stairs can be progressed by increasing the difficulty of the task, for example by increasing the height of the step

shortening is responsible for a loss of dorsiflexion range of motion if the patient feels a stretch in the region of the soleus as the ankle is dorsiflexed or if the tendon and belly of the soleus muscle become palpably very taught as the ankle is dorsiflexed to plantargrade with knee flexed. When these conditions are met it is reasonable to hypothesize that the soleus muscle is short. However, even in these rather restrictive circumstances it is not possible to definitively implicate a short soleus muscle because it is still possible that the major limitation to joint range lies in other muscles or periarticular connective tissues.

In contrast, useful measures of the degree of shortening can be made on muscles that cross two or more mobile joints. These muscles can be stretched over one joint (e.g. the knee can be extended to lengthen gastrocnemius) so that the muscle becomes the sole or dominant restraint to movement at its other joint (i.e. with the knee extended the gastrocnemius can become the major restraint to dorsiflexion). If the muscle does provide the dominant limitation to range of motion at the second joint, the test can logically be said to be a test of the muscle's length.

Note that, almost by definition, these tests can be performed in two ways. For example, the length of the hamstring muscles can be tested by measuring either hip flexion with the knee extended or knee extension with the hip flexed (in this particular example the therapist would need to differentiate between the limitation provided by the hamstring muscles and those due to neural tension). In either case, the position of one joint must be standardized before the range of motion at the other joint can be measured. Thus, if hamstring length is measured by flexing the hip and then measuring the amount of knee extension range, the hip must first be placed in a reproducible position (say, 90° of flexion), or else the final measure of knee extension range will not be reproducible.

In able-bodied people or people with only subtle muscle shortening, the logic of these tests does not necessarily hold up – it may not be possible to sufficiently lengthen the muscle over one joint to cause it to become the major limitation to range of motion at the second joint. Then the test is no more rigorous a test of muscle length than the tests of single joint muscles discussed above. Fortunately it is possible to ascertain whether the test does sufficiently lengthen the muscle of interest. This is done after measuring the length of the muscle, by releasing the stretch from the first joint (e.g. after measuring dorsiflexion with the knee extended as a measure of gastrocnemius shortening, flex the knee). If this causes the measured range to increase substantially (e.g. if there is then an increase in dorsiflexion range) the tester can be confident that the test did put sufficient stretch on the muscle to cause it to become the major limitation to the measured movement, and therefore that the measured range was a reasonable measure of the length of the muscle. This is an important part of the procedure for measuring muscle length, because the test is valid only if the muscle can be shown to be a major limitation to the movement tested.

The reliability of many commonly used procedures for measuring muscle length has received little attention in the experimental literature. However there is little reason to suspect that they should be any less reliable than other joint range of motion measures. Most joint range of motion measures have an acceptable to high level of reliability [for reviews see Miller (1985) and Gadjosik and Bohannon (1987)]. Any measure of joint range can be made more reliable by using a standardized procedure (Gadjosik and Bohannon, 1987), marking bony landmarks (Fish and Wingate, 1985), and (where practical and for passive measures) by standardizing the force applied by the therapist to the joint (Brand, 1985; Ada and Herbert, 1988).

Motor performance: evaluation and intervention

J. Carr and R. Shepherd

Lesions of the musculoskeletal system affect the motor apparatus, i.e. the effector part of the system through which we act to achieve our goals. Such lesions affect the way movements are performed. The effect can be far-reaching because of the natural coupling between body segments, i.e. if a

lesion affects one segment or the link between two segments (a joint), then the movement of other segments along the linkage will also be affected. In this way, during walking for example, a stiff ankle joint will affect not only movement at the ankle but will also affect movement at other joints, such as hip extension toward the end of the stance phase. The evaluation of human movement is made complex not only by the dynamics of the segmental linkage but also by the action of monoarticular and biarticular muscles and by the synergic relationships between muscle groups. Furthermore, muscle activation patterns (both postural and task-related) are specific to both task and the context in which the action is performed. The only way one can be certain that treatment directed toward local signs and symptoms (e.g. pain, joint stiffness or muscle weakness) is effective in improving the performance of a functional action (e.g. walking, stair ascent) is by measuring performance of that action in some way.

Indications for testing

Evaluation of functional actions is used both as a guide to intervention and as a measure of outcome. Individuals who experience musculoskeletal lesions, whether as a result of a sporting injury, a car accident, a back injury at work, a degenerative disease or surgery, attend the physiotherapist for relief of pain or stiffness as a means of improving the performance of actions critical to their daily lives. A major objective of physiotherapy for these individuals is, therefore, to regain optimal performance of actions that have become dysfunctional.

Physiotherapy, however, has traditionally utilized methods for relieving pain, increasing joint range and strengthening muscles with the assumption that improved motor performance would naturally follow. Initial evaluation has been concentrated in assessments of relatively local phenomena such as range of pain-free motion and strength of individual muscles. Tests of changes occurring during and at the conclusion of treatment have been similarly based. We would argue that measuring performance of an action in its entirety is more relevant to functional ability than testing an isolated muscle or group of muscles as they act over one joint. The effect of intervention to decrease pain and stiffness, therefore, is examined in the context of the actions the individual has to or wishes to carry out: for example, walking, stair climbing and descent, jogging, swimming, standing up and sitting down, reaching toward an object, grasping and manipulating different objects in order to carry out specific intentions.

Test procedures

Evaluation of motor performance involves an analysis of any critical actions with which the individual is having difficulty because of the musculoskeletal or peripheral neurological lesion. The patient's performance is matched with a normal biomechanical model of that action, if available. Evaluation is either based on observation (qualitative) or it involves some form of measurement, in which case it is quantitative.

Qualitative evaluation

This involves observing the individual performing some relevant action. In order to match this person's performance against a normal model, the physiotherapist needs knowledge of the biomechanics and control features of the action. Only the kinematic features of an action, such as angular displacements at joints and linear displacements of body parts, are readily observable and it is these that can be matched against what would normally be expected. The physiotherapist has to infer the velocity, acceleration and force components underlying the displacements, as well as the muscle-activation patterns.

Simple visual observations lack reliability and some validity, although in the hands of a therapist with a sufficient understanding of biomechanics, they can provide valid information for the development of a treatment or training strategy for that individual. However, when the clinician needs to demonstrate a change in a patient's performance, observational methods of evaluation can provide only suspect conclusions and will rarely be attended to by either patient or other interested party such as physician or health service provider.

A critical future development in scientific rehabilitation practice will be the more general use of reliable measurement devices to provide the therapist with detailed and objective information. This information provides a more effective guide to treatment and training as well as quantitative methods of assessing outcome.

Quantitative evaluation

The biomechanics of an action can be examined using a variety of tools. Smith (1990) describes many of the methods of kinematic, kinetic and muscle activation measurement that have value in the clinical evaluation of motor performance. He illustrates how the equipment needed for measurement ranges from the simple and inexpensive (tape measure, stopwatch, camera) to the complex and expensive (electrogoniometers, accelerometers, forceplates, two- and three-dimensional imaging systems).

In the absence of equipment for complex motion analysis, components of locomotor actions, such as stride length or width, can be measured using non-permanent marking pens on the patient's heels, or by chalking the soles of the feet and having the patient walk on a darker surface. Time taken to walk a certain distance can be measured with a stopwatch. These are somewhat indirect measures of locomotion, in that improvement in these measurements is assumed to reflect improvement in performance. Nevertheless, such methods constitute, if reliably performed, valid measures of change.

Although motion analysis utilizing videotaping of performance is often used to generate extensive and complex data about kinematic and (if used with a forceplate) kinetic components, the use of videotape also enables quite simple measurements to be taken. Transparency paper placed over a still image on a videoscreen enables joint angles to be measured, and, when measured frame-by-frame, angular velocity can be calculated. Van Vliet (1988) describes the methodological details of this technique of deriving kinematic details of walking. Still photography can also be used to measure joint angles and changes over time (e.g. Ada and Canning, 1990). Of course, standardization of measurement technique is necessary for these values to be reliable.

Interpretation of test results and implications for treatment

Evaluation of motor performance involves a comparison between the patient's performance and a normal model of that action. Increasing numbers of biomechanical and motor control studies enable the collection of normative data about common everyday, work-related and sporting actions, for example walking (e.g. Winter, 1987), stair climbing (e.g. Andriacchi *et al.*, 1980), sit-to-stand (e.g. Pai and Rogers, 1991; Carr and Gentile, 1994; Shepherd and Gentile 1994), running (e.g. Mann and Hagy, 1980; Hinrichs, 1990), squat-lifting (e.g.

Scholz, 1993) and jumping (e.g. Hay, 1975; Depena and Chung, 1988).

The analytical process also involves consideration of the typical performance deficits reported in studies of disabled individuals as they perform various actions. Such information clarifies the nature of the movement dysfunction associated with different types of lesion and lesion site. It enables the therapist to predict the nature of the dysfunction resulting from particular injuries or surgical interventions and, where possible, institute procedures to prevent unwanted adaptations.

At this time, few actions apart from walking have been studied in the disabled population. Studies of disabled motor performance include reports of walking and running patterns of individuals with lower limb amputations (Inman *et al.*, 1981; Enoka *et al.*, 1982; Winter and Sienko, 1988). Walking, stair ascent and descent, and sit-to-stand have been studied in individuals after knee replacement surgery (Andriacchi *et al.*, 1982; Weinstein *et al.*, 1986; Jevsevar·*et al.*, 1993) and medial meniscectomy (Moffet *et al.*, 1993) and in subjects with anterior cruciate ligament-deficient knees (Andriacchi *et al.*, 1993).

The qualitative and quantitative evaluation of motor performance, together with input from the patient, gives the physiotherapist an idea of the motor deficit and any adaptive motor behaviours the individual may be using, for example, to avoid pain or lessen the force to be produced over a joint. This information is a guide both to treatment and to change occurring over time. Using quantitative measures, Westwood (1993) described both the biomechanical deficits and the adaptive motor behviours during the action of sit-to-stand in a group of individuals who had been discharged from rehabilitation after total hip replacement (THR). The fact that these individuals were taking little weight through their affected lower limb and could only stand up using their arms to augment vertical propulsion suggests that discharge without follow-up training was premature. After THR surgery it is not typical to test performance of such actions as walking and sit-to-stand, nor is it typical to train such actions specifically (Kerslake *et al.*, 1987; Harris and Sledge, 1990). It is assumed that performance of functional activities will spontaneously improve once pain and stiffness at the hip have been reduced. Improvement may not, however, be so straightforward. The individual may have spent many years developing adaptive motor behaviours to enable some form of mobility to be maintained in the presence of pain and stiffness, and these habitual adaptations are likely to be maintained after surgery.

Measures of functional performance also provide a method of evaluating the relative outcomes of different rehabilitative strategies and the effects of training programmes. Westwood (1993) reported, for example, that after 6 weeks specific training of sit-to-stand, subjects who had used their arms to assist in the action were no longer doing so. Some had also increased the amount of weight taken through the affected leg. This suggests that training resulted in an increase in the ease with which subjects could use their lower limbs during the extension phase of the action.

The maintenance of adaptive and usually relatively inefficient motor patterns may predispose the individual to subsequent episodes of pain and stiffness and may provoke repeated injury. Evaluation of critical actions may, by ensuring that motor performance is significantly improved, be one means of preventing re-injury or subsequent episodes of disability.

Baker and colleagues (1991) have reported the use of a footswitch system, myometer and goniometer in analysing the gait of subjects recovering from fractured neck of femur who had completed a period of gait training on a treadmill. This study illustrates the value of measuring functional motor performance as a means of testing the effectiveness of task-specific training. The trained group was significantly superior to the control group in measures of double-support phase, stance/swing ratio, strength of hip flexion and abduction, and of knee extension. This information provides a valuable measure of outcome, suggesting that treadmill training should become part of the rehabilitation programme of such individuals, with a high degree of probability that any individual with motor dysfunction following hip surgery may also benefit. Such a hypothesis can of course be tested in the clinic, providing further information of relevance to the planning of training programmes.

References

Introduction

Buckley, R.A. (1988). *The Modern Law of Negligence*. London; Butterworths.

Gam, A., Thorsen, H. and Lonnberg, F. (1993). The effect of low-level laser therapy on musculoskeletal pain: a meta-analysis. *Pain*, **52**, 63–6.

Giesen, D. (1988). *International Medical Malpractice Law*. Dordrecht: Martinus Nijhoff Publishers.

Grieve, G.P. (1984). *Mobilisation of the Spine* (4th edn.) London: Churchill Livingstone.

Magee, D.J. (1987). *Orthopedic Physical Assessment*. London: W.B. Saunders.

Maitland, G.D. (1986). *Vertebral Manipulation* (5th edn.) London: Butterworth-Heinemann.

McCloskey, D.I. (1978). Kinesthetic sensibility. *Physiol. Rev.*, **58**, 763–820.

O'Sullivan, J. (1983). *Law for Nurses and Allied Health Professionals in Australia* (3rd edn). Sydney: The Law Book Company.

Siegler, M., Toulmin, S., Zimring, F.E. and Schaffner, K.F. (1987). *Medical Innovation and Bad Outcomes: Legal, Social, and Ethical Responses*. Ann Arbor: Health Administration Press.

Observation

Braun, B. and Amundson, L. (1989). Quantitative assessment of head and shoulder posture. *Arch. Phys. Med. Rehabil.*, **70**, 322–9.

Bullock, J.E., Jull, G.A. and Bullock, M.I. (1987). The relationship of low back pain to postural changes during pregnancy. *Austr. J. Physiother.*, **33**, 10–17.

Dalton, M.B. (1989). The effect of age on cervical posture in a normal female population. In *Proceedings of the 6th Biennial Conference of the Manipulative Therapists Association of Australia*, Adelaide, pp. 34–44.

Diek, G., Kelsey, J., Goel, V. *et al.*, (1985). An epidemiological study of the relationship between postural asymmetry in the teen years and subsequent back and neck pain. *Spine*, **10**, 872–7.

During, H., Goudfrooij, H., Keeson, W. *et al.*, (1985). Towards standards for posture. *Spine*, **10**, 83–7.

Feldman, N., Refshauge, K.M., Goodsell, M. and Adams, R. (1994). The effect of chin retraction exercises on cervical and cervicothoracic posture in an asymptomatic population. In *Proceedings of 4th International Physiotherapy Congress*. 51–3.

Gerrard, B. (1989). The patello-femoral pain syndrome: A clinical trial of the McConnell programme. *Austr. J. Physiother.*, **35**, 71–80.

Griegel-Morris, P., Larson, K., Mueller-Klaus, K. and Oatis, C. (1992). Incidence of common postural abnormalities in the cervical, shoulder, and thoracic regions and their association with pain in two age groups of healthy subjects. *Phys. Ther.*, **72**, 425–30.

Grieve, G.P. (1986). Bony and soft-tissue anomalies of the vertebral column. In *Modern Manual Therapy of the Vertebral Column*, (Grieve, G., ed.), pp. 3–20. London: Churchill Livingstone.

Harms-Ringdahl, K. and Ekholm, J. (1986). Intensity and character of pain and muscular activity levels elicited by maintained extreme flexion position of the lower-cervical–upper-thoracic spine. *Scand. J. Rehabil. Med.*, **18**, 117–26.

Hart, D.L. and Rose, S.J. (1986). Reliability of a noninvasive method for measuring the lumbar curve. *J. Orthop. Sports Phys. Ther.*, **8**, 180–4.

Link, C.S., Nicholson, G.G., Shaddeau, S.A. *et al.*, (1990) Lumbar curvature in standing and sitting in two types of chairs: relationship of hamstring and hip flexor muscle length. *Phys. Ther.*, **10**, 611–18.

Magee, D.J. (1987). *Orthopedic Physical Assessment*. Philadelphia: W.B. Saunders.

Magee, D.J. (1992). *Orthopedic Physical Assessment*, (2nd edn.), pp. 120–2. Philadelphia: W.B. Saunders.

McConnell, J. (1986). The management of chondromalacia patellae: a long term solution. *Austr. J. Physiother.*, **32**, 215–23.

McKenzie, R.A. (1981). *The Lumbar Spine – Mechanical Diagnosis and Therapy*. New Zealand: Spinal Publications.

Milne, J.S. and Lauder, I.J. (1974). Age effects in kyphosis and lordosis in adults. *Ann. Hum. Biol.*, **1**, 327–37.

Pope, M.H., Bevins, T., Wilder, D.G. and Frymoyer, J.W. (1985). The relationship between anthropometric, postural, muscular and mobility characteristics of males aged 18–55. *Spine*, **10**, 644–8.

Raine, S. and Twomey, L. (1994). Posture of the head, shoulders and thoracic spine in comfortable errect standing. *Austr. J. Physiother.*, **40**, 25–32.

Refshauge, K.M., Bolst, L. and Goodsell, M. (1995). The relationship between cervicothoracic posture and the presence of pain. *J. Man. Manip. Ther.*, **3**, 21–4.

Refshauge, K.M., Goodsell, M. and Lee, M. (1994a). Consistency of natural cervical and cervicothoracic posture in standing. *Aust. J. Physiother.*, **40**, 235–40.

Refshauge, K.M., Goodsell, M. and Lee, M. (1994b). The relationship between surface contour and vertebral body measures of upper spine curvature. *Spine.*, **19**, 2180–5.

Soukka, A., Alaranta, H., Tallroth, K. and Heliovaara, M. (1991), Leg-length inequality in people of working age: the association between mild inequality and low-back pain is questionable. *Spine*, **16**, 429–31.

Twomey, L.T. (1992). A rationale for the treatment of back pain and joint pain by manual therapy, *Phys. Ther.*, **72**, 885–92.

Watson, D. and Trott, P. (1993). Cervical headache: an investigation of natural head posture and upper cervical flexor muscle performance. *Cephalalgia*, **13**, 272–84.

Williams, M.M., Hawley, J.A., McKenzie, R.A. and Wijmen, P.M. (1991). A comparison of the effects of two sitting postures on back and referred pain. *Spine*, **16**, 1185–90.

Testing of active movements

Beattie, P., Rothstein, J. and Lamb, R. (1987). Reliability of the attraction method for measuring lumbar spine backward bending. *Phys. Ther.*, **67**, 364–9.

Edwards, B. (1987). Clinical assessment: the use of combined movements in assessment and treatment. In *Physical Therapy of the Low Back* (L. Twomey, and J. Taylor, eds), pp. 175–98. New York: Churchill Livingstone.

Edwards, B. (1988). Combined movements of the cervical spine in examination and treatment. In *Physical Therapy of the Cervical and Thoracic Spine*, (R. Grant, ed.) pp. 125–51,

New York: Churchill Livingstone.

Garrett, T.R., Youdas, J.W. and Madson, T.J. (1993). Reliability of measuring forward head posture in a clinical setting. *J. Orthop. Sports Phys. Ther.*, **17**, 155–60.

Grieve, G.P. (1984). *Mobilisation of the Spine*. Edinburgh: Churchill Livingstone.

Hsieh, C. and Yeung, B. (1986). Active neck motion measurement with a tape measure. *J. Orthop. Sports Phys. Ther.*, **8**, 88–92.

Maitland, G.D. (1986). *Vertebral Manipulation* (5th edn). London: Butterworth-Heinemann.

Matyas, T.A. and Bach, T.M. (1985). The reliability of selected techniques in clinical arthrometrics. *Austr. J. Physiother.*, **5**, 175–99.

McKenzie, R.A. (1981). *The Lumbar Spine – Mechanical Diagnosis and Therapy*. New Zealand: Spinal Publications.

Twomey, L.T. and Taylor, J. (1979). A description of two new instruments for measuring the ranges of sagittal and horizontal plane motions in the lumbar region. *Austr. J. Physiother.*, **25**, 201–4.

Williams, P.L. and Warwick, R. (eds) (1980). *Gray's Anatomy* (36th edn). London: Churchill Livingstone.

Youdas, J.W., Carey, J.R. and Garrett, T.R. (1991). Reliability of measurements of cervical spine range of motion – comparison of three methods. *Phys. Ther.*, **71**, 98–104.

Testing adequacy of cerebral blood flow

Abrahams, V.C. (1981) Sensory and motor specialization in some muscles of the neck. *Trends in Neurosciences*, Jan., 24–27.

Australian Physiotherapy Association (1988). Protocol for premanipulative testing of the cervical spine. *Austr. J. Physiother.*, **34**, 97–100.

Barton, J.W. and Margolis, M.T. (1975). Rotational obstruction of the vertebral artery at the atlantoaxial joint. *Neuroradiology*, **9**, 117–20.

Bogduk, N. (1986). Cervical causes of headaches and dizziness. In *Modern Manual Therapy of the Vertebral Column* (G.P. Grieve, ed.), chapter 27, London: Churchill Livingstone.

Bolton, P.S., Stick, P.E. and Lord, R.S.A. (1989). Failure of clinical tests to predict cerebral ischaemia before neck manipulation. *J. Manip. Physiol. Ther.*, **12**, 304–7.

Brown, B. and Tatlow, W.F.T. (1963). Radiographic studies of the vertebral arteries in cadavers. *Radiology*, **81**, 80–8.

Burton, A.C. (1965). *Physiology and Biophysics of the Circulation – An Introductory Text*, pp. 95–101, Chicago: Year Book Medical Publishers.

Coman, W.B. (1986). Dizziness related to ENT conditions. In *Modern Manual Therapy of the Vertebral Column* (G.P. Grieve, ed.) pp. 303–14. London: Churchill Livingstone.

de Jong, P.T.V.M., de Jong, J.M.B.V., Cohen, B. and Jongkees, L.B.W. (1977). Ataxia and nystagmus induced by injection of local anaesthetics in the neck. *Ann. Neural.*, **1**, 240–6.

Fields, W.S., Brustman, M.E. and Weibel, J. (1965). *Collateral Circulation of the Brain*. Baltimore: Williams and Wilkins.

Fisher, C.M., Gore, I., Okabe, N. and White, P.D. (1965). Atherosclerosis of the carotid and vertebral arteries: extracranial and intracranial. *J. Neuropathol. Exp. Neurol.*, **10**, 92–4.

Frumkin, L. and Baloh, R.W. (1990). Wallenberg's syndrome following neck manipulation. *Neurology*, **40**, 611–15.

Goldberg, M.E., Eggers, H.M. and Couras, P. (1991). The ocular motor system. In *Principles of Neural Science* (3rd edn), (E.R. Kandel, J.H. Schwartz and T.M. Jessel, eds), pp. 660–78 Connecticut: Prentice-Hall International.

Grant, R. (ed) (1988). Dizziness testing and manipulation of the cervical spine. *Physical Therapy of the Cervical and Thoracic Spine, Clinics in Physical Therapy*, vol. 17, chapter 7, New York: Churchill Livingstone, pp. 111–14.

Grant, E.R. (1987). Clinical testing before cervical manipulation – can we recognize the patient at risk? In *Proceedings of the Tenth International Congress of the World Confederation for Physical Therapy*, Part 1, Sydney.

Hardesty, W.H., Whiteacre, W.B., Toole, J.W. *et al.* (1963). Studies on vertebral artery flow in man. *Surge. Gynecol. Obstet.*, **116**, 662–4.

Hart R.G. and Easton, J.D. (1986). Dissections and trauma of cervico-cerebral arteries. In *Stroke: Pathophysiology, Diagnosis and Management* (H.J.M. Barnett, J.P. Mohr and F.M. Yatsu, eds), New York: Churchill Livingstone.

Horn, S.W. (1983). The 'locked-in' syndrome following chiropractic manipulation of the cervical spine. *Ann. Emerg. Med.*, **12**, 648–50.

Hosek, R.S., Schram, S.B., Silverman, H. *et al.* (1981). Cervical manipulation. *J. Austr. Med. Assoc.*, **245**, 922.

Hutchinson, M.S. (1989). An investigation of pre-manipulative dizziness testing. In *Proceedings of 5th Biennial Conference of Manipulative Physiotherapists of Australia*, Sydney, pp. 104–12.

Kanshepolski, J., Danielson, H. and Flynn, R.E. (1972). Vertebral artery insufficiency and cerebellar infarct due to manipulation of the neck. *Bull. L.A. Neurol. Soc.*, **37**, 62–5.

Kelly, J.P. (1991). The sense of balance. In *Principles of Neural Science* (E.R. Kandell, J.H. Schwartz and T.M. Jessell, eds), Connecticut: Prentice-Hall, pp. 500–11.

Krueger, B.R. and Okazaki, H. (1980). Vertebral-basilar distribution infarction following chiropractic cervical manipulation. *Mayo Clin. Proc.*, **55**, 322–32.

Loeb, C. and Meyer, J.S. (1965). *Strokes due to Veretebrobasilar Disease.* Springfield, Illinois: Charles C. Thomas Publishers.

Lord, R.S.A. (1986). *Surgery of Occlusive Cerebrovascular Disease.* St Louis: C.V. Mosby.

Lyness, S.S. and Wagman, A.D. (1974). Neurological deficit following cervical manipulation. *Surg. Neurol* **2**, 121–3.

Maitland, G.D. (1986). *Vertebral Manipulation* (5th edn). London: Butterworth-Heinemann.

Mishkin, M.M. and Schreiber, M.N. (1974). Collateral circulation. In *Radiology of the Skull and Brain: Angiography* (T.H. Newton and D.G. Potts, eds), vol. 2, book 4, St Louis: C.V. Mosby.

Nagler, W. (1973). Vertebral artery obstruction by hyperextension of the neck: report of three cases. *Arch. Phys. Med. Rehabil.*, **54**, 232–40.

Okawarra, S. and Nibbelink, D. (1974). Vertebral artery occlusion following hyperextension and rotation of the head. *Stroke*, **5**, 640–2.

Osol, A. (ed.) (1972). *Blakiston's Gould Medical Dictionary* (3rd edn.) New York: McGraw-Hill.

Patjin, J. (1991). Complications in manual medicine: a review of the literature. *J. Man. Med.*, **6**, 89–92.

Refshauge, K. (1994). Rotation: a valid pre-manipulative dizziness test. Does it predict safe manipulation? *J. Manip. Physiol. Ther.*, **17**, 15–19.

Rowell, L.B. (1986). *Human Circulation Regulation During Physcial Stress*, New York: Oxford University Press.

Rowland, L.P. (1991). Clinical syndromes of the spinal cord and brain stem. In *Principles of Neural Science* (E.R. Kandell, J.H. Schwartz and T.M. Jessell, eds) pp. 711–30, Connecticut: Prentice-Hall International.

Schellhas, K.P., Latchaw, R.E., Wendling, L.R. and Gold, L.H.A. (1980). Vertebrobasilar injuries following cervical manipulation. *J. Med. Assoc. Austr.*, **244**, 1450–3.

Schmitt, H.P. (1991). Anatomical structure of the cervical spine with reference to pathology of manipulation complications. *J. Man. Med.*, **6**, 93–101.

Stevens, A. (1991). Functional Doppler sonography of the vertebral artery and some considerations about manual techniques. *J. Manual Med.*, **6**, 102–5.

Stopford, J.S.B. (1916). The arteries of the pons and medulla. *J. Anat.*, **5**, 255–80.

Terrett, A.G. (1987). Vascular accidents from cervical spine manipulation: the mechanisms. *J. Austr. Chiropract. Assoc.*, **17**, 131–144.

Thiel, H.W. (1991). Gross morphology and pathoanatomy of the vertebral arteries. *J. Manip. Physiol. Ther.*, **14**, 133–41.

Tissington-Tatlow, W.F. and Bammer, H.G. (1957). Syndrome of vertebral artery compression. *Neurology*, **7**, 331–40.

Toole, J.F. and Tucker, S.H. (1960). Influence of head position upon cerebral circulation. *Arch. Neurol.*, **2**, 616–23.

Williams, P.R. and Warwick, R. (eds) (1980). *Gray's Anatomy* (36th edn.) London: Churchill Livingstone.

Zweibel, W.J. (1986) *Introduction to Vascular Ultrasonography* (2nd edn). New York: Harcourt Brace Jovanich.

Tension tests

Beel, J.A., Groswald, D.E. and Luttges, M.W. (1984). Alterations in the mechanical properties of peripheral nerve following crush injury. *J. Biomech.*, **17**, 185–93.

Bell, A. (1987). The upper limb tension test – bilateral straight leg raising – a validating manoeuvre for the upper limb tension test. In *Proceedings of the 5th Biennial Conference of the Manipulative Therapists Association of Australia*, Melbourne, pp. 106–14.

Bogduk, N. and Twomey, L.T. (1991). *Clinical Anatomy of the Lumbar Spine* (2nd edn). London: Churchill Livingstone.

Brieg, A. (1978). *Adverse Mechanical Tension in the Central Nervous System: An Analysis of Cause and Effect by Functional Neurosurgery.* Stockholm: Almquist and Wiksell International.

Brieg, A. and Marions, O. (1963). Biomechanics of the lumbosacral nerve roots. *Acta Radiol.: Diagnosis*, **1**,

1141–60.

Brieg, A. and Troup, J.D. (1979). Biomechanical considerations in the straight leg raising test: cadaveric and clinical studies of the effects of medial hip rotation. *Spine*, **4**, 242–50.

Brudzinski (1909) cited in O'Connell, J.E. (1946) The clinical signs of meningeal irritation. *Brain*, **69**, 9–21.

Butler, D. (1991) *Mobilisation of the Nervous System* Melbourne: Churchill Livingstone.

Charnley, J. (1951). Orthopaedic signs in the diagnosis of disc protrusion – with special reference to the straight-leg-raising test. *Lancet*, **4**, 186–92.

Christodoulides, A.N. (1989). Ipsilateral sciatica on femoral nerve stretch test is pathognomonic of an L4/5 disc protusion. *J. Bone Joint Surg.*, **71B**, 88–9.

Davidson, S. (1987). Prone knee bend – an investigation into the effect of cervical flexion and extension. In *Proceedings of the 5th Biennial Conference of the Manipulative Therapists Association of Australia*, Melbourne, pp. 106–14.

Dyck, P. (1976). The femoral nerve traction test with lumbar disc protrusions. *Surg. Neurol.*, **6**, 163–6.

Dyck, P. (1984). Lumbar nerve root: the enigmatic eponyms. *Spine*, **9**, 3–6.

Elvey, R.L. (1979). Brachial plexus tension tests and the pathoanatomical origin of arm pain. In *Aspects of Manipulative Therapy* (R.M. Idczack, ed.), pp. 105–10, Melbourne: Lincoln Institute of Health Sciences.

Elvey, R.L. (1981). Brachial plexus tension tests and the pathoanatomical origin of arm pain. In *Aspects of Manipulative Therapy* (R.M. Idczack, ed.), pp. 116–22, Melbourne: Lincoln Institute of Health Sciences.

Elvey, R.L. (1983). The need to test the brachial plexus in painful shoulder and upper quadrant conditions. In *Proceedings of Neck and Shoulder Symposium*. Brisbane, pp. 39–52.

Estridge, M.N., Rouhe, S.A. and Johnson, N.G. (1982). The femoral stretching test – a valuable sign in diagnosing upper lumbar disc herniations. *J. Neurosurg.*, **57**, 813–17.

Fahrni, W.H. (1966) Observations on straight leg-raising with special reference to nerve root adhesions. *Can. J. Surg.*, **9**, 44–8.

Fung, Y.C. (1981). *Biomechanics – Mechanical Properties of Living Tissues*. New York: Springer-Verlag.

Goddard, M.D. and Reid, J.D. (1965). Movements induced by straight leg raising in the lumbo-sacral roots, nerves and plexus, and in the intrapelvic section of the sciatic nerve. *J. Neurol. Neurosurg. Psychia.*, **28**, 12–18.

Grieve, G.P. (1984). *Mobilisation of the Spine* (4th edn). London: Churchill Livingstone.

Herbert, R. (1988). The passive mechanical properties of muscle and their adaptations to altered patterns of use. *Austr. J. Physiother.*, **34**, 141–9.

Howe, J.F., Loeser, J.D. and Calvin, W.H. (1977). Mechano-sensitivity of dorsal root ganglia and chronically injured axons: a physiological basis for the radicular pain of nerve root compression. *Pain*, **3**, 25–41.

Hsieh, C.-Y., Walker, J.M. and Gillis, K. (1983). Straight leg raising test: comparison of three instruments. *Phys. Ther.*, **63**, 1429–33.

Hudgins, W.R. (1975). The crossed straight leg raising test. *N.*

Engl. J. Med., **297**, 1127.

Kenneally, M. (1985) The upper limb tension test. In *Proceedings of the 4th Biennial conference of the Manipulative Therapists Association of Australia*, Brisbane, pp. 259–73.

Landers, J. (1987). The upper limb tension test. In *Proceedings of the 5th Biennial Conference of the Manipulative Therapists Association of Australia*, Melbourne, pp. 1–12.

Lerman, V.I. and Drasnin, H.V. (1975). Adhesive lesions of the nerve root in the dural orifice as a cause of sciatica. *Surg. Neurol.*, **4**, 229–32.

McNab, I. (1971). Negative disc exploration – an analysis of the causes of nerve-root involvement in sixty-eight patients. *J. Bone Joint Surg.*, **53A**, 891–903.

Maitland, G.D. (1978). Movement of pain sensitive structures in the vertebral canal in a group of physiotherapy students. In *Proceedings of the Inaugural Congress of the Manipulative Therapists Association of Australia*, pp. 37–52.

Maitland, G.D. (1979). Negative disc exploration: positive canal signs. *Austr. J. Physiother.*, **25**, 129–33.

Maitland, G.D. (1985). The slump test: examination and treatment. *Austr. J. Physiother.*, **31**, 215–19.

Maitland, G.D. (1986). *Vertebral Manipulation* (5th edn). London: Butterworths.

Matyas, T. and Bach, T. (1985). The reliability of selected techniques in clinical arthrometrics. *Austr. J. Physiother.*, **31**, 175–299.

Pullos, J. (1986). The upper limb tension test. *Austr. J. Physiother.*, **32**, 258–9.

Quintner, J. (1989). A study of upper limb pain and paraesthesia following neck injury in motor vehicle accidents: assessment of the brachial plexus test of Elvey. *Br. J. Rheumatol.*, **28**, 528–33.

Rubenach, H. (1985). The upper limb tension test – the effect of the position and movement of the contralateral arm. In *Proceedings of the 4th Biennial Conference of the Manipulative Therapists Association of Australia*, Brisbane, pp. 274–83.

Selveratnam, P., Glasgow, E. and Matyas, T. (1987). The discriminative validity of the brachial tension test. In *Proceedings of the 5th Biennial Conference of the Manipulative Therapists Association of Australia*, Melbourne, pp. 325–50.

Selveratnam, P., Glasgow, E. and Matyas, T. (1989). Differential strain produced by the brachial plexus tension test on C5 to T1 nerve roots. In *Proceedings of 6th Biennial Conference of the Manipulative Therapists Association of Australia*, Adelaide, pp. 167–72.

Selveratnam, P., Glasgow, E. and Matyas, T. (1994). Non-invasive discrimination of Brachial Plexus involvement in upper limb pain. *Spine*, **19**, 26–33.

Simionato, R., Stiller, K. and Butler, D. (1988). Neural tension signs in Guillan Barre syndrome: 2 case reports. *Austr. J. Physiother.*, **34**, 257–9.

Smyth, M.J. and Wright, V. (1958). Sciatica and the intervertebral disc – an experimental study. *J. Bone Joint Surg.*, **40A**, 1401–18.

Sunderland, S. and Bradley, K.C. (1961a). Stress–strain phemomena in human peripheral nerve trunks. *Brain*, **84**, 102–19.

Sunderland, S. and Bradley, K.C. (1961b). Stress–strain phenomena in human spinal nerve roots. *Brain*, **84**, 120–7.

Troup, J.D.G. (1981). Straight-leg-raising (SLR) and the qualifying tests for increased root tension. Their predictive value after back and sciatic pain. *Spine*, **6**, 526–7.

Wasserman, S. (1918). Uber ein neues Schenkelnervneuritis nebst Bemerkungen aus diagnostik der Schenkelnerverkrankungen. *Dtsh. Z. Schft, Nervenhk*, **63**, 140–3. In Dyck, P. (1984) Lumbar nerve root: the enigmatic eponyms. *Spine*, **9**, 3–6.

Woodhall, B.H. and Major, G.J. (1950). The well-leg-raising test of Fajersztajn in the diagnosis of ruptured lumbar intervertebral disc. *J. Bone Joint Surg.*, **32A**, 786–92.

Yaxley, G.A. and Jull, G.A. (1991). A modified upper limb tension test: an investigation of responses in normal subjects. *Austr. J. Physiother.*, **37**, 143–54.

The Neurological examination

Appelberg, B., Hulliger, M., Johansson, H. and Sojka, P. (1983). Actions on gamma motor neurons by electrical stimulation of group I muscle afferents in the hind limb of the cat. *J. Physiol.*, **335**, 275–92.

Bannister, R. (ed.) (1992) *Brain and Bannisters Clinical Neurology* (7th edn). Oxford: Oxford University Press.

Barr, M. (1974) *The Human Nervous System*. Maryland: Harper and Row.

Bickerstaff, E.R. (1980). *Neurological Examination in Clinical Practice* (4th edn). Melbourne: Blackwell Scientific Publications.

Bogduk, N. (1987). Innervation, pain patterns and mechanisms of pain production. In *Clinics in Physical Therapy, Physical Therapy of the Low Back* (L.T. Twomey and J.R. Taylor, eds), Melbourne: Churchill Livingstone.

Bogduk, N. and Twomey, L.T. (1987). *Clinical Anatomy of the Lumbar Spine*. London: Churchill Livingstone.

Bohannon, R. (1986). Manual muscle test scores and dynamometer test scores of knee extension strength. *Arch. Phys. Med. Rehabil.*, **4**, 390–2.

Bohannon, R. and Gajdosik, R. (1987). Spinal nerve compression – some clinical implications. *Phys. Ther.*, **67**, 376–81.

Bouchier, I.A.D. and Morris, J.S. (1982). *Clinical Skills – A System of Clinical Examination*. London: W.B. Saunders.

Burke, D., Gracies, J.M., Mazevet, D. *et al.* (1992a). Convergence of descending and various peripheral inputs onto common propriospinal-like neurones in man. *J. Physiol.*, **449**, 655–71.

Burke, D., Gracies, J.M., Meunier, S. and Pierrot-Deseilligny, E. (1992b). Changes in presynaptic inhibition in man during voluntary contractions. *J. Physiol.*, **449**, 673–87.

Coscia, M., Leipzig, T. and Cooper, D. (1994). Acute cauda equina syndrome: Diagnostic advantage of MRI. *Spine*, **19**, 475–8.

Davis, A., Bolin, T. and Ham, J. (1985) *Symptom Analysis and Physical Diagnosis*. Sydney: Pergamon Press.

De Palma, A.F. and Rothman, R.H. (1970). *The Intervertebral Disc*. London: W.B. Saunders.

Dillon, W., Booth, R., Cuckler, J. *et al.* (1986). Cervical radiculopathy: a review. *Spine*, **11**, 988–91.

Falconer, M.W., Patterson, H.R., Gustafson, E.A. and Sheridan, E. (1978). *Drug Handbook*. London: W.B. Saunders.

Finsterbush, A., Frankel, V., Pharu, B. and Arnon, R. (1983). Quantitative power measurement of extensor hallucis longus: a simple objective test in evaluation of low back pain with neurological involvement. *Spine*, **8**, 206–9.

Foreman, S.M. and Croft, A.C. (1988) *Whiplash Injuries – the Cervical Acceleration/Deceleration Syndrome*. Sydney: Williams and Wilkins.

Ganong. W.F. (1975) *Review of Medical Physiology*. Los Altos: Lang Medical Publications.

Gelberman, R., Szabo, R., Williamson, R. and Dimick, M. (1983). Sensibility testing in peripheral nerve compression syndromes. *J. Bone Joint Surg.*, **65-A**, 632–8.

Hagbath, K.-E., Wallin, G., Burke, D. and Lofstedt, L. (1975). Effects of Jendrassic manoeuvre on muscle spindle activity in man. *J. Neurol. Neurosurg. Psychiat.*, **38**, 1143–53.

Hart, D. and Rose, S. (1986). Reliability of a non-invasive method for measuring the lumbar curve. *J. Orthop. Sports Physiother.*, **8**, 180–4.

Helfet, A.J. and Gruebel, L. (1978) *Disorders of the Lumbar Spine*. Philadelphia: J.B. Lippincott.

Janig, W. (1978). The autonomic nervous system. In *Fundamentals of Neurophysiology* (R.F. Schmidt, ed.), New York: Springer Verlag.

Kandell, E.R., Schwartz, J.H. and Jessell, T.M. (1991). *Principles of Neural Science* (3rd edn). Connecticut: Prentice-Hall International.

Knutsson, E., Skoglund, C.R. and Natchev, E. (1988). Changes in voluntary muscle strength, somatosensory transmission and skin temperature concomitant with pain relief during autotraction in patients with lumbar and sacral root lesions. *Pain*, **33**, 173–9.

Kortelainen, P., Puranen, J., Koivisto, E. and Lahde, S. (1985). Symptoms and signs of sciatica and their relation to the localization of the lumbar disc herniation. *Spine*, **10**, 88–92.

Lance. J.W. and McLeod, J.G. (1975). *A Physiological Approach to Clinical Neurology* (2nd edn). London: Butterworths.

Lieberman, J., Corkill, G. and Taylor, R. (1983). Fatiguing weakness; an initial symptom in clinical compressive radiculopathy. *Surg. Neurol.*, **19**, 354–7.

Loeser, J.D. (1985). Pain due to nerve injury. *Spine*, **10**, 232–5.

Luhan, J. (1968) *Neurology, a Concise Clinical Textbook*. Baltimore: Williams and Wilkins.

Magee, D.J. (1987). *Orthopaedic Physical Assessment*. London: W.B. Saunders.

Maitland, G.D. (1986) *Vertebral Manipulation* (5th edn). London: Butterworths.

Matyas, T. and Bach, T. (1985). The reliability of selected techniques in clinical arthrometrics. *Austr. J. Physiother.*, **31**, 175–99.

McCall, I.W., Park, W.M. and O'Brien, J.P. (1979). Induced pain referral from posterior lumbar elements in normal subjects. *Spine*, **4**, 441–6.

McNab, I. (1972). The mechanism of spondylogenic pain. In

Cervical Pain (C. Hirsch and Y. Zotterman, eds), Oxford: Pergamon.

McCulloch, J.A. and Waddell, G. (1980). Variations of the lumbosacral myotomes with bony segmental anomalies. *J. Bone Joint Surg.*, **62A**, 475–80.

Mooney, V. and Robertson, J. (1976). The facet syndrome. *Clin. Orthop. Relat. Res.*, **115**, 149–56.

Neidre, A. and McNab, I. (1983) Anomalies of lumbar spine nerve roots. *Spine*, **8**, 294–9.

Olmarker, K., Rydevick, B. and Holm, S. (1989). Edema formation in spinal nerve roots induced by experimental, graded compression. *Spine*, **14**, 569–73.

Osol, A. (1972). *Blakiston's Gould Medical Dictionary* (3rd edn), New York: McGraw-Hill.

Pandya, S., Florence, J., King, W. *et al.* (1985). Reliability of gonimetric measurements in patients with Duchenne muscular dystrophy. *Phys. Ther.*, **5**, 1339–42.

Rydevick, B., Myer, R. and Powell, H. (1989). Pressure increases in the dorsal root ganglion following mechanical compression. Closed compartment syndrome in nerve roots. *Spine*, **14**, 574–6.

Skre, H. (1972). Neurological signs in a normal population. *Acta Neurol. Scand.*, **48**, 575–606.

Smyth, M.J. and Wright, V. (1958). Sciatica and the intervertebral disc: an experimental study. *J. Bone Joint Surg.*, **40A**, 1401–8.

Sunderland, S. (1978) *Nerve and Nerve Injuries* (2nd edn). London: Churchill Livingstone.

Thorn, G.W. (1977) *Harrison's Principles of Internal Medicine*. Tokyo: McGraw-Hill Kogadusha Ltd.

Viikari-Juntura, E., Porras, M. and Laasonen, E.M. (1989). Validity of clinical tests in the diagnosis of root compression in cervical disc disease. *Spine*, **14**, 253–7.

Viikari-Juntura, E. (1987). Inter-examiner reliability of observations in physical examinations of the neck. *Phys. Ther.*, **67**, 1526–32.

Weiss, M.D., Garfin, S.R., Gelberman, R.H. *et al.* (1985). Lower extremity sensibility testing in patients with herniated lumbar intervertebral discs. *Spine*, **9**, 1219–24.

Williams, P.R. and Warwick, R. (1980) *Gray's Anatomy* (36th edn). London: Churchill Livingstone.

Young, A., Getty, J., Jackson, A. *et al.* (1983). Variations in the pattern of muscle innervation by the L5 and S1 nerve roots. *Spine*, **8**, 616–24.

Zimmerman, M. (1978). Regulatory functions of the nervous system as exemplified by the spinal motor system. In *Fundamentals of Neurophysiology* (R.F. Schmidt, ed.), New York: Springer-Verlag.

Palpation and passive motion tests

Cibulka, M., Delitto, A. and Koldehoff, R. (1988). Changes in innominate tilt after manipulation of the sacroiliac joint in patients with low back pain. An experimental study. *Phys. Ther.*, **68**, 1359–63.

DiFabio, R. (1992). Efficacy of manual therapy. *Phys. Ther.*, **72**, 853–64.

Doran, D. and Newell, D. (1975). Manipulation in the treatment of low back pain: a multicentre study. *Br. Med. J.*, **ii**, 161–4.

Farrell, J.P., and Twomey, L.T. (1982). Acute low back pain: comparison of two conservative treatment approaches. *Med. J. Austr.*, **i**, 160–4.

Fleiss, J. (1986). *The Design and Analysis of Clinical Experiments*. New York: John Wiley and Sons.

Grieve, G. (1984). *Mobilisation of the Spine* (4th edn). New York: Churchill Livingstone.

Hardy, G. and Napier, J. (1991). Inter and intratherapist reliability of passive accessory movement technique. *N.Z. J. Physiother.*, 22–4.

Harryman, D.T., Sidles, J.M., Clark, J.M. *et al.* (1990). Translation of the humeral head on the glenoid with passive glenohumeral motion. *J. Bone Joint Surg.*, **72A**, 1334–43.

Howell, S., Galinat, B., Renzi, A. and Marone, P. (1988) Normal and abnormal mechanics of the glenohumeral joint in the horizontal plane. *J. Bone Joint Surg.*, **70A**, 227–32.

Jull, G. and Bullock, M. (1987). A motion profile of the lumbar spine in an ageing population assessed by manual examination. *Physiother. Pract.*, **3**, 70–81.

Jull, G., Bogduk, N. and Marsland, A. (1988). The accuracy of manual diagnosis for cervical zygapophysial joint pain syndromes. *Med. J. Austr.*, **148**, 233–6.

Kaltenborn, F. (1980). *Mobilization of the Extremity Joints*. Oslo: Olaf Noris Bokhandel Universitetsgaten.

Keating, J.C., Bergman, T.F., Jacobs, G.E. *et al.* (1990). Interexaminer reliability of eight evaluative dimensions of lumbar segmental abnormality. *J. Manipulative Physiol. Ther.*, **13**, 463–70.

Kettle, D. (1991). The effects of manipulative physiotherapy on chronic cervical dysfunction. *Physiother. Theory Pract.*, **7**, 23–31.

Koes, B., Bouter, L., Van Mameran, H. *et al.* (1992). A blinded randomised clinical trial of manual therapy and physiotherapy for chronic back and neck complaints: physical outcome measures. *J. Manipulative Physiol. Ther.*, **15**, 16–23.

Koes, B., Bouter, L., Van Mameren, H. *et al.* (1993). A randomized clinical trial of manual therapy and physiotherapy for persistent back and neck complaints: subgroup analysis and relationship between outcome measures. *J. Manipulative Physiol. Ther.*, **16**, 211–17.

Lee, M., Latimer, J. and Maher, C. (1993). Manipulation: investigation of a proposed mechanism. *Clin. Biomech.*, **8**, 302–6.

Lee, M. and Moseley, A. (1991). *Dynamics of the Human Body* (2nd edn) pp. 153–6. Sydney: Zygal.

MacConaill, M. and Basmajian, J. (1969). *Muscles and Movements: A Basis for Human Kinesiology*. Baltimore: Williams and Wilkins.

Magee, D.J. (1987). *Orthopaedic Physical Assessment*. Philadelphia: WB Saunders.

Maitland, G. (1986). *Vertebral Manipulation* (5th edn). London: Butterworths.

Maher, C. and Adams, R. (1994). Reliability of pain and stiffness assessments in clinical manual lumbar spine examination. *Physical Therapy*, **74**, 801–11.

Maher, C. and Latimer, J. (1992). Pain or resistance – the manual therapists' dilemma. *Austr. J. Physiother.*, **38**, 257–60.

Matyas, T. and Bach, T. (1985). The reliability of selected techniques in clinical arthometrics. *Austr. J. Physiother.*, **31**, 175–99.

McClure, P. and Flowers, K.R. (1992). Treatment of limited shoulder motion: a case study based upon biomechanical considerations. *Phys. Ther.*, **72**, 929–36.

Mealy, K., Brennan, M. and Fenelon, G. (1986). Early mobilization of acute whiplash injuries. *Br. Med. J.*, **292**, 656–7.

Nachemson, A.L. (1992). Newest knowledge of low back pain. *Clin. Orthop. Relat. Res.*, **279**, 8–20.

Nwuga, V. (1982). Relative therapeutic efficacy of vertebral manipulation and conventional treatment in back pain management. *Am. J. Phys. Med.*, **61**, 273–8.

Penning, L. (1992). Functional pathology of lumbar spinal stenosis. *Clin. Biomech.*, **7**, 3–17.

Phillips, D.R. and Twomey, L. (1993). Comparison of manual diagnosis with a diagnosis established by a uni-level lumbar spinal block procedure. In *Integrating Approaches. Proceedings of the Eigth Biennial Conference of the Manipulative Physiotherapists Association of Australia* November 24–27, Perth, Western Australia, pp. 55–61.

Poppen, N. and Walker, P. (1976). Normal and abnormal motion of the shoulder. *J. Bone Joint Surg.*, **58A**, 195–201.

Rothstein, J., Campbell, S., Echternach, J.L. *et al.* (1991). Standards for tests and measurements in physical therapy practice. *Phys. Ther.*, **71**, 589–97.

Scott-Blair, G.W. and Coppen, F.M. (1939). The subjective judgements of the elastic and plastic properties of soft bodies; the 'differential thresholds' for viscosities and compression moduli. *Proc. R. Soc.*, **128B**, 109–25.

Sidor, M.L., Zuckerman, J.D., Lyon, T. *et al.* (1993). The Neer classification system for proximal humeral fractures. *J. Bone Joint Surg.*, **75A**, 1745–50.

Siebenrock, K.A. and Gerber, C. (1993). The reproducibility of classification of fractures of the proximal end of the humerus. *J. Bone Joint Surg.*, **75A**, 1751–5.

Spitzer, W.O. (1987). Scientific approach to the assessment and management of activity-related spinal disorders. A monograph for clinicians. Report of the Quebec task force on spinal disorders. *Spine*, **12**, S1–S59.

Sturesson, B., Selvile, G. and Uden, A. (1989). Movements of the sacroiliac joints. A roentgen stereophotogrammetric analysis. *Spine*, **14**, 162–5.

Trott, P., Evans, D. and Frick, R. (1989). Accuracy of manual palpation skills: the ability of manipulative physiotherapists to detect changes in force and displacement on a palpation simulator. *Proceedings of the 6th Biennial Conference of Manipulative Physiotherapists Association of Australia*, Adelaide, pp. 207–14.

Viner, A., Mackey, C., Porter, D. and Lee, M. (1991). Perception of stiffness in spinal assessment. *7th Biennial Conference of the Manipulative Physiotherapists Association of Australia*, Blue Mountains, New South Wales, pp. 238–43.

Ward, M. (1988). Unpublished Research Project. GradDip-AppSc (ManipPhty) Cumberland College of Health Sciences, University of Sydney, Australia.

Muscle testing

Ada, L. and Herbert, R. (1988). Measurement of joint range of motion. *Austr. J. Physiother.*, **34**, 260–2.

Bohannon, R.W. (1990). Testing isometric limb muscle strength with dynamometers. *Crit. Rev. Phys. Rehabil. Med.*, **2**, 75–86.

Brand, P.W. (1985). *Clinical Mechanics of the Hand*. St Louis: C.V. Mosby.

Corrigan, B. and Maitland, G.D. (1983). *Practical Orthopaedic Medicine*. London: Butterworths.

Daniels, L. and Worthingham, C. (1986). *Muscle Testing* (5th edn). Philadelphia: W.B. Saunders.

Fish, D.R. and Wingate, L. (1985). Sources of goniometric error at the elbow. *Phys. Ther.*, **65**, 1666–70.

Gadjosik, R.L. and Bohannon, R.W. (1987). Clinical measurement of range of motion. Review of goniometry emphasizing reliability and validity. *Phys. Ther.*, **67**, 1867–72.

Gravel, D., Richards, C.L. and Filion, M. (1988). Influence of contractile tension development on dynamic strength measurements of the plantarflexors in man. *J. Biomech.*, **21**, 89–96.

Herzog, W. (1988). The relation between the resultant moments at a joint and the moments measured by an isokinetic dynamometer. *J. Biomech.*, **21**, 5–12.

Hortobagyi, T., Katch, F. and LaChance, P.F. (1989). Inter-relationships among various measures of upper body strength assessed by different contraction modes. *Eur. J. Physiol.*, **58**, 749–55.

Kendall, F.P., McCreary, E.K. and Provance, P.G. (1993). *Muscles, Testing and Function* (4th edn), Baltimore, Williams and Wilkins.

Lamb, R.L. (1985). Manual muscle testing. In *Measurement in Physical Therapy* (J.M. Rothstein, ed.), New York: Churchill Livingstone, pp. 47–56.

Mayhew, T.P. and Rothstein, J.M. (1985). Measurement of muscle performance with instruments. In *Measurement in Physical Therapy* (J.M. Rothstein, ed.), New York: Churchill Livingstone, pp. 57–102.

McDonagh, M.J.N. and Davies, C.T.M. (1984). Adaptive response to mammalian skeletal muscle to exercise with high loads. *Eur. J. Appl. Physiol.*, **52**, 139–55.

Miller, P.J. (1985). Assessment of joint motion. In *Measurement in Physical Therapy* (J.M. Rothstein, ed.), New York: Churchill Livingstone, pp. 103–36.

Munsat, T.L. (1990). Clinical trials in neuromuscular disease. *Muscle Nerve* (Suppl.), S3–S6.

Sapega, A.A., Nicholas, J.A., Sokolow, D. and Saraniti, A. (1982). The nature of torque 'overshoot' in Cybex isokinetic dynamometry. *Med. Sci. Sports Exerc.*, **14**, 368–75.

Winter, D.A., Wells, R.P. and Orr, G.W. (1981). Errors in the use of isokinetic dynamometers. *Eur. J. Appl. Physiol.*, **46**, 397–408.

Motor performance: evaluation and intervention

Ada, L. and Canning, C. (1990). Anticipating and avoiding muscle shortening. In *Key Issues in Neurological Physio-*

therapy (L. Ada and C. Canning, eds), pp. 219–36, Oxford: Butterworth-Heinemann.

Andriacchi, T.P. and Birac, D. (1993). Functional testing in the anterior cruciate ligament-deficient knee. *Clin. Orthop. Relat. Res.*, **288**, 40–7.

Andriacchi, T.P., Andersson, G.B.J., Fermier, R. *et al.* (1980). A study of lower limb mechanics during stairclimbing. *J. Bone Joint Surg.*, **62A**, 749–57.

Andriacchi, T.P., Galante, J.O. and Fermier, R.W. (1982). The influence of total knee-replacement design on walking and stair-climbing. *J. Bone Joint Surg.*, **64A**, 1328–35.

Baker, P.A., Evans, O.M. and Lee, C. (1991). Treadmill training following fractured neck-of-femur. *Arch. Phys. Med. Rehabil.*, **72**, 649–52.

Carr, J.H. and Gentile, A.M. (1994). The effect of arm movement on the biomechanics of standing up. *Hum. Movement Sci.*, **13**, 175–93.

Depena, J. and Chung, C.S. (1988). Vertical and radial motions of the body during the take-off phase of high jumping. *Med. Sci. Sports Exerc.*, **20**, 290.

Enoka, R.M., Miller, D.I. and Burgess, E.M. (1982). Below-knee amputee running gait. *Am. J. Phys. Med.*, **62**, 66–84.

Harris, W.H. and Sledge, C.B. (1990). Total hip replacement. *N. Engl. J. Med.*, **323**, 725–31.

Hay, J.G. (1975). Biomechanical aspects of jumping. In *Exercise and Sports Sciences* (J.H. Wilmore and J.F. Keogh, eds), pp. 135–61. New York: Academic Press.

Hinrichs, R.N. (1990). Whole body movement: coordination of arms and legs in walking and running. In *Multiple Muscle Systems* (J.M. Winters and S.L-Y. Woo, eds), pp. 694–705, New York: Springer-Verlag.

Inman, V.T., Ralston, H.J. and Todd, F. (1981). *Human Walking.* Baltimore: Williams and Wilkins.

Jevsevar, D.S., Riley, P.O., Hodge, W.A. and Krebs, D.E. (1993). Knee kinematics and kinetics during locomotor activities of daily living in subjects with knee arthroplasty and in healthy control subjects. *Phys. Ther.*, **73**, 229.

Kerslake, J.M., Catton, L. and Ford, S.G. (1987). Functional activities following cementless isoelastic total hip replacement. *Proceedings of the Tenth International Congress of the World Confederation for Physical Therapy*, Sydney, pp. 451–5.

Mann, R. and Hagy, J. (1980). Biomechanics of walking, running and spring. *Am. J. Sports Med.*, **8**, 345–50.

Moffet, H., Richards, C., Malouin, F. and Bravo, G. (1993). Impact of knee extensor strength deficits on stair ascent performance in patients after medial meniscectomy. *Scand. J. Rehabil. Med.*, **25**, 63.

Pai, Y.-C. and Rogers, M.W. (1991). Segmental contributions to total body momentum in sit-to-stand. *Med. Sci. Sports Exerc.*, **23**, 225–30.

Scholz, J.P. (1993). Organizational principles for the coordination of lifting. *Hum. Movement Sci.*, **12**, 537.

Shepherd, R.B. and Gentile, A.M. (1994). Sit-to-stand: functional relationship between upper body and lower limb segments. *Hum. Movement Sci.*, **13**, 817–40.

Smith, A. (1990). The measurement of human motor performance. In *Key Issues in Neurological Physiotherapy* (L. Ada and C. Canning, eds), pp. 51–79, Oxford: Butterworth-Heninemann.

van Vliet, P. (1988). Kinematic analysis of videotape to measure walking following stroke: a case study. *Austr. J. Physiother.*, **34**, 48–51.

Weinstein, J.N., Andriacchi, T.P. and Galante, J.O. (1986). Factors influencing walking and stair climbing following unicompartmental knee arthroplasty. *J. Arthropl.*, **1**, 109.

Westwood, P. (1993). An investigation into the effects of task-specific training on the biomechanics of standing up in patients following total hip replacement. MAppSc Thesis, School of Physiotherapy, University of Sydney, Australia.

Winter, D.A. (1987). *The Biomechanics and Motor Control of Human Gait.* Waterloo: University of Waterloo Press.

Winter, D.A. and Sienko, S.E. (1988). Biomechanics of below-knee amputee gait. *J. Biomech.*, **21**, 361–7.

Chapter 7

Selection and application of treatment

N. Bogduk and S. Mercer

Introduction

Be it in medicine at large, in musculoskeletal medicine, or in musculoskeletal physiotherapy, any form of treatment can be appraised against three distinct, but complementary, axes. These are *convention, biological basis* and *empirical proof* (Figure 7.1). A good therapy would score highly on all three axes. However, this is rarely the case; most therapies manage to score perhaps along one or two axes. In that event, the merit of a therapy is judged not only by its score along any particular axis but also by the relative value of that axis. To be professionally responsible, a therapist selecting or prescribing a therapy should be conscious of the basis for their selection – whether they are simply conforming to convention, using a biologically sound therapy or applying a proven remedy.

Axis I: convention

Convention is a socially powerful but intellectually weak dimension. It pertains to influences such as 'we have always used this' and 'everyone does it'. When seeking a therapeutic armamentarium, new students are particularly vulnerable to being swayed by assertions from lecturers or in textbooks that a particular therapy or a particular combination of therapies is good for a particular condition. After all, it is difficult for students to question the implicit authority of lecturers or textbooks. Even the professional journals are replete with assertions and recommendations that a particular therapy or some new twist works for a particular problem.

Examples of therapies endorsed by convention are exercise, the so-called 'modalities', mobilization and manipulation. These are the hallmarks of physiotherapy. Notwithstanding how physiotherapy may be evolving towards other means of treatment, these remain the core of the therapeutic armamentarium of physiotherapy and the basis for the image and reputation of physiotherapy.

The power of convention lies in peer pressure and role modelling. Individuals seeking to be part of a profession are reluctant and unlikely to dispute what the established and ostensibly authoritative members of that profession do and have been accustomed to doing. Meanwhile, young trainees are more likely to want to emulate leaders rather than challenge them, particularly when the trainee has no personal professional experience with

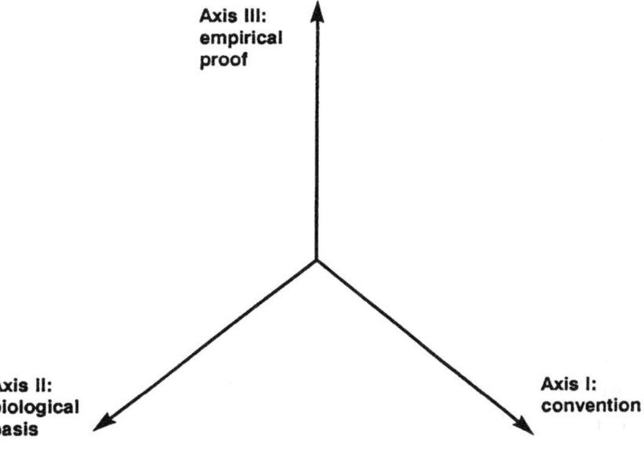

Figure 7.1 A graphical representation of the three axes against which the propriety of any therapy might be considered.

which to compete with the leader. Convention is also a resort when there is no other legitimate basis for a therapy.

Convention, however, is scientifically and intellectually weak. To challenge it does not require clinical experience; it requires only certain principles of critical reasoning. Responsible students do not need to compete with matching experience; they need only to ask the pertinent questions. If these questions remain unanswered, the weakness of convention as a justification for therapy will automatically be revealed.

Convention is often defended by reference to 'clinical experience'. The implication is that someone who has been practising a particular therapy for a long time would know what is best. The telling argument in this context is that every craft group uses the same defence. Surgeons claim success; acupuncturists and naturopaths claim success; chiropractors as well as physiotherapists claim success. All defend their claims with 'clinical experience'. Yet they cannot all be right, for why then do so many patients continue to languish with musculoskeletal problems?

The reason why convention is an intellectually flawed basis for therapy is that it is confounded by factors such as patient bias, recall bias, misperception, outcome measures and lack of controls.

Patient bias operates when a patient likes the therapist and for that reason is reluctant to disappoint them by reporting that the treatment did not work. Rather than confront or threaten the therapist's obvious dedication and kindness, they deny failure, fail to report it or tell a white lie by reporting modest success. As a result, the therapist, through no fault of their own, gains the impression that the therapy is not failing and therefore may, indeed, be quite good.

In the pursuit of truth, patient bias is reduced, if not eliminated, by having independent observers to evaluate the therapy. Since they lack any contractual relationship with an independent observer, patients are less inclined to fabricate a benevolent response when it is not due. Any study or any claim that lacks an independent observer can, therefore, be challenged in principle, for it is likely to be compromised by patient bias.

Recall bias operates when a therapist, in recounting their experience, remembers only the 'good' cases. Psychologically it is only natural for a therapist to suppress unpleasant memories of 'bad' experiences such as failures. Moreover, a therapist is actually likely to continue to see patients who are satisfied with their treatment and come back for more; dissatisfied patients simply do not return. Therefore, the therapist's memories of their experience are dominated by the 'good' cases.

Recall bias is eliminated by studying all consecutive cases over a predetermined time-frame. This eliminates intellectual cheating such as 'that case doesn't count because they did not come back to finish therapy'. The chances are that such patients did not finish therapy because they were dissatisfied with it. The effect of monitoring all consecutive patients is to dilute, but render more realistic, the reported or claimed percentage success rate.

Outcome measures is a vexatious issue. A success might be claimed by a therapist if the patient simply feels 'better'. A more cynical interpretation would be that 'better' does not count if the patient still has the problem and is continuing to seek therapy. Another consideration is the temporal stability of outcome. A patient may feel totally relieved of their symptoms upon rising from the plinth, but that does not count as a success if upon leaving the front door of the practice the patient suffers a total recurrence of their complaint.

There is no single or absolute outcome measure. Any therapist is entitled to declare their own; but they must do so honestly. It is fair, legitimate and acceptable for a therapist to declare that their intended or attained outcome was simply to make the patient feel better. That outcome, however, cannot be declared to constitute a 'cure'. The critical issue is that whatever success a therapy achieves should not be misrepresented or overplayed. In teaching a therapy a therapist should be obliged to declare clearly what outcome honestly can be expected. There is no justification for portraying a therapy as 'good' (because it makes the patient feel 'better') but implying that it will 'cure'. Nor should students be allowed to infer that a treatment will cure when in reality it will at best be only palliative.

Black and white outcome measures are easy to apply and to interpret: 'the patient either has pain or has no pain'. Such outcome measures are severe, and many therapies are likely to fail if pitted against such demanding standards. Less demanding outcome measures, however, may be difficult to quantify and calibrate. For example, how big is a 25% reduction in pain? How worth while is a 25% loss? After all, the patient still has 75% of their pain.

It is important for any consumer of outcome data to be assured that the instruments used to measure outcome are appropriate. The size of inter-observer errors should be known, lest their magnitude be greater than that of the purported therapeutic benefit. Natural variance must also be taken into account. Some patients improve more than others yet at the same time, patients who do not undergo therapy will nonetheless show variations in the severity of their complaint. Random variations between or within patients should not be misrepresented as being due to the therapy. For this reason, before any claim about the success of therapy can be sustained, it must be based on a sample-size that takes into account natural variation. In formal statistical terms, the study must have the power to detect what it purports to show.

Misperception pertains to when a therapist noticing a genuine success ascribes that success erroneously to a particular therapy when in fact the result was due to some other factor. Of particular concern here are the covert or accidental psychotherapeutic dimensions of physiotherapy treatment. The patient may feel better not because of the exercise or manipulation but because the therapist appeared to care, spent time with them and tried to help. This effect has not been quantified in physiotherapy at large, but has attracted attention with respect to preventive measures for low back pain. It has been recognized that a public caring attitude achieves greater success than training in lifting techniques or a back school programme (Wood, 1987; Gundewall *et al.*, 1993).

Related to misperception are *extrapolation* and *generalization*. Therapies useful for one region of the body may be erroneously extrapolated as useful for another homologous region. For example, although the neck and back are both regions of the vertebral column, therapies worthwhile for one are not necessarily equally efficacious for the other; the two regions differ sufficiently in anatomy, biomechanics and pathology for this caveat to apply. Similarly, therapies that might work for acute problems will not necessarily apply to chronic problems of the same body part. Acute back pain, for example, may have a different pathology from that of chronic back pain, and be responsive to different interventions. Or it may be that the biology (and psychology) of the same, original pathology evolves as the condition changes from acute to chronic, rendering it less responsive to therapy. Success with acute problems, therefore, does not constitute a basis for claiming or predicting success with chronic disorders.

Controls are ubiquitously the missing factor in 'clinical experience'. Therapists in conventional practice are unlikely to be able to submit themselves or their patients to controlled studies. In institutional practice, the demand for services is usually too great to allow therapists either to double or to halve their workload in order to submit a cohort of age-matched and gendermatched patients to parallel sham therapy as a control. In private practice, ethical restrictions would apply to charging patients for control therapy, and therapists are unlikely to be able to afford to treat free of charge equal numbers of 'active' and 'control' patients. Controls, however, are crucial if illusions are to be eliminated.

Consider the claim 'my therapy has a 75% success rate' (Figure 7.2). Are you impressed? Would you be inclined to adopt this treatment for your own patients? What if we now unveil a control (Figure 7.3)? Are you still impressed? What if the control results are somewhat more modest (Figure 7.4). Are you yet convinced? How much difference should there be between the rows before you are 'sold' on the efficacy of the therapy?

Outcome

Success	Failure
75	25

Figure 7.2 Hypothetical observed results of treatment of 100 patients.

Outcome

	Success	Failure
Treatment	75	25
Control	75	25

Figure 7.3 Hypothetical observed results of treatment of 100 patients and 100 matched controls.

Outcome

	Success	Failure
Treatment	75	25
Control	65	35

Figure 7.4 Hypothetical observed results of treatment of 100 patients and 100 matched controls

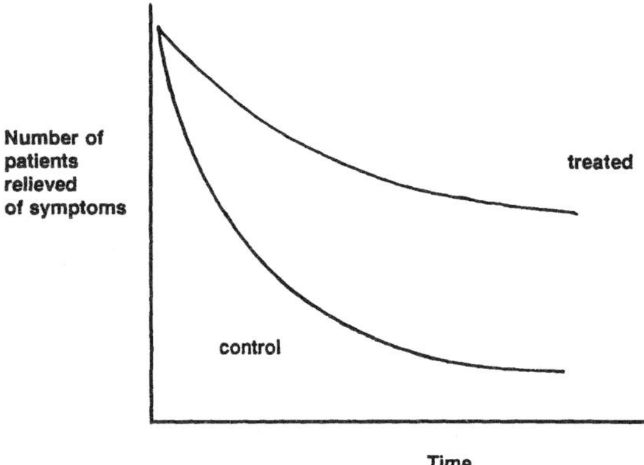

Figure 7.5 The difference in outcome over time between a hypothetical treatment and a control displayed graphically by a pair of survival curves

When time is a factor in outcome, results may be displayed graphically in the form of survival curves (Figure 7.5). These show the number of patients, or the proportion of patients, persisting with relief of symptoms over time. The superiority of a treatment over control is displayed by the difference between the survival curves of the treated and control groups.

The formality of deciding statistically significant, and therefore convincing, differences between therapy and control lies in tests like chi-squared, the *t* test and various rank tests (Sackett, *et al.* 1985). In the case of graphic data, tests such as the Mantel–Haenszel procedure may be used (Kirkwood, 1988); these constitute a series of chi-squared tests looking for significant differences between the two curves along their entire length. Familiarity with these statistical tests is critical for consumers to be able to tell whether or not purported differences between therapy and control are significant. However, no truth is evident if the therapist fails to provide the second row in a two-by-two table or the second curve in a survival analysis.

Axis II: biological basis

This axis is a seductive one; it appeals to common sense and logic, and is attractive, for instead of requiring a therapist to learn individualized recipes for every possible condition it allows the therapist to apply principles. If one determines the mechanism of a symptom it is appealing to apply a therapy that is known to reverse that mechanism. The implication and legitimate expectation is that by reversing the mechanism the therapy will reverse the symptom. The philosophical strength here is that it is immaterial if controlled trials have not proven that the intended therapy works for the condition in question; what has been proven is that the intervention works for the mechanism of the symptom. The advantage is that this principle can be applied to a diversity of conditions some of which may be so uncommon as to never attract a randomized double-blind controlled trial.

Thus, it would be worthwhile if physiotherapy had at its disposal a selection of generic techniques of known physiological effect that could be applied to conditions with discernible mechanisms that could be reversed by these techniques. The problem here, however, is threefold.

First, for which therapies do we properly know the physiological effect? Secondly, to what extent are physiotherapists able reliably to discern the actual mechanism of a symptom? Thirdly, even if there is a match between therapy and mechanism, is that match at all appropriate for the cardinal complaint of the patient?

For some therapies there is an obvious or unquestioned biological effect. Strong exercise strengthens muscles. No-one disputes that. How much exercise and which regimen is best might be contested but the principle is not in dispute. Less convincing are the mechanisms of effect of mobilization and manipulation. Even though theories have been advanced, the biological basis of these therapies has not been demonstrated.

This raises a critical point. Many explanations of the effect of physical therapies are *post hoc*. Instead of explicitly determining the mechanism of a therapy, physiotherapists have been accustomed to inferring what must be the biological basis of the therapy. This, however, is not proof. Rather, it is creating a model (retrospectively) to explain why a therapy must work. This may be satisfying as an allegory when teaching students, but it is not the same as proving a generic biological mechanism that might legitimately be applied to any circumstance that warrants it.

A distinction must be drawn between a *plausible* explanation and a *proven* one. Thus, a physiotherapist may believe that selective contraction of a particular band of the multifidus muscle may selectively mobilize or stabilize a given segment of the lumbar spine. This is a plausible mechanism, but it has never been objectively demonstrated. Until such a mechanism has been demonstrated (e.g. radiographically) it remains only a plausible hypothesis, and does not constitute a demonstrated biological mechanism.

Even if it is accepted that a treatment has a sound biological basis, it behoves the therapist to be able to determine that the pertinent mechanism is operating in a given patient. Teachers and experts may adduce a model to explain a patient's complaint but that is not evidence that those mechanisms actually operate in the patient. Model-making and model fitting is common in health practice; reliable detection is rare.

A physiotherapist may interpret as follows: 'the patient has back pain and a list because the proprioceptive output from the left L4–5 zygapophyseal joint has been disturbed and has recruited an increased gamma outflow to the psoas major, resulting in an increased la discharge from that muscle and consequent shortening'. An acupuncturist seeing the same patient might deduce 'a disturbance of the balance between Yin and Yang expressed along the bladder meridian'.

To be believed the physiotherapist must be able to show that they can reliably detect 'disturbed proprioceptive output' or 'increased gamma outflow', or have recourse to biological data that show that the model proffered above operates in all patients with a list. Only then are they justified in applying a therapy that corrects 'disturbed proprioceptive output' or reduces 'increased gamma outflow' (assuming that such techniques are available).

By the same token, to be credible, the acupuncturist must show that Yin and Yang exist and can be quantified, and that the bladder meridian does exist and has something flowing along it. Without such connections to reality, elaborate models are nothing but attractive word-play.

When faced with rigorous scientific challenges to their biological theories, therapists are prone to avoidance, and retort that the mechanism does not matter because (anyhow) the treatment works; but this changes the argument from axis II to axis III.

Next, even though the biological basis may be sound, and even though the appropriate clinical signs may be detectable, the concordance may not be relevant. In a patient with back pain, muscle weakness may be found; and it is known that exercise will strengthen muscles. Hence, there is an invitation to treat back pain with exercise. The flaw lies in that the weakness may only be an epiphenomenon and has little to do with the primary complaint. Exercise may strengthen the muscles but do nothing for the pain. The imperative should be that therapy should be directed to the primary mechanism and not to epiphenomena. At best, failing to do so is implicit defeatism – 'we can't treat the pain, so let us treat something we can treat'. At worst, it creates an illusion – 'we treat back pain with exercise because exercise has a sound biological basis, and therefore (!), it will relieve pain'.

These various principles can be illustrated by examining several of the more commonly applied therapies. Under consideration is not whether the therapy works but, in terms of axis II, whether or not the therapy has a reliably proven biological basis that allows it to be applied in a generic manner.

The foremost effect of *cryotherapy* is vasoconstriction which reduces blood flow and decreases metabolic activity (Stillwell, 1971; Basford, 1988). In principle, therefore, therapeutic cold has a place in the treatment of acute injuries to reduce swelling and minimize tissue damage. That, however, does not give it a place for chronic pain or when there is no evidence of tissue damage.

Therapeutic cold also has a variety of effects on motor nerves that offer it a place in the treatment of spasticity (Hartviksen, 1962; Abramson *et al.*, 1966; Stillwell, 1971; Basford, 1988). It is not clear, however, that these effects justify a role for therapeutic cold for musculoskeletal complaints.

In the cat, cooling blocks conduction along nerve fibres, particularly along small diameter A fibres (Douglas and Malcolm, 1962). This most likely underlies the observation that in humans therapeutic cold produces a loss in perception first of light touch and cold, and later of pain and gross pressure (Fox, 1961). Therapeutic cold may, therefore, be applied as an analgesic. There is no evidence, however, that these effects have any lasting influence on musculoskeletal pain. Analgesia occurs only as long as the cold is applied.

Combining these observations offers a legitimate place for the use of therapeutic cold in the treatment of acute injuries; the patient appreciates the temporary analgesia, and hopefully the decreased metabolic activity minimizes tissue damage.

Superficial heat, produced by hot packs, heat lamps or warm hydrotherapy, is portrayed as producing increased local temperature, increased local metabolic rate, arteriolar dilatation and increased capillary blood flow (Stillwell, 1971). These effects, however, occur in the skin, and there is no explicit evidence of analogous effects in deeper tissues.

Concurrently, superficial heat appears to offer an analgesic effect (Grana, 1993), but the mechanism of this effect is not known. The use of superficial heat as an analgesic, therefore, is based on empirical observation and not on an established physiological precept.

Ultrasound is believed to operate by the production of heat in deep tissues, but may also operate by a variety of non-thermal effects such as cavitation, acoustic streaming and the production of standing waves (Lehman, 1971; Dyson and Suckling, 1978; Basford, 1988; Gann, 1991). It is used for its deep heating and pain-relieving effects (Sweitzer, 1994).

The deep-heating effects are believed to increase blood flow and to increase local metabolic rate. These effects are desirable when tissue repair is the objective, and the beneficial effects of ultrasound have been demonstrated in the case of varicose ulcers (Dyson and Sucking, 1978). These data, however, do not constitute evidence of an analogous effect in deeper tissues.

Ultrasound alters the physical properties of fibrous tissues, rendering them more yielding to stretch (Gersten, 1955; Lehman, *et al.*, 1970; Lehman, 1971). This offers it a place in the treatment of joint contractures and muscle fibrosis.

When applied to a nerve, ultrasound raises the pain threshold in the territory of that nerve (Lehman *et al.*, 1958). This effect is probably due to temporary blockade of conduction along C fibres (Lehman *et al.*, 1971). Ultrasound may, therefore, be legitimately used, in principle, as an analgesic. Ultrasound, however, is not an anaesthetic; it does not abolish pain; it simply increases the threshold for perception of pain. Experimental studies in normal volunteers indicate that the increase in threshold is dependent on the intensity of ultrasound, but is only of the order of 20% (Williams *et al.*, 1987).

Notwithstanding their valid biological basis, none of these effects indicate that ultrasound may alone be curative of musculoskeletal conditions. Softening fibrous tissue only provides a window of opportunity for mobilization of the affected tissue; the analgesia provided by ultrasound is only temporary and so, too, only provides a window of opportunity.

Interferential therapy is a clever application of physics. Two high-frequency currents can be passed across a selected region of the body such that they intersect at a chosen target site or region. If the two frequencies are unequal, a beat frequency will be established at the point of intersection. This manoeuvre allows relatively low-frequency currents to be delivered to deep sites without irritation of the overlying skin and other tissues.

Interferential is believed to improve deep venous and lymphatic circulation, break down muscular adhesions, and provide pain relief by some form of mechanism involving the sympathetic nervous system (Nelson, 1981). Its mechanism and biological effects, however, have not been explicitly demonstrated. It is, therefore, an empirical therapy whose mechanisms are inferred. It does not qualify as a therapy that can be prescribed on the basis of established biological principles.

There is no established biological basis for the therapeutic effects of *low energy laser* therapy (Kitchen and Partridge, 1991; Beckerman *et al.*, 1992). Some of the proposed physiological effects attributed to low-power laser energy are accelerated collagen synthesis, increased vascularization of healing tissues, a decrease in microorganisms, and pain reduction (Synder-Mackler and Seitz, 1990). But none of these effects has been explicitly demonstrated. Studies on the superficial radial nerve have shown no effect of laser on conduction velocity (Greathouse *et al.*, 1985; Kramer and Sandrin, 1993). Concepts such as *biostimulation* or *photoacceptance* do not constitute a valid explanation of the biological basis for laser therapy and do not provide a logical basis for the application of laser for conditions such as epicondylitis or radicular pain. The utility of laser therapy therefore rests solely on empirical data.

Spinal traction is a therapy steeped in history and tradition. Its biological basis, however, is very limited. Traction is believed to separate vertebrae (Geiringer *et al.*, 1988); however, in the lumbar spine much of the elongation observed arises from flattening of the lumbar lordosis (Twomey, 1985). In the cervical spine 30 pounds of traction achieves only fractions of a millimetre separation between vertebral bodies, amounting to 2 mm total elongation anteriorly and 6 mm posteriorly between C2 and T1 (Colachis and Strohm, 1966).

One rationale for traction is that separating the vertebrae relieves compression of spinal nerve roots. There may be other effects such as stretching spinal muscles, but this has not been documented biologically. Decompression of nerve roots is the only pathophysiological effect consistent with the mechanical effect of separating vertebrae; but this rationale is flawed in two ways.

Despite earlier beliefs to the contrary, there is no evidence that nerve root compression underlies complaints of spinal pain. It may be the basis for some cases of radicular pain, but not the basis for somatic spinal pain and somatic referred pain (Bogduk and Twomey, 1991). Hence, there is a potential mismatch between perceived effect of therapy and the actual mechanism of pain.

Secondly, traction is bound to be futile. Even if traction succeeds in separating vertebrae, when the patient leaves the traction table and stands upright they are immediately exposed to the compression loads of the head and trunk, which must immediately reverse any effect of therapeutic traction. Indeed, it has been shown that, without rising, after simply resting on the traction table for 20 min, the effects of cervical traction are all but lost (Colachis and Strohm, 1966).

Spinal traction, therefore, lacks a valid biological basis or is inconsistent with the mechanism of complaint. Whether or not it works empirically is another issue, addressed below. But without an established rationale, traction resembles little more than offering the patient a good stretch, for whatever that is worth.

There is no evidence that *collars* and *corsets* prevent movement of the treated region of the vertebral column. Studies have expressly shown that soft collars have no effect on cervical mobility (Colachis *et al.*, 1973); no studies have addressed the biological effect of lumbar corsets. One can deduce only that collars and corsets have a behavioural effect in that they remind the patient not to move the affected part. Unlike splints of the appendicular skeleton, collars and corsets do not have a generic biomechanical basis.

Exercises may be prescribed for a variety of purposes. The classical role of exercise has been to strengthen the target muscle. That this can be achieved is not in doubt. Therefore, exercise is a legitimate generic tool if the goal is increased strength.

Another effect of exercise is mobilization. By using the muscles around a joint the patient will achieve movement of that joint. The range achieved depends only on the degree of shortening achieved on the muscle used. In this case, strengthening is not necessarily the objective; what is desired is the execution of the movement. Such exercises may be prescribed for prophylactic purposes to prevent contractures of joints that might not be moved because of pain, or to restore the range of movement of afflicted joints. Perhaps the classical example is moving a painful shoulder after injury. There is no evidence, however, that mobilization has any direct biological effect on pain. Pain may improve coincidentally or as a result of mobilization, but as a generic principle, the only legitimate rationale for exercise is to improve range of movement.

Exercise may also be used to achieve particular motor skills. The principle and experience stems from neurological practice where patients have lost a particular function but one which can be re-established by learning to perform a movement using different muscles. In musculoskeletal practice the analogue lies in training individuals to co-ordinate their muscles differently, for example to remember to co-contract the abdominal muscles when lifting in order to enhance the stability of the lumbar spine (Jull and Richardson, 1994). However, as foreshadowed above, it is important to distinguish between plausible hypotheses and established mechanisms. Retraining may be plausible and desirable, but physiotherapists need to demonstrate that retraining does have explicit biological effects.

Exercise may also be used as a 'vehicle' for intervention. Patients may be encouraged to improve general fitness by undertaking exercise, but in this case, achieving fitness is the operant factor; not the specific exercise itself.

Theories abound for the biological basis of *manipulative therapy*. The proposed mechanisms include restoration of vertebral movement by overcoming capsular, ligamentous or muscular shortening, or by breaking intra-articular adhesions, repositioning a subluxated vertebra, a zygapophyseal meniscoid or a disordered intervertebral disc, or altering the neural output of the affected segment or joint (Geiringer *et al.* 1988; Zusman, 1986).

None of these mechanisms has been demonstrated in experimental animals, nor has their relationship to pain been established. They are but theories, and do not constitute a valid biological basis that justifies the application of manipulative therapy. Moreover, there is no evidence that a physiotherapist can tell in a given patient whether their pain is due to capsular stiffness, or subluxation, or a trapped meniscoid or a disordered disc. Therefore, there can be no legitimate match between operant pathology and purported mechanism of therapy. Manipulation cannot be portrayed as being based on sound biological grounds; it is a therapy that rests only on convention and alleged empirical proof.

Mobilization is the gentle cousin of manipulation. Its attraction is that by intention and by experience it carries less risk of morbidity than manipulation. However, like manipulation it lacks any demonstrated biological mechanism. Clinically, mobilization involves moving a joint passively but slowly within its immediately available range of motion or slightly beyond the limit of that range. What this achieves biologically is unknown.

On the one hand, mobilization may be perceived to stretch fibrous tissues in or around a joint. On the grounds that stretching fibrous tissue may cause it to creep, mobilization is sound in principle if the objective is to increase range of motion. It is contentious, however, that any gains achieved by this means are sustained. With respect to relief of pain, it has been postulated that mobilization promotes adaptation of capsular nerve endings, essentially decreasing their threshold for mechanical activation (Zusman, 1986). However, while attractive in theory this mechanism of pain relief has not been expressly demonstrated.

Like manipulation, mobilization cannot be justified on the basis of a sound proven biological mechanism; its justification rests solely on convention and empirical data.

Spinal *posture* is often addressed by physiotherapists for patients with neck pain or back pain, but there is no basic biological data that defines what constitutes a 'bad' posture; nor has it been shown that a physiotherapist can discriminate between normal variations and a posture that causes symptoms. Therapies addressing posture are therefore simply based on hypotheses, and have no established biological basis.

Axis III: empirical proof

It is purveyed by some and believed by others that no therapy is 'scientific' unless it has a known physiological basis. This is not true. It is satisfying to know the biological basis for a therapy but not essential for it to be scientific.

A therapy could be regarded as a 'black box'; in as much as the mechanism of the therapy is not known, just as the contents of the box are unknown. But the utility of the box can nonetheless be evaluated scientifically without knowing its contents. A therapy can be tested and proven without regard to its mechanism, and thereby become scientifically proven, provided that the appropriate rigour has been applied. The science lies in the testing and not in knowledge of the mechanism.

Indeed, logistically it is far more worthwhile to prove a therapy empirically beforehand rather than exploring its mechanism. Research effort should not be squandered exploring the mechanism of a therapy that in due course is proven not to work. Proponents of a particular therapy would serve journals better by reporting the results of proper therapeutic trials instead of consuming time and publication space by manufacturing and contesting factitious theories to explain the mechanism of clinically unproven therapies.

Axis III relates to valid empirical clinical evidence. Irrespective of how popular a therapy may or may not be, irrespective of whether its mechanism is known or not, a therapy becomes legitimate only if and once its efficacy is proven. Conversely, irrespective of its popularity a therapy can be outrightly condemned if it fails to be vindicated in a properly conducted controlled trial.

In the past, physiotherapy as a profession has been reluctant to subject its therapeutic armamentarium to scrutiny. It has been satisfied that convention and peer endorsement were enough, or that an attractive biological basis was enough to justify teaching, implementing and perpetuating a therapy. Moreover, because physiotherapy was never subjected to authorities such as the Food and Drug Administration it has lacked a traditional familiarity with the process and obligation of validation. These conditions have changed.

In recent years, investigators have sought to evaluate the physiotherapy literature according to contemporary standards of critical reasoning and clinical epidemiology, to determine what, if anything, really works. The principles and means by which any form of therapy (not just physiotherapy) can be evaluated are outlined in various textbooks and journal articles (Sackett *et al.*, 1985; Koes *et al.*, 1991a, b; Beckerman *et al.*, 1992, 1993). In particular, checklists of the components of a properly conducted clinical trial of physical therapies have been published, against which any or all of the literature and any belief can be evaluated (Koes *et al.*, 1991a, b; Beckerman *et al.*, 1993).

The news is not good. Despite the enthusiasm of physiotherapists and despite any political defensiveness, validation of musculoskeletal physiotherapy is conspicuously lacking. Either therapeutic benefit has been denied or the literature is of such poor quality that it offers little or no support for perpetuated beliefs.

It is not the place nor the ambition of this chapter to survey and evaluate each and every study that has ever been conducted on physiotherapy. By and large that has been done by others, to date (Koes *et al.*, 1991a, b; Beckerman *et al.*, 1993; Shekelle, *et al.*, 1992). Instead, only some of the highlights will be outlined.

A review of exercises for back pain found most studies to be of poor quality, allowing no conclusion to be drawn about the efficacy of exercises for this condition or whether a specific type of exercise was more effective (Beckerman *et al.*, 1993). Studies published since that review have found exercises to offer no specific therapeutic benefit for acute low back pain (Faas *et al.*, 1993).

Collars and corsets for patients with grossly stable spines offer no benefit greater than placebo (Huston, 1988).

The poor quality of available literature precludes any conclusions about the value of physical therapy for disorders of the shoulder or knee (Beckerman *et al.*, 1993).

No trials have validated a therapeutic value of ultrasound for musculoskeletal disorders (Beckerman *et al.*, 1993). Although one study purported to show a benefit from ultrasound for prolapsed lumbar intervertebral disc (Nwuga, 1983), it was also apparent that only 40% of patients responded. A similar finding pertains to the treatment of epicondylitis; although significantly better than placebo, ultrasound benefited only 63% of cases (Binder *et al.*, 1985). Ultrasound was found not to be beneficial for ankle sprains (Williamson *et al.*, 1986).

The literature on laser therapy is mixed. Positive and negative results have been reported for a variety of disorders of joints, tendons and muscles; but overall, the literature is poor (Beckerman *et al.*, 1992). The better quality studies suggest that laser does have a therapeutic effect greater than placebo (Beckerman *et al.*, 1992).

Several contrasting conclusions have stemmed from reviews of the efficacy of manipulative therapy. Strikingly, none endorses this form of therapy with the same enthusiasm expressed by its clinical proponents. A review by Dutch epidemiologists lamented the poor quality of literature and concluded that, although some results are promising, the efficacy of manipulation had not yet been convincingly shown (Koes *et al.*, 1991a). Their

subsequent clinical trial did little to alter this situation (Koes *et al.*, 1992a, b).

A meta-analysis by chiropractors, tended to support manipulative therapy but recognized that statistically the effect was small (Anderson *et al.*, 1992). A similar meta-analysis by American epidemiologists found that for patients with acute low back pain the difference in probability of recovery at 3 weeks favouring manipulative therapy was 0.17, with 95% confidence intervals of 0.07 to 0.28 (Shekelle *et al.*, 1992). This is a very modest benefit, amounting to a 67% chance of recovery compared with 50%. For chronic low back pain, these investigators found insufficient data worthy of analysis (Shekelle *et al.*, 1992). The use of manipulation for chronic low back pain, therefore, rests entirely on convention.

Trials of lumbar traction have found it to be no better than placebo (Matthews and Hickling, 1975; Pal *et al.*, 1986). Studies of cervical traction have found it to be no better than placebo (British Association of Physical Medicine, 1966; Tan and Nordin, 1992) or no better than isometric exercises (Goldie and Landquist, 1970). Another study, comparing cervical traction with instruction only, found significant improvements in some ranges of movement as a result of traction, but no significant improvement in pain (Zylbergold and Piper, 1985).

In the treatment of neck pain, traction, positioning, collars and advice were all found in one study to be no better than placebo tablets (British Association of Physical Medicine, 1966). Physiotherapy, described as 'standard physiotherapy with short-wave diathermy and intermittent mechanized neck-halter traction', has been found to be inferior to acupuncture (Loy, 1983); yet acupuncture is no better than sham transcutaneous electrical nerve stimulation (TENS) (Petrie and Langley, 1983). This sequence of results raises serious doubts about the propriety of that form of physiotherapy for neck pain and its status relative to other therapies.

With respect to neck pain following whiplash injury, physiotherapy and traction has been found to be no better than a collar and analgesics (Pennie and Agambar, 1990); short-wave diathermy appears to promote a faster resolution of symptoms but offers no benefit over control at 12 weeks follow-up (Foley-Nolan *et al.*, 1992); and outpatient physiotherapy offers no greater benefit than a home exercise programme (McKinney *et al.*, 1989). Of some solace, however, is the demonstration that when compared with rest and a collar, mobilization achieves significant improvements in cervical movement and pain, but only in patients with acute pain following whiplash (Mealy *et al.*, 1986). No studies have demonstrated similar benefits in patients with chronic pain after whiplash.

There has been a fashion in recent years for therapists to rely less on traditional modalities and manual therapy, and to participate instead in more behavioural or holistic therapeutic approaches, such as *back school, neck school* and *functional restoration* or work-hardening.

The original trial of back school for low back pain (Berquist-Ullman and Larsson, 1977) itself demonstrated only a modest clinical benefit and for only some parameters; yet this has not prevented this study from being held as proof of the utility of back school. Subsequent studies have failed to substantiate this conviction. Controlled studies have found only marginal (Moffet *et al.*, 1986) or no benefits (Lankhorst *et al.*, 1983) of back school for chronic low back pain. Another controlled study found no differences between 'back school' and control, but superior to both was a simple programme of callisthenics (Donchin *et al.*, 1990). The one published trial of neck school found it no better than no intervention (Kamwendo and Linton, 1991).

In the face of such nihilistic data, it is not unusual for physiotherapists to respond by pointing out the shortcomings of trials with negative results, implying that the results are not valid; yet implying at the same time that, therefore, the therapy is not bad and by exclusion, must be as good as it is believed by the profession. This is an understandable emotional argument but is an unacceptable intellectual argument. If a therapy were as good as it is believed, it is unlikely to have failed a clinical trial. Furthermore, if the therapy really is as good as believed, what is preventing the defenders of the faith from mounting their own trial? If they have the perspicacity to identify the flaws in the published literature, then they must have the skills to design a proper trial which should vindicate their conviction. But unless such trials are forthcoming, the suspicion prevails that perhaps the results of the negative trials may indeed be correct.

Functional restoration programmes remain popular in those countries that can afford them. Initial studies announced astounding success in achieving return to work amongst patients with chronic low back pain (Mayer *et al.*, 1985, 1987). These studies were met with some degree of scepticism for they did not include a convincing control group.

However, a subsequent study by an independent group reproduced the results (Hazard *et al.*, 1989). These studies indicated that instead of treatment delivered by a sole physiotherapist, success in the management of back pain was contingent upon an intensive multidisciplinary approach focused on work-related rehabilitation rather than treatment of a presumed source of pain. As such they challenge the precepts of sole practice in physiotherapy.

Selection of therapy

Table 7.1 lists many of the available therapies in musculoskeletal practice. In the Table the status of each therapy is evaluated against each of the three axes. Therapists wishing to select a therapy might consult this Table to determine how justified their selection is and on what grounds.

It is axiomatic that the therapies in Table 7.1 will all carry some form of peer endorsement and so will score well on the convention axis. It is on the other axes, particularly on axis III, that most therapies come to grief.

Therapists may choose to implement a therapy because it is available, because it is conventional or because there is no other legitimate option. That is their prerogative. But in doing so they must recognize the frailty of the basis of their selection. Notwithstanding its popularity, the therapy may have no legitimate scientific merit. That is not to say that no unproven therapy should be used. All that is called for is the recognition that the therapy may not work, but if it appears to work, there is no evidence that the effect was due to the therapy itself and not to some other influence such as placebo effect, natural resolution or the enthusiasm of the therapist.

A survey of the columns of axis II and axis III of Table 7.1 provides conspicuously little solace for physiotherapists. Although all carry some degree of peer endorsement, few of the therapies have a legitimate generic biological basis, few have been vindicated in controlled trials, while others have been refuted or denied for specified conditions.

The least controversial therapies tend to be those applied to the appendicular skeleton, for acute conditions or for conditions with a clear pathological basis. Thus, the use of continuous passive motion for surgical disorders of the knee is not in question. No one disputes the apparent utility of ice, compression, elevation and rest for the treatment of acute sprains of the joints of the appendicular skeleton. Nor is the propriety in question of

Table 7.1   Ratings of various physical therapies against the axes of (I) convention, (II) biological basis and (III) empirical proof

Therapy	Axis I: convention	Axis II: biological basis	Axis III: empirical proof
Exercise	Very fashionable	Some	Unproven, questionable value
For neck pain	Commonly used	Unstated	No evidence
For back pain	Commonly used	Unclear	Conflicting evidence
For joints	Commonly used	Unclear, various concepts about objectives and rationale	No evidence
Back school	Fashionable in some quarters	Nil	Questionable for acute pain, denied for chronic pain
Neck school	Not as common as back school	Nil	Value denied
Collars	Commonly used	Nil, probably behavioural	Nil
Corsets	Fashionable	Nil	Nil
Ultrasound	Commonly used	Limited	Limited to doubtful
Laser	Not standard	None known	Perhaps useful
Traction	Commonly used	Nil	No supportive proof, value denied
Posture	Often addressed	Nil	No evidence
Manipulation	Used judiciously	Nil	Questionable, marginal benefit for acute back pain, no evidence for chronic back pain, no evidence for neck pain
Mobilization	Commonly used	Nil	As for manipulation, proven benefit for acute neck pain

active or passive exercises to prevent muscle contractures in arthritis or joint injuries.

But none of these 'flagships' of musculoskeletal physiotherapy constitute or provide evidence of efficacy in other spheres. Success in the management of acute problems does not dictate or predict success in chronic problems. There is no evidence that physical therapies significantly relieve the pain of peripheral arthritis. With respect to spinal pain, the record of physiotherapy has been conspicuously poor.

Resolution

Ultimately the responsibility for the scientific state of physiotherapy lies with its academics – not to keep teaching the doctrines but to evaluate them. The dividend will be that the useless can be discarded thereby no longer filling and confounding undergraduate curricula, while the useful can be highlighted. With greater curriculum time consequently available better training in the useful can be achieved.

In the meantime, practising physiotherapists will need to make decisions. They can continue to select therapies on a random or *ad hoc* basis, or on the basis of their perceived 'clinical experience', but in doing so they should not perpetuate any illusions or possible illusions that what they are doing is correct. It is only through the conduct of controlled trials that the truth will eventually emerge and reveal which facets of physiotherapy are genuinely reliable.

References

Abramson, D.I., Chu, L.S.W., Tuck, S. *et al.* (1966). Effect of tissue temperature and blood flow on motor nerve conduction velocity. *J. Am. Med. Assoc.*, **198**, 1082–8.

Anderson, R., Meeker, W.C., Wirick, B.E. *et al.* (1992). A meta-analysis of clinical trial of spinal manipulation. *J. Manip. Physiol. Ther.*, **15**, 181–94.

Basford, J.R. (1988). Physical agents and biofeedback. In *Rehabilitation Medicine. Principles and Practice* (J.A. DeLisa, ed.), pp. 257–75, Philadelphia: J.B. Lippincott.

Beckerman, H., de Bie, R.A., Bouter, L.M. *et al.* (1992). The efficacy of laser therapy for musculoskeletal and skin disorders: a criteria-based meta-analysis of randomised clinical trials. *Phys. Ther.*, **72**, 483–91.

Beckerman, H., Bouter, L.M., van der Heijden, G.J.M.G. *et al.* (1993). Efficacy of physiotherapy for musculoskeletal disorders: what can we learn from research? *Br. J. Gen. Pract.*, **43**, 73–7.

Berquist-Ullman, M. and Larsson, U. (1977). Acute low back pain in industry. *Acta Orthop. Scand. Suppl.*, **170**, 1–117.

Binder, A., Hodge, G. Greenwood, A.M. *et al.* (1985). Is therapeutic ultrasound effective in treating soft tissue lesions? *Br. Med. J.*, **290**, 512–14.

Bogduk, N. and Twomey, L.T. (1991). *Clinical Anatomy of the Lumbar Spine*, (2nd edn), pp. 151–9, Melbourne: Churchill Livingstone.

British Association of Physical Medicine (1966). Pain in the neck and arm: a multicentre trial of the effects of physiotherapy. *Br. Med. J.*, **1**, 243–58.

Colachis, S.C. and Strohm, B.R. (1966). Effect of duration of intermittent cervical traction on vertebral separation. *Arch. Phys. Med. Rehabil.*, **47**, 353–9.

Colachis, S.C., Strohm, B.R. and Ganter, E.L. (1973). Cervical spine motion in normal women: radiographic study of the effect of cervical collars. *Arch. Phys. Med. Rehabil.*, **54**, 161–9.

Donchin, M., Woolf, O., Kaplan, L. and Floman, Y. (1990). Secondary prevention of low-back pain. A clinical trial. *Spine*, **15**, 1317–20.

Douglas, W.W. and Malcolm, J.L. (1962). The effect of localized cooling on conduction in cat nerves. *J. Physiol.*, **130**, 53–71.

Dyson, M. and Suckling, J. (1978). Stimulation of tissue repair by ultrasound: a survey of the mechanisms involved. *Physiotherapy*, **64**, 105–8.

Faas, A., Chavannes, A.W., van Eijk, J.T.M. and Gubbels, J.W. (1993). A randomized, placebo-controlled trial of exercise therapy in patients with acute low back pain. *Spine*, **18**, 1388–95.

Foley-Nolan, D., Moore, K., Codd, M. *et al.* (1992). Low energy high frequency pulsed electromagnetic therapy for acute whiplash injuries. *Scand. J. Rehabil. Med.*, **24**, 51–9.

Fox, R.H. (1961). Local cooling in man. *Br. Med. Bull.*, **17**, 14–18.

Gann, N. (1991). Ultrasound: current concepts. *Clin. Manag.*, **11**, 64–9.

Geiringer, S.R., Kincaid, C.B. and Rechtien, J.J. (1988). Traction, manipulation, and massage. In *Rehabilitation Medicine. Principles and Practice* (J.A. DeLisa, ed.), Philadelphia: J.B. Lippincott. pp. 276–94.

Gersten, J.W. (1955). Effect of ultrasound on tendon extensibility. *Am. J. Phys. Med.*, **34**, 362–9.

Goldie, I. and Landquist, A. (1970). Evaluation of the effects of different forms of physiotherapy in cervical pain. *Scand. J. Rehabil. Med.*, **2–3**, 117.

Grana, W.A. (1993). Physical agents in musculoskeletal problems: heat and cold therapy modalities. In *Instructional Course Lectures* (J.D. Heckman, ed.), pp. 439–42. Park Ridge: American Academy of Orthopaedic Surgeons.

Greathouse, D.G., Currier, D.P. and Gilmore, R.L. (1985). Effects of clinical infrared laser on superficial radial nerve conduction. *Phys. Ther.*, **65**, 1184–7.

Gundewall, B., Lijequist, M. and Hansson, T. (1993). Primary prevention of back symptoms and absence from work. A prospective randomized study among hospital employees. *Spine*, **18**, 587–94.

Hartviksen, K. (1962). Ice therapy in spasticity. *Acta Neurol. Scand.*, **38**, 79–84.

Hazard, R.G., Fenwick, J.W., Kalisch, S.M. *et al.* (1989). Functional restoration with behavioural support: a one-year prospective study of patients with chronic low-back pain. *Spine*, **14**, 157–61.

Huston, G.J. (1988). Collars and corsets. *Br. Med. J.*, **296**, 276.

Jull, G.A. and Richardson, C.A. (1994). Rehabilitation and active stabilization of the lumbar spine. In *Physical Therapy of the Low Back* (2nd end) (L.T. Twomey and J.R. Taylor, eds.), pp. 251–73, New York: Churchill Livingstone.

Kamwendo, K. and Linton, S.J. (1991). A controlled study of the effect of neck school in medical secretaries. *Scand. J. Rehabil. Med.*, **23**, 143–52.

Kirkwood, B.R. (1988). *Essentials of Medical Statistics*, p. 121, Oxford: Blackwell.

Kitchen, S.S. and Partridge, C.J. (1991). A review of low-level laser therapy. *Physiotherapy*, **77**, 161–8.

Koes, B.W., Assendelft, W.J., van der Heijden, G.J.M.G. *et al.* (1991a). Spinal manipulation and mobilisation for back and neck pain: a blinded review. *Br. Med. J.*, **303**, 1298–303.

Koes, B.W., Bouter, L.M., Beckerman, H. *et al.* (1991b). Physiotherapy exercises and back pain: a blinded review. *Br. Med. J.*, **303**, 1572–6.

Koes, B.W., Bouter, L.M., van Mameren, H. *et al.* (1992a). The effectiveness of manual therapy, physiotherapy, and treatment by the general practitioner for nonspecific back and neck complaints: a randomized clinical trial. *Spine*, **17**, 28–35.

Koes, B.W., Bouter, L.M., van Mameren, H. *et al.* (1992b). Randomised clinical trial of manipulative therapy and physiotherapy for persistent back and neck complaints: results of one year follow up. *Br. Med. J.*, **304**, 601–5.

Kramer, J.F. and Sandrin, M. (1993). Effect of low-power laser and white light on sensory conduction rate of the superficial radial nerve. *Physiother. Can.*, **45**, 165–70.

Lankhorst, G.J., van de Stadt, R.J., Vogelar *et al.* (1983). The effect of the Swedish back school in chronic idiopathic low back pain. *Scand. J. Rehabil. Med.*, **15**, 141–5.

Lehman, J.F. (1971). Diathermy. In *Handbook of Physical Medicine and Rehabilitation* (2nd edn) (F.H. Krusen, ed.) pp. 273–345, Philadelphia: W.B. Saunders.

Lehman, J.F., Brunner, G.D. and Stow, R.W. (1958). Pain threshold measurements after therapeutic application of ultrasound microwaves and infrared. *Arch. Phys. Med.*, **39**, 560–5.

Lehman, J.F., Masock, A.J., Warren, C.G. and Koblanski, J.N. (1970). Effects of therapeutic temperatures on tendon extensibility. *Arch. Phys. Med.*, **51**, 481–7.

Loy, T. (1983). Treatment of cervical spondylosis. Electro-acupuncture versus physiotherapy. *Med. J. Austr.*, **2**, 32–4.

Matthews, J.A. and Hickling, J. (1975). Lumbar traction: a double-blind controlled study for sciatica. *Rheumatol. Rehabil.*, **14**, 222–5.

Mayer, T.G., Gatchel, R.J., Kishino, N. *et al.* (1985). Objective assessment of spine function following industrial injury: a prospective study with comparison group and one-year follow-up. *Spine*, **10**, 482–93.

Mayer, T.G., Gatchel, R.J., Mayer, H. *et al.* (1987). A prospective two-year study of functional restoration in industrial low back injury: an objective assessment proce-dure. *J. Am. Med. Assoc.*, **258**, 1763–7.

McKinney, L.A., Dornan, J.O. and Ryan, M. (1989). The role of physiotherapy in the management of acute neck sprains following road-traffic accidents. *Arch. Emerg. Med.*, **6**, 27–33.

Mealy, K., Brennan, H. and Fenelon, G.C. (1986). Early mobilisation of acute whiplash injuries. *Br. Med. J.*, **292**, 656–7.

Moffett, J.A.K., Chase, S.M., Portek, I. and Ennis, J.R. (1986). A controlled, prospective study to evaluate the effectiveness of a back school in the relief of chronic low back pain. *Spine*, **11**, 120–2.

Nelson, B. (1981). Interferential therapy. *Austr. J. Physiother.*, **27**, 53–6.

Nwuga, V.C.B. (1983). Ultrasound in treatment of back pain resulting from prolapsed intervertebral disc. *Arch. Phys. Med. Rehabil.*, **64**, 88–9.

Pal, B., Mangion, P, Hossain, M.A. and Diffey, B.L. (1986). A controlled trial of continuous lumbar traction in the treatment of back pain and sciatica. *Br. J. Rheumatol.*, **25**, 181–3.

Pennie, B.H. and Agambar, L.J. (1990). Whiplash injuries. A trial of early management. *J. Bone Joint Surg.*, **72B**, 277–9.

Petrie, J.P. and Langley, G.B. (1983). Acupuncture in the treatment of chronic cervical pain. A pilot study. *Clin. Exp. Rheumatol.*, **1**, 333–5.

Sackett, D.L., Haynes, R.B. and Tugwell, P. (1985). *Clinical Epidemiology. A Basic Science for Clinical Medicine.* Boston: Little, Brown.

Shekelle, P.G., Adams, A.H., Chassin, M.R. *et al.* (1992). Spinal manipulation for low-back pain. *Ann. Intern. Med.*, **117**, 590–8.

Stillwell, G.K. (1971). Therapeutic heat and cold. In *Handbook of Physical Medicine and Rehabilitation* (2nd edn) (F.H. Krusen, ed.), pp. 259–72, Philadelphia: W.B. Saunders.

Sweitzer, R.W. (1994). Ultrasound. In *Physical Agents. A Comprehensive Text for Physical Therapists* (B. Hecox, T.A. Mehretab, J. Weisberg, eds.), chapter 13, Norwalk, Connecti-cut: Appleton and Lange.

Synder-Mackler, L. and Seitz, L. (1990). Therapeutic uses of light in rehabilitation. In *Thermal Agents in Rehabilitation* (2nd edn) (S.L. Michlovitz, ed.), chapter 9, Philadelphia: F.A. Davis.

Tan, J.C. and Nordin, M. (1992). Role of physical therapy in the treatment of cervical disk disease. *Orthop. Clin. N. Am.*, **23**, 435–49.

Twomey, L. (1985). Sustained lumbar traction. An experimental study of long spine segments. *Spine*, **10**, 146–9.

Williams, A.R., McHale, J. Bowditch, M. *et al.* (1987). Effects of MHz ultrasound on electrical pain threshold perception in humans. *Ultrasound Med. Biol.*, **13**, 249–58.

Williamson, J.B., George, T.K., Simpson, D.C. *et al.* (1986). Ultrasound in the treatment of ankle sprain. *Injury*, **17**, 176–8.

Wood, D.J. (1987). Design and evaluation of a back injury prevention program within a geriatric hospital. *Spine*, **12**, 77–82.

Zusman, M. (1986). Spinal manipulative therapy: review of some proposed mechanisms, and a new hypothesis. *Austr. J. Physiother.*, **32**, 89–99.

Zylbergold, R.S. and Piper, M.C. (1985). Cervical spine disorders: a comparison of three types of traction. *Spine*, **10**, 867–71.

Chapter 8

The use of information in clinical practice

E.M. Gass and K.M. Refshauge
with contributions from R. Boland, M. Goodsell, L. Harmond, D. Larsen and D. Shirley

The preceding chapters have evaluated the theory and principles of musculoskeletal physiotherapy practice on the basis of current knowledge. This chapter demonstrates how some of this information is used in clinical practice. The integration of theory with clinical practice has proved to be extremely difficult: many of our treatment strategies affect the body and tissues in ways not currently understood; decisions made are often based on clinical experience rather than scientific 'fact'; much pathology is not yet clearly defined; and clinical diagnoses sometimes appear unsatisfactory when subjected to rigorous scrutiny. The difficulties encountered in attempting to integrate theory with practice raise many issues about the foundation of our practice as musculoskeletal physiotherapists. Current practice is poorly documented with few case studies appearing in the literature to demonstrate effectiveness. We therefore considered it valuable to describe selected examples of common musculoskeletal physiotherapy practice, and attempt to explain the rationale behind examination and treatment decisions. Some practitioners and teachers of orthopaedic and manual physiotherapy may disagree with certain specific aspects of examination and treatment decisions in the following cases. Such controversy, however, highlights the lack of uniformity in our practice and the justification of the various management approaches. Until randomized controlled clinical trials are conducted, all approaches should probably be considered equally effective. As long as the measured treatment outcomes are valid and carefully monitored using reproducible measurement tools, we can be certain of the effect of intervention on individual patients.

Research activity is rapidly increasing, ensuring that many issues at present not understood will become clear in the future. The authors of the following clinical cases are manipulative physiotherapists who have engaged in further formal education. They have based the following cases on patients who presented to them for treatment.

Several approaches have been taken to illustrate the salient points. On some occasions, two cases with similar presentations are described with a key piece of information that differs between cases. This information is heavily weighted because it suggests that different pathology is responsible for the signs and symptoms and/or that a different management strategy is required. Unusual cases are also presented to highlight signs and symptoms that might alert physiotherapists to the presence of serious pathology. In all cases, the reader is taken through the treating physiotherapist's processing of information as diagnoses and treatment plans are formulated.

A number of abbreviations are used in the case studies. For ease of reference the full terms and abbreviations are displayed in Table 8.1.

Posture

The means of examining posture and the relevance of findings are discussed in Chapter 6. One of the recommendations from this discussion is that the physiotherapist should relate postural 'abnormalities' to the presence of signs and symptoms. In other words, if 'abnormal' posture increases signs

Table 8.1 Abbreviations used in case studies

Term	Abbreviation
Movements and directions	
Extension	E
Flexion	F
Rotation	Rot
Lateral flexion	LF
Right	R
Left	L
Techniques and procedures	
Computerized tomography	CT
Localized manipulation	L(v)
Magnetic resonance imaging	MRI
Passive accessory intervertebral movement	PAIVM
Passive neck flexion	PNF
Passive physiological intervertebral movement	PPIVM
Posteroanterior mobilisation	PA
Prone knee bend	PKB
Straight leg raise	SLR
Anatomical and clinical terms	
As required	PRN
First or fifth lumbar vertebra	L1 or L5
First or seventh cervical vertebra	C1 or C7
Intermittent	I/T
No abnormality detected	NAD
Posterior cruciate ligament	PCL
Remained the same (in status quo)	ISQ
Sacroiliac joint	SIJ
Spiral nerve/nerve roots	SN/NR

and symptoms, then it should be possible to decrease these signs and symptoms by altering posture. If this relationship can be demonstrated, altering posture may form an appropriate part of the management plan. The two following case studies illustrate this point.

Case 1

A young woman presented with suboccipital headaches and pain in the right cervical spine. The neck pain and headache were aggravated by prolonged periods of office work. While taking the history the physiotherapist noticed that the patient appeared to sit in a position of lumbar spine flexion, thoracic kyphosis and upper cervical spine extension. The physiotherapist wondered whether this sitting position was aggravating the symptoms and whether this was how the patient sat at work. When the patient's position was adjusted so that the lumbar spine was in a more neutral position, the thoracic kyphosis became less marked and the upper cervical spine appeared to be less extended. After maintaining this position for a short period the patient felt a decrease in the intensity of the cervical pain.

In this case a relationship was established between the cervical spine pain and the posture the patient adopted when sitting. As part of the treatment, the therapist advised the patient to use a lumbar support when sitting. The patient was asked to use the lumbar support over the next 24 h, and to monitor the intensity of the neck pain over this period, to determine the effect of modifying sitting position on the cervical symptoms.

Case 2

A 16-year-old schoolboy complained of a 4-week history of diffuse occipital and frontal headaches associated with a stiff uncomfortable feeling in the right cervical and suprascapular region. These symptoms were associated with an increase in the amount of time spent studying. The neck discomfort was aggravated by long periods of reading or writing at his desk. The headaches were virtually constant and tended to be worse at the end of the day. On observation of the patient's sitting posture during the physical examination, the physiotherapist noted that he had a slightly increased thoracic kyphosis, and slightly increased upper cervical spine extension. The patient did not have neck pain at the time of the examination and the slight headache present was not affected by altering his sitting position. The patient's description of the positions adopted when studying suggested that, although his chair had a lumbar support and was appropriately adjusted, he spent prolonged periods of time with his neck in flexion when reading and writing at his desk. He also tended to study for periods of about 3 h without having a break.

In this case there did not appear to be a clear relationship between the patient's posture during relaxed sitting and the symptoms. The history of onset and the aggravating factors, however, suggested that the position he adopted when studying was implicated in the production and perpetuation of these symptoms. Therefore suitable aims of treatment might be to modify the positions adopted while studying [for example modify the height and inclination of the patient's desk or chair (Rodgers and Eggleton, 1983)], decrease the time spent in flexion, and to evaluate the effect of such modification on the patient's symptoms.

Diagnosis and treatment selection

The guidelines and rationale for making a physiotherapy diagnosis and deciding the most appropriate treatment dose are evaluated and presented in detail in other sections of this book, particularly Chapters 4, 5, 6 and 7. It is sometimes difficult to imagine how this information will be utilized in one's own clinical practice.

The following cases have been chosen to emphasize the steps involved in the diagnostic process and the methods used to select an appropriate treatment. Each case study presents the key features from the history and physical examination, the physiotherapist's comments on the importance of these findings, their clinical diagnosis, aims of treatment and rationale for the treatment selected. A summary of treatment results and progress is provided as well as an indication of the number of treatments needed, the patient's role in their management and the eventual result.

The following case study is an example of someone who probably has a non-specific mechanical disorder of the cervical spine.

Case 3. A non-specific mechanical disorder of the cervical spine (Fig 8.1)

Key findings from the history (Visit 1)

A 28-year-old woman presented for treatment with a constant dull ache on the right side of her neck. A sharp pain was experienced if she attempted to turn her head to the right or extend her neck. The pain had started 4 days previously while the patient was serving in a tennis game, and had been present since. The patient found it difficult to carry out her work as a receptionist particularly as she often talked on the telephone with the receiver wedged between her head and shoulder. This aggravated the pain.

The patient experienced one similar episode 2 years ago which resolved over a few days with some physiotherapy treatment. The treatment consisted of some passive mobilizations, ice and exercises.

The patient's general health was excellent and X-rays were normal.

Immediate clinical impressions

The problem presented as a 'mechanical' cervical spine problem (Magarey, 1988) most likely

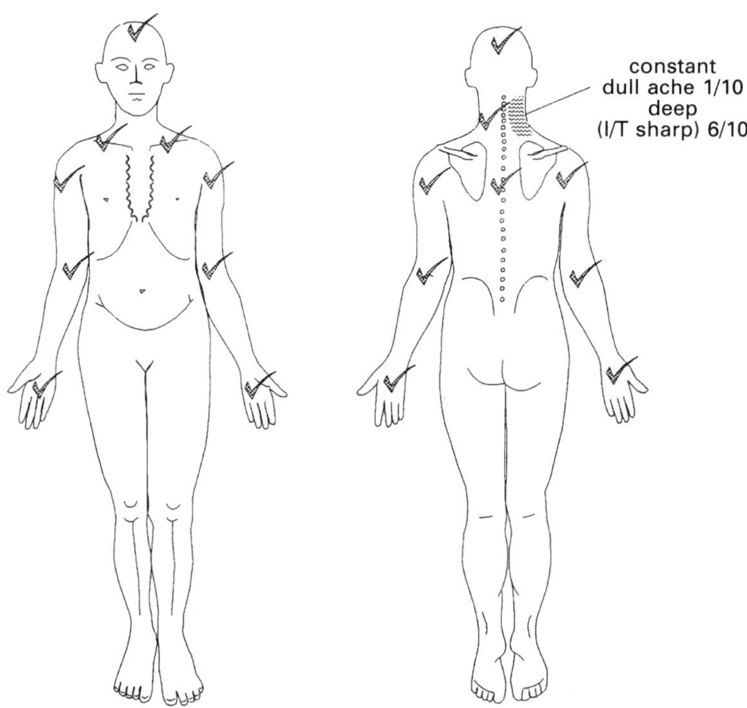

Figure 8.1 Case 3. A non-specific mechanical disorder of the cervical spine

involving damage to a cervical somatic structure (Bogduk and Twomey, 1991). The physiotherapist expected to reproduce the symptoms with some single plane active movements, e.g. Rot, LF and/or E, because these are the movements the patient suggested provoked the pain. As the symptoms appear to be consistent with a non-specific mechanical disorder, the physiotherapist also expected to reproduce the symptoms on passive accessory examination.

Key physical examination findings (Visit 1)

Observation
The patient was holding her head in a slightly flexed position.

Active movements
R LF was limited by pain at one-third range of movement. Rot to the R and E were also limited by pain at half range of movement.

PAIVM testing
R unilateral PA pressure on C2 reproduced the sharp neck pain; R unilateral PA on C3 was slightly painful.

PPIVM testing
R LF between C2 and C3 was restricted at one-third range of movement and reproduced some pain.

Reassessment after examination
After PAIVM examination LF had increased to half range and there was less pain. There was no further change on reassessment after PPIVMs.
[See Maitland, (1986) for description of PPIVM and PAIVM testing].

Clinical impressions

The physical findings were consistent with information from the history and suggested that the source of the symptoms was likely to be a somatic

structure of the cervical spine (Bogduk and Twomey, 1991).

Specifically the examination suggested that:

1. *The signs and symptoms indicated a mechanical disorder of non-specific pathology.*
2. *Somatic structures at C1/2 or C2/3 could be responsible for the symptoms because:*
   (a) *pain was reproduced, and range of movement was reduced, during movements which would involve C1/2 and C2/3;*
   (b) *the area of pain could be referred from C2.*
3. *There appears to be a single source of pain.*
4. *Reassessment after manual examination indicated that use of PAIVMs increased range of movement and decreased pain more than use of PPIVMs.*

The immediate goals of treatment were to:

1. *increase range of R LF (as well as E and Rot);*
2. *decrease pain during movement.*

Treatment (Visit 1)

To achieve the treatment goals a R unilateral PA on C2 was selected.

Dose: Oscillation just short of pain for 45 s, repeated three times

Results: Absence of constant dull ache;
R LF: two-thirds range with mild sharp pain and mild feeling of stiffness;
R Rot and E were less painful and had increased range.

Clinical impressions

These results were slightly better than the physiotherapist had expected. The patient was asked to take careful note of behaviour of symptoms and signs over the next 48 h, and advised to avoid holding the telephone between her ear and shoulder as far as possible. If the activity had to be performed in this way then she was advized to use a wedge on the telephone receiver.

Visit 2 (2 days later)

Key findings from the history
The patient returned 2 days later reporting 60% improvement compared with the status before treatment. She still had moderate pain while holding the telephone between her neck and shoulder, although she had avoided doing this as much as possible. The constant ache had not returned. The patient had noticed that her neck felt a bit stiff in the morning but the stiffness eased after her morning shower.

Key findings from the physical examination
Active movements
R LF was still the most restricted active movement and reproduced mild pain at two-thirds range.
E was three-quarters normal range with some pain on overpressure.
R Rot was full range, with mild pain on overpressure.
A combined movement of R LF and E reproduced the symptoms to the extent experienced by the patient when talking on the telephone.

PAIVM testing
A R unilateral PA on C2 articular pillar with cervical spine in neutral reproduced mild pain.
A unilateral PA on C2 when cervical spine was in R LF reproduced the pain to the same extent as when talking on the telephone.

PPIVM testing
R LF between C2 and C3 felt restricted (approximately three-quarters range of movement).

Reassessment
After PAIVMs in R LF there was less pain on combined LF and E.

Clinical impressions

The immediate response to treatment at the first visit and the improvement in signs and symptoms 2 days later tend to confirm the diagnosis that the disorder was mechanical.

There was improved range of R Rot and E and LF. Further examination with combined movements was carried out at the second visit because there was only mild pain on single plane movements, and the movements had greater range. The most painful activity, i.e. talking on the telephone, was likely to involve a combination of R LF and E therefore this combination was examined. PAIVMs were examined in R LF for the same reasons. It was noted that there was a greater improvement in the combined movement after the PAIVM was performed in R LF than when performed in neutral.

Treatment (Visit 2)

R unilateral PA on C2 was performed in one-third range of R LF.
Dose: Three repetitions of approximately 60 s. Large oscillations were performed towards the end of the range.
Reassessment: Performance of the combined movement R LF and E produced only mild pain and slight restriction of range.

Visit 3

Two days later the patient returned reporting 85% improvement since treatment began. The only symptoms now experienced were after talking on the telephone for more than 5 min with the telephone held between neck and shoulder, and mild pain during serving at tennis.

Physical examination (Visit 3)

R LF was slightly stiff and produced mild pain on overpressure. The combined movement of R LF and E also produced mild pain. A R unilateral PA on C2 in R LF was slightly stiff and produced mild pain at end of range. There was slight restriction on C2/3 R LF PPIVM.

Treatment (Visit 3)

R LF PPIVM at C2/3 (Maitland, 1986)
Dose: Three repetitions of approximately 60 s. Large oscillations were performed towards the end of the range.
Active movements were reassessed after each repetition to ensure that force and duration of treatment dose were appropriate.

Reassessment (after completion of three repetitions): Combined movement (R LF and E) was full range with no pain. There was a very slight feeling of stiffness on a. R unilateral PA on C2 (repeated as for day 1). The patient was advised to perform stretches and active movements 30 min daily to ensure regaining normal range and function. The patient was asked to ring the physiotherapist 1 week later to report on recovery. The patient was provisionally discharged, full discharge to occur after results of self-management known.

Summary of clinical impressions

The patient responded well to treatment and would be expected to remain symptom free, as the active movements and passive movements were now only slightly restricted. It would be expected that these mild restrictions would resolve with normal activities. Treatment was progressed to include a passive physiological procedure as the R LF had remained slightly restricted; this movement was involved in the activity of talking on the telephone and PAIVM treatment had failed to fully restore this movement.

This case study demonstrates a progression of assessment and treatment as the patient improves. Progression of examination procedures was necessary because both the single plane movements and PAIVMs became less painful with a greater range of movement. Failure to progress treatment is likely to result in much slower progress or a less satisfactory result of treatment.

Headaches

Headache is a common complaint in our society, usually constituting no more than a nuisance. Headaches, however, can be a manifestation of vascular or serious intracranial pathology such as cerebral aneurysm or tumour. As primary-contact practitioners, therefore, physiotherapists need to be able to recognize the more serious presentations.

Various classification systems have been developed, representing weighting of information used as diagnostic indicators. The classification system currently employed is that devised by the International Headache Society (IHS) (Olesen, 1988). Most recurring headaches are classified as migraine or tension headaches (Marcus, 1992).

Migraine headaches

The IHS system defines migraine as recurrent headache without aura and lasting 4–72 h with either (a) nausea and/or vomiting or (b) photophobia *and* phonophobia, and two of the following:

1. unilateral location,
2. pulsating pain,
3. inhibition of daily activities,
4. worsening with routine activities.

There are additional criteria describing migraine with aura. The neurological aura must have three of the following four features:

1. reversible neurological symptoms suggesting cerebral or brainstem dysfunction;
2. evolution of the aura over 4 min or two or more symptoms occurring in succession;
3. no single aura symptom lasting longer than 1 h;
4. an interval between aura and beginning of head pain of no more than 1 h.

'Typical' auras include unilateral visual, motor or sensory disturbances and speech disturbance.

Tension headaches

Headaches traditionally classified as arising from muscle contraction are termed tension headaches in the IHS classification system (Olesen, 1988). Episodic tension headaches are defined as recurring headaches lasting from 30 min to 1 week, with chronic tension headaches occurring at least 15 days per month for a period of at least 6 months. Both types of tension headache are characterized by the *absence* of nausea and/or vomiting and *absence* of the combination of photophobia and phonophobia. In addition, two of the following features should be present:

1. bilateral location,
2. non-pulsating pain,
3. no prohibition of daily routine,
4. no worsening with routine daily activities.

Cervicogenic headaches

Cervicogenic headache has not yet been included in the IHS classification system (Sjaastad *et al.*, 1990). Preliminary diagnostic criteria for cervicogenic headache were suggested in 1987

(Fredriksen *et al.*, 1987; Pfaffenrath *et al.*, 1987) following the accumulation of considerable clinical data. However, further clinical trials are probably required before the criteria can be incorporated into the classification system.

Major signs and symptoms are:
1. unilateral head pain without sideshift;
2. symptoms and signs of neck involvement, including:
   (a) head pain triggered by neck movement and/ or sustained awkward head positioning;
   (b) head pain, similar in distribution and character to the spontaneously occurring pain elicited by external pressure applied over the ipsilateral upper posterior neck region or occipital region;
   (c) ipsilateral neck, shoulder, and arm pain of vague non-radicular nature;
   (d) reduced range of motion of the cervical spine.

It is strongly recommended that physiotherapists become familiar with these classifications of headache so that they can recognize headaches that may have a serious pathological cause, and refer the patient for appropriate investigation and intervention. In general, severe unremitting pain is a cause for concern. Headaches that are cervical in origin (i.e. referred from upper cervical spine) can generally be appropriately treated by physiotherapy. Other pathologies must be excluded, and a relationship established between the headache and other cervical signs and symptoms.

Case 4. Mechanical cervicogenic headache (Fig. 8.2)

Key features of the history

A 22-year-old waitress presented with a 6-month history of left-sided suboccipital headache related to mild left supraorbital pain (Figure 8.2). There were no arm or right-sided symptoms. The headaches occurred twice weekly although they did not follow any identifiable diurnal pattern or relationship to activity. She did not experience any dizziness, aura or any other symptoms.

The patient could not identify any aggravating factors that precipitated the headaches although she thought they were more likely to occur during

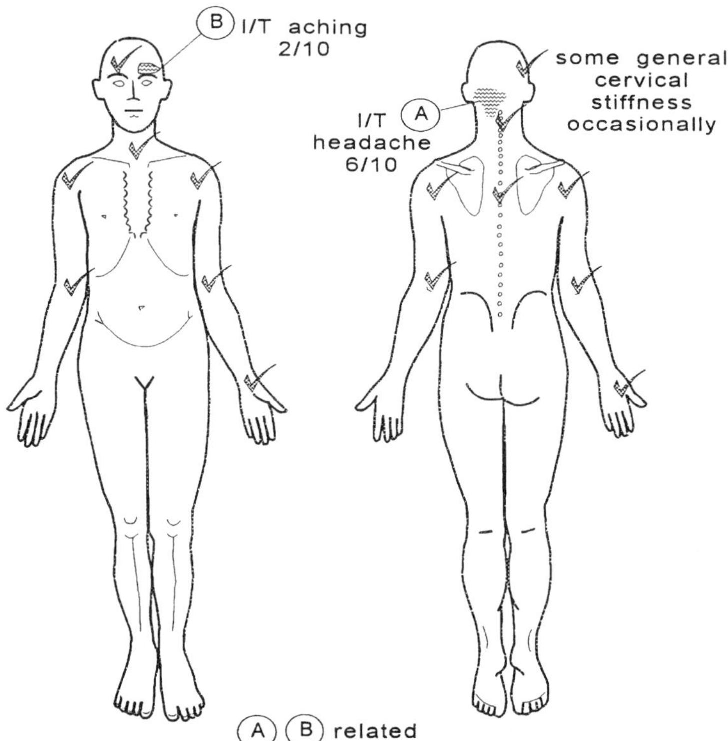

Figure 8.2 Case 4. Cervicogenic headache

a particularly busy shift at work. She could only relieve the headaches by resting in bed. She noticed some generalized cervical stiffness when she had a headache. There was no past history of injury or precipitating factors.

Her general health was otherwise excellent. X-rays were NAD.

Clinical impressions

This patient presented with a history of headaches not unlike cervicogenic headache. There was no apparent activity that aggravated the headache. The regularity of the two headaches per week raised the possibility of migraine headaches; however, the absence of aura and any other features such as photophobia, nausea or vomiting reduced this likelihood. In the physical examination, the physiotherapist intended to determine whether the head symptoms could be referred from the cervical spine by examining the upper cervical spine (Braaf and Rosner, 1975). If the headache were cervicogenic, the physiotherapist would expect to find reproduction of the same pain on active movements and on PAIVM, and perhaps on PPIVM. There may also be some pain on muscle testing. If none of these signs were found, then the physiotherapist would have to consider other possible origins for the headache and possible referral for other investigations.

Key features of the physical examination (Visit 1)

Observation
The patient tended to sit with a more forward head position [commonly associated with headache, (Watson and Trott, 1993)]. This position was reversible when facilitated by the physiotherapist, but did not alter symptoms.

Active movements
Cervical active movements were unrestricted and pain-free.

Overpressure of R upper cervical side flexion and R upper cervical quadrant (described in Maitland, 1986) produced R suboccipital discomfort. This was less intense than and of different quality from the patient's reported symptoms although in the same distribution. The physiotherapist could not reproduce the

---

supraorbital pain with active movements or overpressure.

PAIVM
R unilateral PA C1 in R Rot (described in Maitland, 1986) reproduced a mild suboccipital headache and appeared to be restricted compared with the L.

Reassessment: R LF with overpressure was unchanged.

PPIVM
Extension and R LF and L LF appeared to be restricted.

Reassessment: R LF with overpressure was unchanged.

Clinical impressions

There did not appear to be a relationship between the patient's posture and symptoms. However, there did appear to be some relationship between symptoms and cervical spine signs: discomfort was produced in the same region as the headaches, by R LF and upper cervical quadrant and on PAIVM testing. Overall, the physical findings were consistent with the history and indicated that physiotherapy treatment may relieve head pain. The source of symptoms could be somatic structures at the atlanto-occipital joint.
The examination suggests that:

1. *Signs and symptoms could be from a mechanical disorder with no specific pathology.*
2. *The occipital–C1 joint could be responsible for symptoms because:*
   (a) mild discomfort was reproduced on PAIVM testing of the atlanto-occipital joint. The joint felt abnormal compared with the left and there appeared to be reduced range on local movement testing.
   (b) the area of pain could be referred from C1.

There was no change in active movement testing after examination, however, indicating that treatment may need to be fairly vigorous. Symptoms need to be carefully monitored since the relationship between the areas of pain although consistent and likely, has not been firmly established.

The goals of treatment were to reduce pain in R LF and upper cervical spine quadrant and reduce the frequency of headaches.

Treatment (Visit 1)

R unilateral PA on C1.

Dose: three repetitions of 30 s. Quite vigorous forces were used, oscillating near end of range.

Reassessment: R LF, F and upper cervical quadrant remained unchanged. The physiotherapist noted that the patient's suboccipital muscles did not seem relaxed during treatment.

The patient was advised to record symptoms and activities in a diary to assist memory recall and to try to establish a pattern in symptoms.

Clinical impressions

The symptomatic mobilization was chosen for treatment but reassessment demonstrated no subsequent change in discomfort. This suggested either that treatment was directed at an inappropriate spinal level or that a different technique might have been more effective.

Progress (Visit 2 to 4)

The patient returned to physiotherapy three times in the following week and reported that her suboccipital headaches had reduced to once weekly and her supraorbital pain had disappeared.

Treatment (Visits 2 and 3)

As for visit 1 with increasing vigour of application.

Physical examination

Upper cervical quadrant had become pain-free but was still restricted in range compared with the left.
R LF was still restricted and caused slight discomfort.

Passive motion testing

PA on C1 still reproduced mild suboccipital headache.

Treatment (Visit 4)

Improvement had continued with treatment of R C1. Pain was still reproduced on active R LF with overpressure. However, the headache could still be reproduced with R unilateral PA on C1, and PPIVM still seemed to indicate restricted movement. The physiotherapist chose to locally manipulate the patient's R atlanto-occipital joint. A LF manipulation towards the left (described in Maitland, 1986) was chosen because the suboccipital headache was reproduced during positioning for manipulation.

Vertebral artery testing NAD

Consent was gained for manipulation.

Reassessment after manipulation

R LF
increased range of movement with no discomfort.

PAIVM
no supraorbital headache was reproduced during palpation.

PPIVM
increased range in extension and R LF.

The patient was advised to return for follow-up in 1 week to report on headache status.

Clinical impressions

The response of symptoms to treatment suggests that the headache was cervicogenic, caused by somatic structures at the atlanto-occipital joint. Mobilization improved symptoms, but did not completely relieve them, therefore localized manipulation was performed to resolve residual symptoms and stiffness.

Visit 5

Follow-up: Seven days later the patient returned and reported that she had not suffered from headache at all in the week since the last treatment.

Assessment: Pain-free unrestricted movement in right upper quadrant, R LF and passive movement testing of C1 on the R.
The patient was discharged from treatment. Movements were full range and pain-free.

Testing adequacy of cerebral blood flow (vertebral artery testing)

The consequences of occluding or damaging the vertebrobasilar system in the absence of adequate collateral cerebral circulation are serious (Patjin, 1991; Terrett, 1987). It is recommended, therefore, that physiotherapists test for adequate cerebral blood flow whenever the patient complains of dizziness (either when specifically questioned, or if onset of dizziness occurs during procedures in the physical examination) and always before cervical manipulation, even when the patient has never previously experienced signs and symptoms of vertebrobasilar insufficiency (VBI) (APA protocol, 1988; see Chapter 6 under Testing adequacy of cerebral blood flow). However, when testing for VBI, caution must be applied to ensure that the tests themselves do not cause consequences of diminished cerebral blood flow.

The tests for VBI are neither specific nor sensitive (Hutchinson, 1989; Bolton *et al.*, 1989), therefore interpretation of results is sometimes difficult. Since errors of judgement about VBI can result in serious injuries, conservative interpretation is usually recommended. This means that if any of the tests are positive (i.e. provoke dizziness or associated symptoms) the results should be interpreted as possible VBI, even if the clinical picture is not completely consistent with such an interpretation. If a patient has complained of dizziness which is not reproduced on any testing, the results are still interpreted as possible VBI. In both situations, however, the clinical picture is re-evaluated on the second visit, after effects of intervention are known. In

this way, serious errors of judgement will be avoided.

When the patient has an irritable condition it is not always possible to test VBI. Since vigorous doses and provocative positions would not normally be used to treat irritable conditions, it is possible to treat safely without knowledge of test results, but with close monitoring of signs and symptoms of VBI. If VBI is suspected, then the patient's medical practitioner should be consulted, further investigations probably being required.

Case 5

Key features from the history

A 50-year-old woman presented with right-sided upper neck pain (in the atlanto-occipital region) and right-sided occipital headache (Figure 8.3). The headache was usually present when she woke in the morning, settled during the day and did not vary in response to activity. The neck pain was aggravated by activities involving rotation and extension e.g. reversing the car and hanging out washing. The pain settled when the activities were ceased.

The episode had started about 1 month previously for no apparent reason, although the patient had spent the previous weekend painting the living room before noticing symptoms. The patient had never experienced neck pain or headaches before. She had not previously sought treatment for this episode. Her symptoms had not changed over the past 2 weeks.

The patient was also extremely concerned that in the past 2 weeks she had experienced three episodes of waking with severe dizziness, disorientation and nausea. The symptoms were so severe that they caused her to vomit and she was unable to walk. She was unable to relate the onset of these symptoms to any particular neck position or movement and had not had dizziness at any other time. Her general health was otherwise excellent. There were no other precautions or contraindications to physiotherapy.

Clinical impressions

Cases of VBI following sustained positioning, such as painting ceilings, have been documented (Nagler, 1973). This was, therefore, a possible injuring position for this patient. Sustained

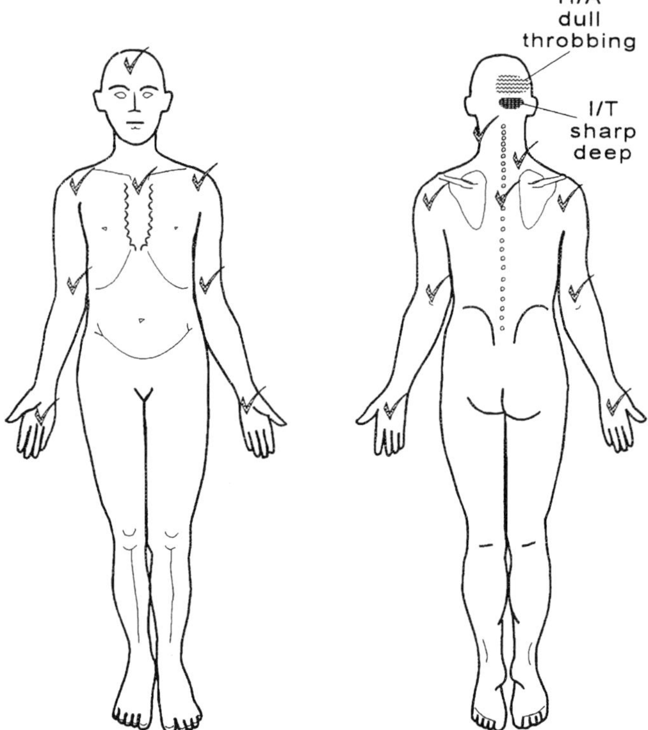

Figure 8.3 Case 5. Headache and dizziness

positioning during sleep (e.g. extension and rotation if she slept prone) could be responsible for the three episodes of dizziness. The symptoms, while suggestive of VBI, could also be caused by somatic structures in the cervical spine or by vestibular dysfunction. The physical examination would therefore include VBI and vestibular tests.

The planned physical examination

Reproduction of symptoms would be closely monitored throughout the physical examination, although it was not expected that they would be reproduced except on sustained postitioning as they had not been reproduced during normal functional activities. The musculoskeletal neck condition was not irritable therefore it was expected that vigorous manoeuvres would be necessary to reproduce head and neck symptoms. VBI testing would be performed before any of these manoeuvres, e.g. combined movements, including quadrant. The results of these tests would determine treatment options, because some positions would be avoided and vigorous forces not used for other procedures.

Key features from the physical examination

Observation

No remarkable findings

Active movements

No reproduction of neck pain, headache or dizziness.

Vertebral artery testing

Dizziness was reproduced on right rotation combined with extension.

Upper cervical quadrant

R quadrant (described in Maitland, 1986) reproduced the headache but no other symptoms.

PAIVM

R unilateral PA on C2 reproduced the neck pain, headache and dizziness.

Clinical impressions

The most likely cause of pain is non-specific mechanical spinal disorder of the right somatic structures at C1–C2. The pain was not reproduced on active movement testing, but the headache was reproduced on positioning in combined extension, rotation and lateral flexion of upper cervical spine. All pains and dizziness were reproduced on PAIVM testing on C2.

The dizziness did not appear to be from vestibular dysfunction, but more likely to be from either VBI or cervical vertigo. The presence of dizziness on VBI testing makes VBI a possible hypothesis, although the low specificity of the tests means a diagnosis of VBI is not definitive. There are currently no sensitive and specific tests to differentiate VBI from cervical vertigo. Differential diagnosis can only be made retrospectively.

The condition is not irritable and therefore would benefit from a vigorous dose of treatment; however, caution must be applied because of the possible existence of VBI. Therefore treatment must be of a dose sufficient to avoid exacerbating dizziness. Combined positions or vigorous end of range procedures should also be avoided.

Aims of treatment

The initial aims of treatment are to:

1. reduce neck pain and headache;
2. monitor dizziness, and determine differential diagnosis on second visit.

Treatment

R unilateral PA on C2.
Dose: the force used was in the part of accessory range of movement that was not producing dizziness.

Three repetitions of 45 s were performed.
Reassessment: decreased pain on quadrant

Visit 2

The patient returned 2 days later having had no further episodes of severe dizziness. VBI testing on Rot combined with E produced only a very mild feeling of dizziness and reduced headache on upper cervical quadrant testing.

PAIVM

R unilateral PA on C2 required a greater force to produce dizziness.

Treatment

Unilateral PA on right C2 (as per treatment on Visit 1)

Reassessment

No dizziness was reproduced on Rot with E. The headache had also improved on upper cervical quadrant testing, and only slight neck pain was elicited during performance of PAIVMs.

Clinical impressions

The dizziness produced by the combined rotation with extension position is most likely to be due to cervical vertigo as the symptoms were improving with manual treatment (Cercut, 1988). It is not clear how the three severe episodes of dizziness related to the dizziness produced by PAIVM testing. It is possible that a sustained end-of-range position during sleep could have stressed cervical somatic structures, stimulating dizziness (Abrahams, 1981). The patient was advised to return to her medical practitioner should dizziness and the associated symptoms recur to have further investigations.

Follow-up Visit 3

After the last treatment the patient had no pain, had full range pain-free upper cervical spine quadrant and had experienced no further episodes of dizziness.

A non-mechanical problem

Occasionally patients present with back pain (and movement restriction) which appears to be mechanical, but has some atypical features. Such atypical features may include unremitting night pain, unusual distribution of pain, unusual pain behaviour and unexpected responses to physiotherapy. The presence of these signs and symptoms arouses suspicion of non-mechanical pathology. Spinal cord or cauda equina neurological symptoms and signs are not always present even in the presence of serious pathology in the region of the spinal cord or cauda equina. Such signs include sphincter disturbance, saddle anaesthesia, positive cord signs or pyramidal or lower motor neuron signs (see Chapter 6 under Neurological testing).

The following case details the clinical presentation of a patient presenting with low back pain who subsequently was diagnosed as having a neurofibroma at the level of the conus medullaris. Standard radiological examination of the lumbar spine failed to identify the problem. Many features of this case study were not typical of a non-specific mechanical musculoskeletal disorder.

Case 6

Key findings in the history

A 35-year-old woman was referred with right lower back and inguinal pain, and anterior thigh and leg pain (Figure 8.4). The referring rheumatologist requested that the physiotherapist confirm his suspicions about the nature of the patient's disorder. He was particularly interested in the physiotherapist's opinion of the status of the SIJ as a possible site of this woman's pain. The source of pain was elusive despite extensive investigation.

The patient reported that the right groin pain began abruptly during the first trimester of her second pregnancy (6 months ago) and increased in severity and distribution during the pregnancy. Her son was delivered at 36 weeks with an uneventful labour. There was no respite from symptoms after delivery and since then she had become increasingly distressed by pain, to the point of needing regular oral opiate and increasing amounts of injected pethidine.

Night pain was severe and unremitting (the patient was unable to find a position of relief or

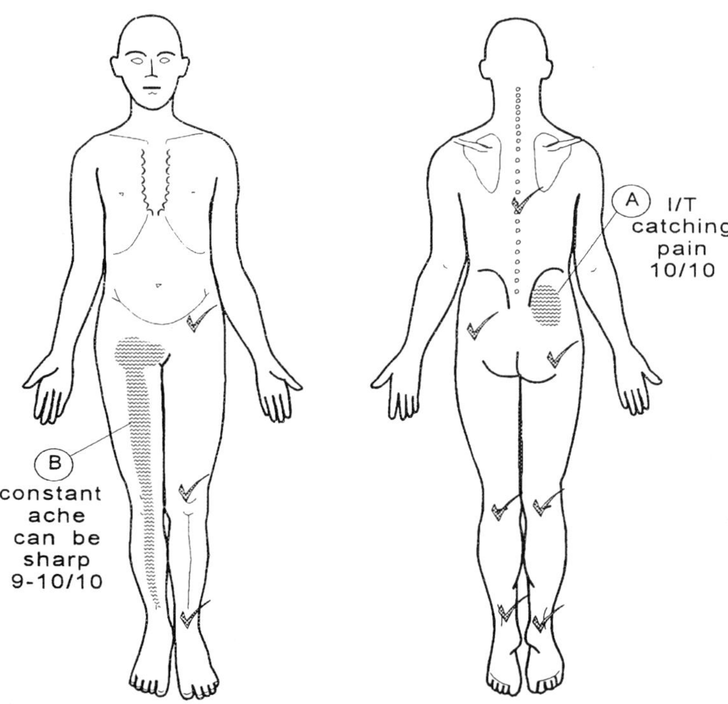

Figure 8.4

ease the pain in any way), despite regular analgesic use. The patient was consequently exhausted when she presented.

Aggravating activites: there was no particular position or movement that worsened symptoms, but the patient was unable to stand or walk for more than 3–4 h. She therefore spent most of her time in bed. At the time of presentation to physiotherapy her pain was so disabling that she required a housekeeper to care for her two children aged 4 years, and 5 months.

The only relief from pain was analgesia from strong medication.

The patient had lost weight (8 kg) in the last 5 months, but had been unable to eat well because of the distressing nature of her pain.

Results of other investigations
Serology testing during pregnancy: increased erythrocyte sedimentation rate.

Radiological investigations could not be performed during pregnancy.

Recent imaging included:
plane radiograph of low lumbar spine and SIJ: NAD;
CT scans of low lumbar spine: NAD;
bone scans of low lumbar spine: NAD;
MRI of pelvis and sacrum: NAD.

Key findings in the physical examination

Observation

The patient was in obvious distress, standing in some hip and lumbar spine flexion.

Active movements

F reproduced pain over the right SIJ when fingertips were 10 cm from the floor.
E was pain-free, but restricted to 20°.
All other movements were full range and pain-free.

Neurological tests

NAD

Tension tests

R SLR reproduced right hip and thigh pain at 60°.

Palpation and passive motion testing

- of lumbar spine was not possible due to severe paravertebral muscle spasm and pain;
- of SIJ reproduced pain into posterior thigh.

Clinical impressions

This patient's problem did not appear to be a typical presentation of an SIJ disorder. The SIJ could have been involved, because inguinal and lower back pain are consistent with referral patterns from the SIJ. The anterior leg pain would be unusual, but possible since innervation of the SIJ is from L1–L3 spinal segments (Williams and Warwick, 1980). The physiotherapist was concerned, however, because the intensity of the pain, the unremitting night pain, the patient's weight loss and the severity of spasm in the paravertebral muscles were unlike a typical mechanical musculoskeletal presentation. The weight loss could be explained by the patient's lack of appetite due to severe pain. The lack of disturbance of active movements was inconsistent with the apparent irritability of the condition and pain intensity. The physiotherapist discussed these issues with the referring rheumatologist, suggesting that other pathology may be responsible for the pain.

The patient was referred for consultation with a neurologist. The neurologist identified the following key features:

1. the severity of the pain;
2. pain commencing during pregnancy;
3. severe night pain;
4. pronounced spasm in the paravertebral muscles.

The neurologist interpreted this information as being suspicious of a neoplasm, potentially in the upper lumbar spine. The patient subsequently had a CT scan of the upper lumbar spine, which demonstrated a neurofibroma at the level of the conus medullaris (Fig. 8.5). All previous scans had been directed at the low lumbar spine and pelvis

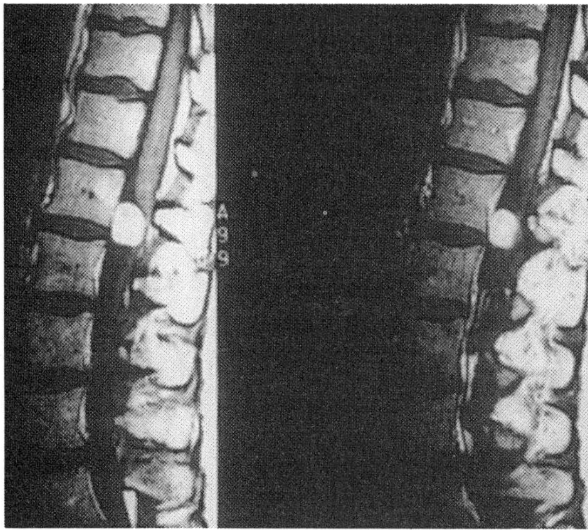

Figure 8.5 Neurofibroma compressing spinal cord in region of lower thoracic/upper lumbar spine

and therefore had missed the tumour. The patient underwent surgical removal of the tumour, and made a good recovery with minimal residual symptoms. Had progress of the tumour not been halted, cord compression and urinary symptoms are likely to have resulted (Mulder and Dale, 1993).

Prevention of chronic low back pain: active approach to managing acute low back pain

Although low back pain is largely self-limiting, 75% of cases resolving within 4 weeks and 90% within 3 months, a small proportion of cases may become chronic, persisting for 6 months or more (Nachemson, 1992). Chronic low back pain accounts for a disproportionate amount of the costs associated with back pain. It also seems that very few patients with chronic low back pain return to work (Spitzer *et al.*, 1987). Therefore, when managing patients with acute low back pain, one important aim of treatment is to prevent the progression of acute or subacute back pain to chronic back pain (see Chapter 9 for further information). It is also important that the procedures we use to treat low back pain do not foster disability or the development of chronic pain syndromes.

Several factors that increase the risk of developing chronic low back pain from an acute episode have been identified. Importantly, there appears to be a strong relationship between job satisfaction and reports of low back pain. It appears that the more satisfied the worker the less likely she/he is to complain of low back pain (Bigos *et al.*, 1991). Violinn *et al.* (1991) in the USA, have identified additional risk factors. These include that the person:

(i)   has been absent from work for more than 14 days,

(ii)   is aged more than 40 years,

(iii)   earns a monthly wage of less than $US1,000, and

(iv)   has a family status of either divorced or widowed with no children.

Psychological variables may also be associated with the development of chronic pain syndromes from acute episodes. Waddell *et al.* (1984) and Main *et al.* (1992) found that the most important psychological trait associated with chronic low back pain was increased bodily awareness. It could be argued that the physiotherapist's focus on pain to guide a patient with low back pain may develop increased bodily awareness, assessment and treatment. This focus may lead to increased disability in some patients, and actually foster the development of chronicity. Physiotherapists should therefore be aware that the thorough system of examination could encourage an abnormal increase in bodily awareness.

Preventing an acute episode of back pain from becoming a chronic pain syndrome may depend on both identifying the presence of risk factors and implementing an approriate approach to treatment. Weiser and Cedraschi (1992) suggest that at the first visit, the clinician should look for unusual signs of psychological distress, including expressed attitudes or behaviours indicating that the patient's recovery may be affected by his or her attitudes or beliefs. These expressed attitudes or behaviours may include excessive pain behaviours, increased bodily awareness and fear avoidance behaviour. Waddell (1992) suggests ways to minimise the patient's anxiety. He recommends that, after ruling out serious pathology, anxiety associated with low back pain should be relieved by reassuring the patient that the problem is one of simple non-specific low back pain that often resolves within 1–2 weeks and almost always by 6 weeks. He stresses the avoidance of words associated with long-term disability, such as rupture, degeneration or arthritis, using instead words associated with short term disability and early recovery. In addition, Weiser and Cedraschi (1992) strongly emphasize that the patient should be an active participant in their own recovery from the first treatment occasion rather than only a recipient of passive treatments.

The measurement of outcome in patients with acute and subacute low back pain needs to include measures that help identify whether a patient is progressing to a chronic pain syndrome. Many authors have stressed the importance of measuring disability, job satisfaction, quality of life, and fear avoidance behaviour (as well as pain and some measures of impairment). Questionnaires are readily available, easy to administer and easily scored (Bigos *et al.*, 1992; Spitzer *et al.*, 1987); Waddell, 1992; Fairbank *et al.*, 1980). Useful clinical measures may include submaximal aerobic testing and muscle endurance tests. Several authors (Berquist-Ullman and Larsson, 1977; Mayer *et al.*, 1985, 1987) have also demonstrated that high aerobic fitness can reduce back pain disability.

Biering-Sorensen (1984) found that subjects with recurrent low back pain had decreased endurance of the back extensors when compared with asymptomatic subjects. He therefore designed a simple test to assess extensor endurance and also provides normative data for this test (Biering-Sorensen 1984).

Treatment of acute and subacute low back pain, when relevant, could focus on active interventions such as exercise to increase fitness, improve trunk endurance, reduce pain, and restore general well being, perhaps by removing the fear of activity. This may include an individually-designed gym circuit programme, swimming, walking and cycling. Passive treatments such as mobilization and manipulation are appropriate for pain relief especially in the acute phase, but should rarely be the only focus of treatment after allowing time for tissue healing and repair. Often treatment will include the retraining of specific tasks such as lifting from different heights, and various loads, and other manual handling procedures. The training programme should be generic rather than job

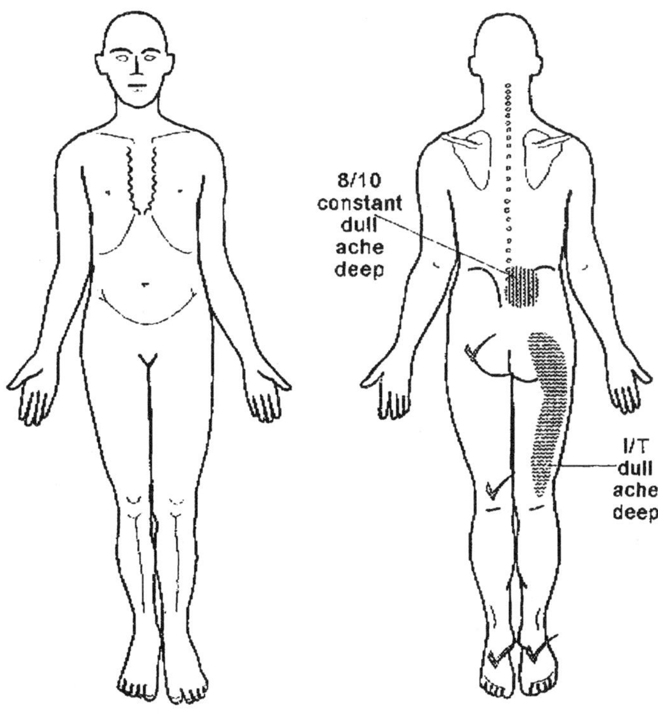

Figure 8.6 Mechanical low back pain

specific, and goal oriented, limited by quota or number of repetitions not pain, and perhaps time limited: patients are re-evaluated and returned to work at 4–6 weeks regardless of their pain status (providing there is no contra-indicating pathology) (Fordyce *et al.*, 1986).

The preceding discussion relates largely to patients with mechanical non-specific low back pain. A major role of the physiotherapist is to identify those patients with non specific low back pain and those with identifiable pathology requiring specific intervention. A thorough assessment should therefore always be completed to ensure appropriate diagnosis and intervention.

Case 7

Key features of the history

A 37-year-old package handler presented with back and leg pain. He felt an immediate sharp, severe pain in the right lumbar spine after lifting a package from a conveyor belt (in flexion and rotation) 3 weeks earlier. He also experienced difficulty straightening up. He continued to work until the end of his shift. The next day he noticed great difficulty getting out of bed and a dull ache in the posterior right thigh. He visited the local doctor who prescribed 10 days of bed rest and heat. He complied with this regimen, but his low back and posterior thigh pain remained ISQ. He consulted a different medical practitioner who referred him for physiotherapy management in preparation for return to work. His work involves much standing and bending. He has never had back problems before.

Currently the back and leg pain are aggravated by most flexion activities, e.g. tying up shoelaces, brushing teeth at the basin and sitting. Coughing markedly increases the pain, as do rotation activities in flexion. He can ease the pain by lying on his left side with his knees flexed, and by crook lying (supine with knees flexed).

He wakes at night when turning because of the pain, and wakes with pain in the morning.

X-rays: NAD. His general health is otherwise excellent.

He is a non-smoker, is single, currently plays little sport – ten pin bowling once weekly. Has had 10 days of physiotherapy treatment, of PA on L5, gentle oscillations, which decreased pain initially, and then plateaued.

Key findings – psychological testing

Quality of life index: Score = 6/10 (10/10 = high quality of life) (Spitzer *et al.*, 1987)

Oswestry Disability Measure: Score 50/90 (the higher the score the greater the disability) (Fairbank *et al.*, 1980).

Fear avoidance behaviour questionnaire: Score = 40/96 (the higher the score the greater the fear avoidance behaviour, and associated risk of developing chronicity).

Clinical impressions

The traumatic onset suggests that the patient has sustained a musculoskeletal injury. The increase in pain caused by flexion, particularly combined with rotation, suggests involvement of the posterior elements of the lumbar spine. The physiotherapist intends to investigate the involvement of injury to the posterior structures by examining the lumbar spine including the spinal nerve/nerve root at L5/S1. The questionnaire results suggest that the patient exhibits high fear avoidance, reduced quality of life, and marked disability. It is possible that the patient may now have reduced fitness and muscle strength following the three weeks bedrest and time off work. These will also be assessed.

Key features of the physical examination

Active movements

Movements were restricted in all directions by pain:

Flexion: 1/2 ROM, marked increase LBP and thigh pain (32° = inclinometer measure);

Ext: 1/2 ROM, marked increase LBP and thigh pain (14° = inclinometer measure);

LLF: mid-femur, marked increase LBP and thigh pain;

RLF: mid-femur, marked increase LBP/thigh pain.

Neurological examination: NAD

Tension tests:
Right SLR: 50° hip flexion caused LBP and leg pain. The addition of DF increased both pains.
Left SLR: 65° hip flexion caused slight LBP. The addition of DF produced no change.

Soft tissue palpation: mid-line tenderness L2–L5.

Strength and endurance testing of trunk extensors: Unable to complete because pain too severe.

Clinical impressions

The patient has sustained an acute injury with no specific pathology. There is no neural involvement, X-rays are clear, and there are no other signs or symptoms suggesting specific pathology. Thus the problem appears to be mechanical non-specific low back pain. However, the marked disability, reduced quality of life, high fear avoidance behaviour noted from the history, as well as the time off work (3 weeks) suggests that with this patient it is important to prevent the development of a chronic pain syndrome.

Aims of treatment are therefore to: reduce pain; decrease his fear of activity; minimize the effects of inactivity; prevent further effects of pain-induced inactivity; and prevent the development of chronic pain. It will also be important to prepare the patient for return to work. The addition of active approach to treatment may therefore be appropriate at this stage.

The treatment plan requires determining a dose of exercise that will demonstrate to the patient his ability to successfully perform resisted exercises, improve or maintain his strength, but will not be detrimental in any way. It is anticipated that 50% of 1RM for his arm and leg muscles will be appropriate for general exercises. His capacity to exercise on a treadmill will also be tested, and a low level used for exercises. This dose will be maintained for 1 week, the dose increasing after 1 week for a further week (Fordyce *et al.*, 1986). The patient will then be reassessed to determine feasibility of discharge back to work on full duties.

Treatment 1

In addition to PA on L5 an exercise programme was instituted to decrease fear of activity and maintain general strength and aerobic fitness.

Treadmill: grade: 0
            speed: 3.5 mph
            duration: 15 min

General exercises in supine, prone and side-lying e.g.: knees to chest, extension exercises, hip abduction, pelvic tilting, trunk rotation, (10 repetitions of each exercise).

Reassessment: Reduced pain and increase in all active movements: F–40°, Ext–20°.

Treatments 2 and 3

Repeated as above.

In addition:
– circuit including stationary cycle for 5 min at low intensity, and resisted exercises for upper and lower limbs e.g. lat pull downs, chest presses, leg presses. Dose: 50% of 1RM, 10 repeats, 2 sets.

Treatment 4: (2 days later)

Improvement maintained.

Repeat Treatment 1 with increased intensity.

1RM reassessed. Exercises performed at 50% of new 1RM, and repeated 20 times. Treadmill time increased to 20 min.

Circuit time and intensity increased: Stationary cycle for 10 min, at higher intensity.

In addition: patient education about lifestyle and other factors affecting LBP.

Reassessment after 10 days:

Patient considered himself much improved as there had been a significant reduction in pain: the only remaining symptoms were slight left ache in lumbosacral junction, 1/10.

Questionnaires:
Oswestry = 8/90 (significant reduction from 50).
Quality of life = 10/10 (significant improvement from 6/10).
Fear avoidance behaviour questionnaire = 0/96 (now absent, significant improvement from 40).

Active movements: NAD except for slight pain at end of range flexion.
Soft tissue palpation: slight tenderness at lumbosaoral junction.
SLR: bilaterally limited 65° (equal pull in both hamstrings, no pain).
1RM improved for all muscles tested in upper and lower limbs.
Capacity for aerobic exercise improved in circuit programme and treadmill exercises.

Clinical impressions

There was a marked decrease in pain and disability, and the patient's fear of activity was removed. His strength improved, and the acute episode did not progress to a chronic pain syndrome. The patient was able to return to full employment without limitation following 2 weeks of supervised exercise. It was suggested that the patient maintain such an exercise programme to prevent further episodes of low back pain.

References

Abrahams, V.C. (1981) Sensory and motor specialization in some muscles of the neck. *Trends Neurosci.*, Jan., 24–27.

Australian Physiotherapy Association (1988). Protocol for pre-manipulative testing of the cervical spine. *Austr. J. Physiother.*, **34**, 97–100.

Berquist-Ullman, M. and Larsson, U. (1977) Acute LBP in industry. *Acta Orthop. Scand.* supplement, **170**, 1–117.

Biering-Sorensen F. (1984) Physical measurement as risk indicators for low-back trouble over a one-year period. *Spine*, **9**, 106–19.

Bigos, S. J., Battie, M. C., Spengler, D.M. *et al.* (1991). A prospective study of work perceptions and psychosocial factors affecting the report of back injury. *Spine*, **16**, 1–6.

Bogduk, N. (1984). The rationale for patterns of neck and back pain. *Patient Manag.*, **13**, 17–28.

Bogduk, N. (1988). Innervation and pain patterns of the cervical spine. In *Physical Therapy of the Cervical and Thoracic Spine*, R. Grant, (ed.), London: Churchill Livingstone.

Bogduk, N. and Twomey, L. (1991). *Clinical Anatomy of the Lumbar Spine* (2nd edn.). Melbourne: Churchill Livingstone.

Bolton, P.S., Stick, P.E. and Lord, R.S.A. (1989). Failure of clinical tests to predict cerebral ischaemia before neck manipulation. *J. Manipulative Physiol. Ther.*, **12**, 304–7.

Braaf, M. and Rosner, S. (1975). Trauma of cervical spine as a cause of chronic headache. *J. Trauma*, **15**, 441–6.

Fairbank, J., Couper, J., Davies, J. and O'Brien, J. (1980). The Oswestry low back pain disability questionnaire. *Physiotherapy*, **66**, 271–3.

Fordyce, W., Brockway, J., Bergman, J. and Spengler, D. (1986). Acute back pain: a control group comparison of behavioral vs traditional management methods. *J. Behav. Med.*, **9**, 127–40.

Fredriksen, T.A., Hovdal, H. and Sjaastad, O. (1987). 'Cervicogenic headache'. Clinical manifestation. *Cephalalgia*, **7**, 147–60.

Grant, R. (1988). Dizziness testing and manipulation of the cervical spine. In *Physical Therapy of the Cervical and Thoracic Spine* (R. Grant, ed.), London: Churchill Livingstone.

Hutchinson, M.S. (1989). An investigation of pre-manipulative dizziness testing. In *Proceedings of 5th Biennial Conference of Manipulative Physiotherapists of Australia, Sydney*, pp. 104–12.

Magarey, M.E. (1988). Examination of the cervical and thoracic spine. In *Physical Therapy of the Cervical and Thoracic Spine.*, (R. Grant, ed.), London: Churchill Livingstone.

Main, C.J., Wood, P.L.R., Hollis, S. *et al.* (1992). The distress and risk assessment method (DRAM): a simple patient classification to identify distress and evaluate the risk of poor outcome. *Spine*, **17**, 42–52.

Maitland, G.D. (1986). *Vertebral Manipulation* (5th edn.), London: Butterworth–Heinemann.

Marcus, D.A. (1992). Migraine and tension type headaches: the questionable validity of current classification systems. *Clin. J. Pain*, **8**, 28–36.

Mayer, T., Gatchel, R., Kishino, N. *et al.* (1985). Objective assessment of spine function following industrial injury: a prospective study with comparison group and one-year follow up. *Spine*, **10**, 482–93.

Mayer, T., Gatchel, R., Mayer, H. *et al.* (1987). A prospective two-year study of functional restoration in industrial low back injury. *J. Am. Med. Assoc.*, **258**, 1763–7.

Mense, S. (1993). Nociception from skeletal muscle in relation to clinical muscle pain. *Pain*, **54**, 241–89.

Mulder, D.W. and Dale, A.J.O. (1993). Spinal cord tumors and disks. In *Clinical Neurology* (R.J. Joynt, ed.), pp. 1–28,

Philadelphia: J.B. Lippincott.

Nachemson, A.L. (1992) Newest knowledge of low back pain. *Clin. Orthopaed. Rel. Res.,* **279**, 8–20.

Nagler, W. (1973) Vertebral artery obstruction by hyperextension of the neck: Report of three cases. *Arch. Phys. Med. Rehabil.,* **54**, 232–40.

Olesen, J. (1988). Classification and diagnostic criteria for headache disorders, cranial neuralgias and facial pain. *Cephalalgia,* **8**, (Suppl. 7), 1–96.

Patjin, J. (1991). Complications in manual medicine: a review of the literature. *J. Man. Med.* **6**, 89–92.

Pfaffenrath, V., Dandekar, R. and Pollmann, W. (1987). Cervicogenic headache – The clinical picture, radiological findings and hypotheses on its pathophysiology. *Headache,* 495–9.

Rodgers, S. and Eggleton, E. (eds) (1983). *Ergonomic Design for People at Work,* vol. 1. New York: Van Nostrand Reinhold.

Sjaastad, O., Fredriksen, T.A. and Pfaffenrath, V. (1990). The headache of challenge in our time: cervicogenic headache. *Funct. Neurol.,* **5**, 155–8.

Spitzer, W.O., Leblanc, F.E., Dupuis, M. *et al.* (1987). Scientific approach to the assessment and management of activity-related spinal disorders: a monograph for physicians. Report of the Quebec Task Force on Spinal Disorders. *Spine,* **13**, (suppl. 7); S1–S59.

Terrett, A.G. (1987). Vascular accidents from cervical spine manipulation: the mechanisms. *J. Austr. Chiropract. Assoc.,* **17**, 131–44.

Violinn, E., Van Koevering, D. and Loeser, J.D. (1991). Back sprain in industry: the role of socioeconomic factors in chronicity. *Spine,* **16**, 542–79.

Waddell, G., Main, C.J., Morris, E.W. *et al.* (1984). Chronic low back pain, psychological distress, and illness behaviour. *Spine,* **9**, 209–13.

Waddell, G. (1992). Biopsychosocial analysis of low back pain. *Clin. Rheumatol.,* **6**, 523–58.

Watson, D. and Trott, P. (1993). Cervical headache: an investigation of natural head posture and upper cervical flexor muscle performance. *Cephalalgia,* **13**, 272–84.

Williams, P. and Warwick, R. (eds) (1980). *Gray's Anatomy.* Edinburgh: Churchill Livingstone.

Weiser, S. and Cedraschi, C. (1992). Psychosocial issues in the prevention of chronic low back pain – a literature review. *Clin. Rheumatol.,* **6**, 657–84.

Chapter 9

The challenging role for physiotherapy in chronic musculoskeletal disorders

E.M. Gass

It is vital that physiotherapists continually question and evaluate their role in improving and maintaining the health of the community in which they work. It is no longer adequate to continue delivery of clinical practices simply because that is the way it has been done in the past. Evaluation of specific physiotherapy practices, the needs of patients and the needs of the health care system must be systematically undertaken.

In Australia, as in many other countries, some of the current factors that influence the context of physiotherapy include:

1. a rapid trend towards shorter hospital admissions;
2. use of technology, such as fibre optic technology, to revolutionize surgical procedures and patient recovery time;
3. the need for cost savings and efficiencies in the health system,
4. the increasing knowledge available about efficacious intervention strategies;
5. the greater proportion of people living to 'old age' and thus the increasing incidence of degenerative and chronic conditions in the community;
6. the role patients play in making decisions about their own health needs.

This context indicates an increasing role for physiotherapists in community-based programmes directed at prevention and management of chronic disorders, and a lessening role in acute, large-hospital-based care. Physiotherapists need to re-evaluate their roles in the health system. Physiotherapy will only continue to progress if physiotherapists are able to adequately predict and meet the health needs of their community.

The emphasis in this chapter is on chronic musculoskeletal disorders, but much of the information applies equally to chronic disorders of other body systems.

Chronic musculoskeletal disorders include:

1. those that are non-specific, e.g. low back or neck pain, chronic shoulder, hip or knee problems;
2. diseases such as rheumatoid disease, Pagets disease and ankylosing spondylitis;
3. degenerative diseases such as osteoarthritis and spondylosis.

Chronicity is often a poorly and imprecisely defined term. Some authors, particularly when describing low back pain, will suggest that chronicity relies on the length of time that the person has had the disorder, usually said to be more than 6 months. Others will state that chronicity means that the patient has been 'unresponsive' to surgical/conservative management (Gottleib *et al.*, 1977). Unfortunately in some studies the definition of chronicity is not even provided (Edwards *et al.*, 1992; Mellin *et al.*, 1993).

Such definitions are inadequate as they fail to address the complex issues that feature in chronic disorders. For example, not all people with back pain lasting for more than 6 months have an intractable problem with associated behavioural changes. A preferable definition of chronic pain is that pain, disability and work loss may be out of proportion to any identifiable disease of pathological diagnosis or objective physical impairment

(Waddell *et al.*, 1992) or that chronic pain, disability or illness are typically dissociated from the original physical basis (Waddell, 1987). This latter definition seems appropriate for the changing knowledge about chronic musculoskeletal disorders.

Other sections in this chapter provide information about possible causes and consequences of the dissociation between signs and symptoms and physical findings in low back pain. It is important that recognition of chronicity of a condition occurs early as this should direct treatment. It has been suggested (De Rosa and Porterfield, 1992) that, if physiotherapists fail to recognize the natural history of low back pain or apply inappropriate treatments, simple low back pain may be converted into chronic low back disability. Examination and treatment approaches for the acute disorder should be different from the strategies employed for a chronic disorder. Once the decision has been made that the patient has chronic pain, the focus should

not be on pain modulation, rather on augmenting function and increasing physical activity. Increasing evidence is available to support the impressive results of such a focus particularly in combination with a multidisciplinary team approach (Waddell, 1987; Cutler *et al.*, 1994).

The physiotherapist needs to be aware that there are two major components to any chronic musculoskeletal disorder:

1. elements related to the musculoskeletal disorder itself;
2. elements related to the associated inactivity and disuse.

This chapter will present information about the desirable role of the physiotherapist in chronic pain disorders in general and in chronic low back pain and arthritis management in particular. In addition, the sequelae of chronic conditions – inactivity and disuse – and the role of the physiotherapist will be explored.

Chronic pain disorders and the multidisciplinary team approach

D. Gronow

Chronic pain can be defined as pain persisting longer than the time that the tissue damage causing the pain would take to heal. Apart from a very few isolated cases, chronic pain is always preceded by an acute pain with a determinable injury. After such injury the body will immediately begin the repair process. The usual expectation is that the acute pain suffered at this time will wane as healing occurs and normal function will then be restored. The evolution of chronic pain therefore is often surreptitious, particularly to the primary-care manager. The physiotherapist will usually encounter patients with chronic pain in two settings, either in an outpatient department or private practice managing acute injuries, or, for a few, it will be in the environment of a chronic pain management team. The roles the physiotherapist plays in these two settings are quite different.

Chronic pain is multimodal in its presentation. How a patient presents with ongoing pain will be determined by their physical, psychological, social and environmental status. Chronic pain causes a cluster of abnormalities that envelop the patient.

Such a patient presents complaining not only of pain but also dysfunctional life style. The need for rest and medication increases while decreases occur in work, recreation and leisure activity, social contacts, independence and physical conditioning. Musculoskeletal changes include muscle contracture and weakness, and alterations in posture and gait. There will be mood changes, sleep disturbances and breakdown in inter-personal relationships. All or some of these features may be present in the patient with chronic pain.

In assessing and managing a patient with chronic pain, all of these needs require consideration and any or all may need individual and collective management to provide a successful outcome. In most instances, patients will not be able to identify the various inputs that affect pain perception, rather they will be concentrating only on the physical aspect. Even when patients recognize that they are having difficulties in other areas of their life, because of the natural tendency to compartmentalize, they will not readily acknowledge the influence that these difficulties may have on their chronic pain. Pain is difficult to measure externally, as it is felt only by the patient. The pain felt by the patient induces a degree of suffering which in turn presents itself as multiple pain behaviours. These pain behaviours include not only the patient's language but such things as sighing, grimacing, limping, protecting, medication taking and cure seeking.

Desirable practice

Our understanding of nociception helps us in managing an acute injury. It is most important that return of function is our primary goal. To achieve this early in the injury, passive therapy must give way to more active therapy. During this time the patient should be taking *adequate* and *regular* analgesia. This may well inhibit the pathological changes developing in the nociceptive system and reduce the likelihood of development of chronic pain. The physiotherapist must be a reinforcer of the patient in complying and understanding the benefits of such management.

The patient with chronic pain presents to the physiotherapist via one of two methods: as an initial referral during an acute phase where, despite ongoing treatment, there has been a failure to make significant gains; or as a referral with a long-standing pain complaint. In the first type of patient it is often difficult to recognize that chronic pain status is beginning to occur. Such patients will often continue to attend treatment, stating that the previous physiotherapy visit was beneficial or 'made them feel good', but this effect was short-lived and was not maintained until the next therapy visit. This encouragement by the patient ensures ongoing therapy and gives a false sense of confidence to the physiotherapist that progress is being made. The patient will be keen to maintain the contact for fear of being abandoned or that their pain will not be believed. It is therefore important that the physiotherapist sets clear goals, continually monitors whether these are being achieved and, if not, puts in place alternative management. This management will shift from a primary goal of alleviating pain to the restoration of function. This will need the concurrence of others treating the patient and establishing this new goal with the patient. Identifying the psychosocial inhibitors to improvement will be part of the management plan. The physiotherapist is in a unique position to contribute because of the strong professional

relationship established with the patient. The options for the physiotherapist could be to suggest referral to a pain clinic or, if this is not possible, to establish a network of communication with other professionals to deal with the situation. The physiotherapist needs to have a good understanding of the psychology involved but should be careful not to practice 'pop-psychology' which, while given in good faith, will undermine the patients progression.

When confronted with a patient with chronic pain the physiotherapist needs to be fully aware of the complexity of the problem. Ideally such patients should be managed in an inter-disciplinary environment. The physiotherapist can become involved in this environment as an outreach member and physiotherapists need to recognize their own skills, biases and limitations in managing such people. Where it is not possible for a patient to be assessed in an inter-disciplinary environment, the physiotherapist should establish a close working relationship with the treating medical practitioner and others involved in the patient's care. The physiotherapist must be aware of the nature of the problem and so, of course, must the treating medical practitioner. Unfortunately this is often not the case. Any treatment programme should aim to re-establish a functional level and will need the combined agreement from all those from whom the patient is seeking treatment. Without this communication treatment is likely to fail. The time involved with managing patients will be extensive, but must not be open-ended.

The physiotherapist as a part of a multidisciplinary team

Being part of a team is often a new experience for any health-care worker. Most training programmes of health professionals address management on a one-to-one basis with each health-care professional making their own judgement about the patient's treatment requirements. In a multidisciplinary team, these decisions need to be shared and a unified management programme presented to the patient. It is often not easy to adjust to this environment where each member of the team is of equal ranking. One of the most important activities is to shift the patient's belief structure and management away from the medical model to the rehabilitation model. As part of the medical model, the patient with chronic pain endlessly searches for the condition that is causing the pain, believing that once this cause is found it can be treated and the pain will be gone. Often this search is reinforced by health-care professionals. During this period of expectancy, increased inactivity occurs with consequences of deconditioning, contractures and fear avoidance behaviours. The prime goal of management of a patient with chronic pain must be to restore function. If improvement of pain levels occurs by methods used, then this is a secondary benefit.

The function of the physiotherapist in the team will be to:

1. Assess the patient's present physical status. This will include examination of posture, gait, range of movement of the affected part, presence of contractures, muscle strength/weakness, level of physical activity, and level of deconditioning.

2. Assess the role of further physiotherapy. Many patients continue to receive inappropriate passive physiotherapy modalities once the acute phase has passed. The physiotherapist will need to determine whether the patient's present physiotherapy, if any, is still appropriate, and if further physiotherapy will help achieve the goals of management. Decisions need to be made as to whether the treatment should be in the form of hands-on therapy or a self-management programme. Hands-on therapy may include: mobilization techniques, assessing segmental level and presence of neural involvement; posture and gait correction; a graduated activity programme of stretches, improvement of muscle balance and improvement of activity levels. Assessing patient compliance can also be extremely important and will determine whether the patient can be managed in an outpatient or inpatient programme.

3. Participate in an informed manner in the patient's total management. An important area of involvement for the physiotherapist relates to the psychological evaluation of the patient. Physiotherapy, because of the close physical contact with the patient, is often non-threatening. The physiotherapist needs to be a good listener and can often identify other psychological and physical stresses that may be important to manage as part of the overall team strategy. The physiotherapist can be a reinforcer of the other components of the patient's programme and can also assess and report on compliance, of their own and other components. Often a joint consultation between the medical officer, the physiotherapist and the patient can be extremely beneficial in assisting the patient to understand the unified team management approach. Discussion amongst the team members remains an important component of patient management.

4. Provide the highest-quality most appropriate physiotherapy management. In the inpatient setting, the physiotherapist's goal will be to establish a graduated programme of activities such as stretches, and physical strengthening and aerobic upgrading including walking programmes. Hydrotherapy may be a useful medium for some of these activities. The physiotherapist will assess the patient's baseline abilities and then set an increasing level of achievement or quota system for the patient. One of the difficulties that most patients with chronic pain find is the amount of 'down time' that they have been told, or believe, that they should undertake whilst waiting for the pain to disappear. One week of rest will lose 20% of muscle strength and endurance and will have widespread effects on a patient's status. The patient must be educated about the importance of maintaining activity even with pain flare-ups. The physiotherapist will also be involved in adapting the patient's disability to their functional requirements, both at work and at home. Thus, improving endurance and a programme of reactivation is absolute. It is important for the physiotherapist and the patient to recognize gains such as reaching the quota level, improvement of gait and posture, improvement of range of movement and strength. Often feedback tools such as graphs can be an important visualization of the patient's gains. Alternatively use of video pre- and post-programme can be a significant reinforcer for gains and progress made. Recognition of positive changes to behaviour and function, however small, are the key to a patient's progress.

As the physiotherapist has a key role in the management of patients with chronic pain, he or she must feel comfortable about dealing with an overtly or covertly stressed patient and their family. The physiotherapist needs to be able to work within a team environment and, if this is not possible, needs to be able to recognize the differences between physiotherapy management for acute and chronic disorders and manage the patient accordingly.

The role of the physiotherapist in management of chronic low back pain

E.M. Gass

In society in general and physiotherapy practice in particular the incidence of people with chronic low back pain is increasing. From 1971 to 1981, for example, in the United States of America the number of people disabled with low back pain grew at a rate 14 times the population growth (Kelsey, 1982). This was also a time of great technological advance in diagnosis, ergonomic knowledge and design although it has been suggested that, unfortunately, these advances have had little effect on the incidence or treatment results of those with chronic low back pain (Bigos and Battié, 1987; De Rosa and Porterfield, 1992).

The majority of people who sustain a low back injury recover. The natural history of the symptoms is variable, possibly explained by the fact that different pathological processes are responsible for the production of back pain symptoms (Roland and Morris, 1983). Efforts to prevent the occurrence of low back injury have included pre-employment screening, education programmes and the application of ergonomic principles at work (Snook *et al.*, 1978). These strategies do not appear to have reduced the incidence of low back injury. Increasingly authors suggest that the focus of management after acute low back injury should be to prevent progression or escalation of the acute problem to a chronic disorder (Bigos and Battié, 1987; Frymoyer and Cats-Baril, 1987) One hypothesis is that intensive rehabilitation early in the course of low back pain can prevent long-term disability. This rehabilitation should involve both controlling the symptoms and avoiding the debilitating effects of bed rest (Bigos and Battié, 1987). Clinical trials are needed to evaluate the results of such an approach, particularly to isolate treatment results from natural improvement of the condition. Such trials need in particular to consider classification and diagnosis of the low back disorder and suitable outcome measures. Physiotherapists have a role in providing active rehabilitation to those with low back injury, documenting the results carefully and establishing the effectiveness of treatment interventions. The trend from previous studies is that education programmes, surgery in specific situations, combinations of endurance training, work evaluation and other strategies can achieve good

functional outcome and prevent chronic back disability (Bergquist-Ullman and Larsson, 1977; Weber, 1978; Cady *et al.*, 1979; Chöler *et al.*, 1985). This approach must be considered by physiotherapists who treat patients with acute low back pain.

In monetary and social terms the larger problem lies with the group of people who sustain a low back injury and develop a chronic condition. In many countries it has been shown that the people with chronic low back disorders are a tiny minority compared with overall low back disorders; however, the former group can account for as much as 85% of the costs (Frymoyer *et al.*, 1983). This probably explains the vast amount written about chronic low back pain!

The role of medical practitioners and other health professionals in the management of chronic low back pain has been evaluated (Waddell, 1987) with the suggestion being made that people with a chronic low back disorder should be treated in a different fashion from those with an acute disorder. This seems logical; however, observation in physiotherapy clinics would indicate that, in the main, this philosophy, although logical in theory, is not being applied in practice. This could be due to the difficulty in actually establishing whether or not a person has a chronic low back disorder. After a back injury has occurred, treatment may continue for many months, or for numerous short periods over months or years, without the treating health professional making the decision that a chronic disorder exists. It has been suggested that this decision is critical if adequate and effective treatment is to be prescribed (Waddell, 1987). Acute pain bears a direct relationship to the tissue damage, hence acute pain, acute disability and acute illness behaviour are generally in proportion to the physical examination findings. Chronic pain, chronic disability and chronic illness behaviour are dissociated from the original tissue damage and from physical examination findings. Instead of being associated with nociceptive input from the injured tissues, the chronic symptoms become associated with emotional distress, failed treatment and adoption of the sick role (Waddell, 1987). If the physiotherapist fails to recognize these latter relationships, then treatment may be prescribed as if the condition is acute. This will be in the main unsuccessful but, more significantly, because of the emphasis on pain, and pain related to physical activity, this approach may reinforce the distress and illness behaviour of the patient with chronic low back pain.

If one accepts that chronic low back pain is fundamentally different from acute low back pain because in the former case the pain has become dissociated from the physical function (Waddell, 1987), then one should also accept that examination and management procedures should be different. This is reinforced by the results of studies which support the view that conventional physiotherapy (such as manual therapy, massage, electrophysical agents) is not adequate to provide satisfactory long-term outcomes for patients with chronic low back pain (Doliber, 1984; Edwards, 1988). It seems, however, that when making a diagnosis and selecting treatment, physiotherapists traditionally weight the presence, distribution and behaviour of pain more heavily than other information from the examination. It is rare to encounter a systematic attempt to evaluate any mismatch between pain, pain behaviour, physical function and disability. When confronted with the challenge of deciding whether a low back problem is chronic or not the physiotherapist may need to add different examination procedures to his or her repertoire, or may need to involve other health professionals in this decision.

Waddell and colleagues (1992), for example, investigated physical impairment in patients with chronic low back pain in order to propose a suitable method of clinical evaluation, and to investigate the relationship between pain, disability and physical impairment. These authors found that pelvic flexion, total flexion, total extension, lateral flexion, straight leg raising, spinal tenderness, bilateral straight leg raise and sit up all discriminated patients with low back pain from healthy subjects and in addition that these manoeuvres were all significantly related to self-report disability in daily activities. On the basis of this study a scale of physical impairment was proposed which could be used for examination and estimation of progress in those with chronic low back pain (Waddell *et al.*, 1992).

Another approach suggested is to use accepted methods of pain assessment to encode information gained from the physical examination (Spratt *et al.*, 1990). Physical tests appropriate to examination of idiopathic low back pain are performed and results

Table 9.1 Questionnaires to measure function in patients with chronic low back pain

Name of questionnaire	Reference
The Sickness Impact Profile (SIP)	Bergner *et al.* (1976)
The Functional Limitations Profile (FLP)	Patrick *et al.* (1982)
Index of Independence in Activities of Daily Living (ADL)	Katz *et al.* (1963)
Functional Status Index (FSI)	Jette (1980)
Disability Questionnaire	Roland and Morris (1983)

noted for pain location (patient self-report) and pain intensity (patient self-report and rater observation of pain behaviours). These outcome measures have been demonstrated as being reliable and valid in assessment of people with chronic pain (Keefe and Block, 1982). Physiotherapists traditionally use measures of pain and physical ability such as range of movement and strength to provide evidence of an improvement in the patient's condition. Patient function could also be evaluated by using questionnaires which have been designed for this purpose. There are a plethora of such instruments. Table 9.1 summarizes some of those that could be used for patients with chronic low back pain.

It may also be desirable to measure illness behaviour, an important aspect of chronic low back pain. Strategies that can be used for this purpose include pain drawing (Ransford *et al.*, 1976), information about the use of walking aids and down time or inactivity time (Rosensteil and Keefe, 1983) and a variety of other behavioural procedures. The physiotherapist should work with members of the team with behavioural science knowledge to administer and interpret such tests.

Once the diagnosis of chronic low back pain is made, the physiotherapist, the patient and other members of the health-care team must decide what the goals of treatment should be, select the appropriate strategies to achieve these goals, select valid baseline and progress measurements, and decide measurement intervals. It is most likely that traditional physiotherapy management structures and outcome measures will be inadequate. The more reliable and valid the outcome measures are, the more likely it is that systematic clinical decisions can be made.

The relationship of diagnosis to treatment

One of the difficult areas in the management of those with chronic low back pain is the question of diagnosis. It is often not possible to make a pathological or structural diagnosis after the onset of low back pain, whether it be acute or chronic. It has been variously estimated that the pathological diagnosis is unknown in some 80–90% of patients with disabling back pain (Dillane *et al.*, 1966; Nachemson, 1982; Valkenburg and Haanen, 1982). It has been suggested that low back pain can be categorized as mechanical, non-mechanical or visceral (Deyo, 1987). Although useful these categories are too broad as a basis for physiotherapy. Given the fact that precise diagnosis of low back disorders is not always possible, it has been suggested that the physiotherapist should use movement and mechanical stress to make an activity-related diagnosis (De Rosa and Porterfield, 1992). This is similar to the philosophy espoused by Maitland (1986). De Rosa and Porterfield (1992) suggest the use of three categories of diagnosis for those with low back pain: acute injury; re-injury or exacerbation of a previous injury; and chronic pain syndrome. If the patient has an acute low back injury, physical stresses applied in the physical examination such as movement or tension tests should lead to signs and symptoms proportional to the time since injury and the amount and type of trauma suffered. The healing and repair of the majority of tissues of the low back should behave as other tissues in the body and should result in decreased symptoms and signs and increased function 6–8 weeks after injury.

To be classified in the second category, i.e. re-injury or recurrent injury, patients will report multiple similar episodes usually increasing in frequency, duration and/or severity over time. The exacerbations occur in response to reapplication of stress to previously injured and possibly incompletely repaired tissues (Troup *et al.*, 1981; Valkenburg and Haanen, 1982). Physical examination utilizing weight-bearing and non-weight-bearing stresses would produce deficits proportional to the injury sustained in these patients.

For a person to be classified into the chronic low back pain category there will no longer be a relationship between application of forces in the physical examination and pain and functional response (De Rosa and Porterfield, 1992). The patient's physical dysfunction is associated with pain behaviour, emotional upheaval, discouragement and sometimes hopelessness (Waddell, 1987). In order to make the decision that a chronic low back disorder exists, the physiotherapist must be able to demonstrate this mismatch between physical stresses applied in examination and resulting functional deficits. This may involve the use of tests that are known to discriminate low back pain patients from healthy people (Waddell *et al.*, 1992), judging the results of physical tests with pain assessment measures (Spratt *et al.*, 1990), combining patient self-report and rater observation measures (Keefe and Block, 1982), evaluating disability with questionnaires (Table 9.1), or measuring illness behaviour (Ransford *et al.*, 1976; Rosensteil and Keefe, 1983).

If the decision is made that the patient has an acute or recurrent low back disorder, then treatment should be directed at alleviation of pain and encouraging an environment conducive to tissue healing and repair (De Rosa and Porterfield, 1992). Treatment should also be directed at minimizing the effects of decreased activity and disuse. This approach should result in an acceptable outcome. For those with recurrent disorders, neuromuscular performance must be enhanced. This could involve specific strategies to make good any residual effects of deconditioning, biomechanical analysis and skill retraining to enable adequate performance of desired tasks and prevent future recurrence, or modification of tasks to enable better performance (De Rosa and Porterfield, 1992). Promotion of self-efficacy techniques is useful to attempt to change the fact of recurrence. Pain modulation procedures have a minor role for the patient with a recurrent disorder.

Pain modulation has little place in the management of the person with chronic low back pain (De Rosa and Porterfield, 1992). The emphasis should be on restoration of physical function, reversing sequelae of inactivity and disuse and promoting an emphasis on health and self-worth. Self-efficacy procedures are vitally important in this group. There is an increasing awareness that this approach, although needing research and refinement, will provide the most satisfactory outcome for patients with chronic low back pain. Some studies have demonstrated that, provided there is careful baseline measurement of physical function, daily activities and behavioural characteristics, programmes of a multidisciplinary nature emphasizing appropriate physical and behavioural management have successful outcome for those with chronic low back pain (Edwards *et al.*, 1992; Lindstrom *et al.*, 1992; Cutler *et al.*, 1994).

Although there is some diversity and debate about selection of outcome measures and there are methodological problems with many of the studies in this area, it does seem that the physiotherapist and the patient with chronic low back pain are more likely to achieve a successful outcome if:

1. the diagnosis of chronic low back pain is made promptly;
2. examination procedures focus on physical ability and disability and are chosen to identify the mismatch between physical function and pain behaviour;
3. health professionals with varied backgrounds such as psychology, medicine and ergonomics collaborate with the physiotherapist and the patient to set treatment goals and plan management;
4. treatment goals are carefully delineated and focus on improvement of function;
5. treatment is positive, goal directed and aimed at improving health and physical ability;
6. behavioural and psychological strategies are used to help minimize pain and fear behaviour;
7. exercise is a component of the treatment programme;
8. a focus on electrotherapeutic modalities and specific manual procedures designed to decrease pain is avoided because it will *not* usually aid symptom resolution;
9. outcome measures should be selected carefully to best represent the goals of treatment. Standard pain measures and movement tests should not be the only measures used.

The De Rosa and Porterfield (1992) model provides a straightforward classification system which can be matched with appropriate treatment strategies. The classification system is based upon applying mechanical forces and measuring resultant function or dysfunction. Although this approach has practical merit, physiotherapists and other health professionals must continue to strive to understand pathologies affecting the low back. If a more accurate clinical diagnosis were possible, i.e. not only naming the structure involved but also quantifying the accompanying signs and symptoms, then treatment and prevention strategies could be better designed and targeted. The physiotherapist thus has a role in diagnosis and treatment of chronic disorders that is different from the role in acute low back disorders. The emphasis is not on

procedures to maximize healing and repair because, by definition, the chronic disorder is not based upon a deficit in this area. Rather the physiotherapist needs to work within a team to ensure adequate expertise to tackle the physical, psychosocial and vocational disability which is characteristic of low back pain (Ganora, 1984). The patient needs support and guidance to be an active participant in an activity outcome-focused rehabilitation programme.

Use of exercise in treatment of chronic low back pain

Exercise is a frequent component of rehabilitation and prevention programmes for the low back. Physiotherapists have a key role in prescribing and evaluating the results of exercise strategies. Exercise can be prescribed specifically for vertebral column muscles or more generally to increase physical function.

Exercise for vertebral column muscles

Physiotherapists commonly prescribe exercise for vertebral column muscles because it is believed that weak muscles, tight muscles or an imbalance between muscle groups can cause the patient's symptoms and signs. A brief review of the basis for such beliefs is worth while to make evident the rôle of exercise in chronic low back pain.

Weak muscles as a source of pain

Many studies suggest that people with low back pain have decreased muscle strength compared with healthy people (McNeill *et al.*, 1980; Kishino *et al.*, 1985; Mayer and Smith, 1985; Mayer *et al.*, 1985; Jull and Janda, 1987; Nouwen, *et al.*, 1987). A typical finding would be that of Mayer *et al.*, (1985) who found significantly lower trunk extension/flexion ratios for female normal controls compared with female patients. These authors also demonstrated: significantly lower isometric and multispeed isokinetic torque/body-weight ratios for male patients compared with male controls during lumbar spine flexion and extension; that normal females have less strength than normal males; and that strength tends to decrease with increasing age.

Most of the studies that have investigated strength in those with low back pain have methodological problems such as lack of random selection of subjects, questionable reliability and validity of measuring instruments, and results that demonstrate a correlational and *not* a causal relationship (although the latter is usually implied or suggested by the authors). In spite of these difficulties, the apparent trend is for those with chronic low back pain to have 'weaker' muscles, whether it is in terms of absolute maximum torque development, maximum torque related to bodyweight, or fatiguability during prolonged exercise. Such results are not surprising in people whose activity is reduced because of back pain and whose muscles and associated structures have, therefore, adapted to the changed, i.e. less physically stressful, environment.

Studies conducted on non-vertebral-column muscles (Sargeant *et al.*, 1977; MacDougall *et al.*, 1980; Klausen *et al.*, 1981) demonstrate that structural changes occur in muscles that have the normal movement stimulus removed or decreased. Leg muscle adaptation was studied in seven people after removal of plaster 15 weeks after unilateral leg fracture (Sargeant; *et al.*, 1977). Given the lack of certainty about the alteration in muscle stress in the limb in plaster, the results are still interesting showing approximately 12% decrease in total leg volume, and 15% decrease in peak oxygen consumption during one leg cycling. There was a reduction in mean cross-sectional area of both Type I and Type II muscle fibres. Other studies have examined the effects of training followed by detraining (MacDougall *et al.*, 1980; Klausen, *et al.*, 1981) and found that detraining can result in up to 40% decrease in strength measured by Cybex dynamometry, decreased fibre area of Type I and Type II fibres, decreased number of capillaries per muscle fibre and decreased oxidative enzyme activity. It would seem likely that similar detraining or disuse effects would be seen in people with chronic vertebral column disorders, the extent and specific muscles involved depending partly on the person's pain distribution and intensity and consequent amount of restriction of daily activity.

Thus it is probably true that those patients with chronic spinal pain have weak muscles. It is also probably true that there is likely to be tissue and enzymic adaptation within the weak muscles. What has not been demonstrated, however, is that the weak muscles are a *causative* factor of the patients

chronic low back disorder. Studies systematically examining muscle-strengthening programmes for such answers are lacking, partly because it is difficult to prove causality and partly because it is more straightforward to demonstrate correlation in what is usually a multifactorial clinical disorder. In general, commonly prescribed strengthening and flexibility exercises have not been found to be helpful. Abdominal strengthening and back flexibility exercises have not decreased patients' symptoms nor increased their functional ability (Kendall and Jenkins, 1968; Lidstrom and Zachrisson, 1970; Bergquist-Ullman and Larsson, 1977).

Logic would suggest that the weak muscles are more likely to be a consequence of the low back disorder, not an antecedent.

Tight muscles as a cause of pain

This concept is related to the belief that poor posture can cause pain because muscle/tendon tightness is usually thought to be an adaptive response to inadequate or incorrect movement or posture. Much literature has been written on such issues but interpretation is difficult. Certainly tightness of muscles such as hamstrings and iliopsoas has been reported in adults and children with low back pain (Kucera, 1986; Máckova *et al.*, 1986; Jull and Janda, 1987). Again methodological difficulties of reliability and validity arise, as well as the inability to demonstrate causality.

The situation is made more complicated by the fact that decisions about what is normal and abnormal are difficult to make, given the range of 'normal' distributed in the population. In one study (During *et al.*, 1985) the author makes comment about a harmonious postural situation being one in which the parts are not deformed beyond their normal range and in which their shape at any instant is governed by rules of mutual dependency. Unfortunately normal range is unknown and rules of mutual dependency remain obscure. These authors examined mathematical relationships between lumbosacral elements and were able to conclude that mean values of postural parameters in a group of patients with spondylolisis differed significantly from healthy volunteers whereas those with disc space narrowing could not be distinguished this way from healthy subjects (During *et al.*, 1985). This seems to suggest, in the lumbosacral region anyway, that severe structural alterations are necessary before departure from 'normal' posture can result. Longitudinal studies have measured postural asymmetry in teenage years, and investigated back and neck pain in the same subjects in later years, and found no evidence of a relationship between simple postural asymmetries and subsequent pain development; and that an increase in frequency of low back pain is not a long-term effect of scoliosis (Dieck *et al.*, 1985). These authors hypothesized that either the asymmetries were not enough to damage tissues, that the damaged tissues did not cause pain or that the asymmetrical load was compensated by adaptation of the body according to Wolff's Law which, paraphrased, states that form follows function.

There is also questionable evidence supporting the need to increase spinal flexibility to aid recovery or to prevent back problems (Lidstrom and Zachrisson, 1970; Biering-Sorensen, 1983) with some studies suggesting that women rowers who regularly stretched their spines had a greater incidence of back pain than rowers who did not stretch (Howell, 1984) or that those with greater spinal flexibility were more likely to suffer back pain (Biering-Sorensen, 1983).

The foundation for the belief that tight muscles or resultant abnormalities of posture can cause low back pain is elusive. This is due to the difficulty in making the decision that lack of movement or 'tightness' is abnormal and identifying the structure(s) responsible for such restriction. The belief is also hard to support because studies proving causality are lacking. On current evidence it would seem 'tight' muscles are a likely adaptive response to altered activity.

Muscle imbalance and pain

Muscle imbalance is variously and imprecisely defined. It can either mean the ratio of respective strengths of two opposing muscle groups, e.g. quadriceps and hamstrings, or can mean the relationship between length and strength of opposing groups. This concept of muscle imbalance is prominent at present, partly because of the availability of isokinetic testing machines which can readily generate values for muscle strength. Many problems arise with this research including validity of testing and generalizability of results. With limb muscles, for example the tester generally has the non-affected limb for comparison; however, this is not possible with vertebral column muscles. More information is needed about how trunk muscles work and their specific structure, including fibre-type distribution, before we rush into comparing

possibly invalid data and establishing 'norms' for muscle group balance. Norms for muscle group balance need to be established before one can define 'imbalance'.

Although localized exercises to increase strength, and range may be used for patients with chronic low back pain, the physiotherapist must be clear about the aims of such interventions. They may make good existing deficits and enable improved overall physical function, but care must be taken not to suggest that the patient's back disorder is being 'cured' by such measures. This would be an inappropriate aim for the patient with chronic low back pain and in addition such a relationship would not be supported by experimental studies.

Exercise for increasing physical function

Given that specific vertebral muscle exercise has an equivocal role in the resolution of chronic low back disorders, there is an increasing trend for the prescription of more generalized exercise. The aims of such exercise are usually to encourage whole body movement and physical activity in a positive way and to overcome the effects of inactivity and disuse.

Exercise to encourage whole body movement and physical activity

This type of exercise is usually one component of a total rehabilitation approach for those with chronic low back pain, thus in most studies it is impossible to isolate the effects of exercise from other interventions. In a typical study, 72 patients with chronic low back pain received a range of treatments designed around the theme of self-regulation (Gottlieb *et al.*, 1977). These treatments included biofeedback training for relaxation, psychological counselling, a patient-regulated medication programme, a physical therapy reconditioning programme and education sessions all conducted in a therapeutic milieu designed for relaxation, recreation and socialization. Success was defined as functional physical activity at discharge and amount of vocational restoration. After this programme of average length 45 days, 50 patients had a satisfactory functional improvement rating on discharge, and 38 of these were employed or in training 6 months after discharge.

Similar results are reported for other studies combining general exercise, work simulation, functional restoration and psychological and educational strategies (Edwards *et al.*, 1992; Mellin *et al.*, 1993; Brady *et al.*, 1994; Mayer *et al.*, 1994). It was noted by some that, although improvement occurred, results were still less than normal when compared with a population-average normative database specific to age and gender (Brady *et al.*, 1994). Unfortunately none of these studies used a control group therefore it is difficult to ascribe causality between interventions used and results obtained. A meta-analysis and review of 164 studies, in which outcomes were measured after all types of non-surgical treatment for chronic pain, chose return to work as the outcome measure (Cutler *et al.*, 1994). The conclusions from this review were that non-surgical treatment (including exercise in some cases) does return patients to work, increased rates of return to work were due to treatment and the benefits of treatment were not temporary.

A complete review of the literature related to back pain and exercise is beyond the scope of this chapter. The major message from current studies, however, is that the most effective approach to minimizing the incidence of chronic low back pain is to prevent the disability that occurs after acute back injury. Early intervention, including patient education, the use of exercise and cardiovascular conditioning to prevent adaptation to disuse, combined with visits to the worksite by health-care professionals has been shown to reduce disability by 50% (Chöler, *et al.*, 1985). Controlled clinical trials will ultimately provide the answers about specific and general exercise as treatment for those with chronic low back pain. The first steps involve careful planning of outcome measures and documentation that exercise has more effect than natural history of the disorder.

Inactivity and disuse – sequelae of chronicity

Unfortunately, physiotherapists have insufficiently recognized the role they can play in preventing and reversing the effects of inactivity and disuse occurring in many chronic conditions. Inactivity and disuse cause functional alterations to the neuromusculoskeletal, cardiopulmonary and related systems. These alterations or adaptations occur in response to decreased use. Many studies have convincingly demonstrated the positive results achievable after an appropriately designed rehabilitation programme for those who have become inactive. Exercise is the major ingredient in these programmes.

Exercise as a stimulus to cause beneficial adaptation in chronic conditions

Although specific and localized therapeutic exercise has been used in various ways by physiotherapists, the potential of general exercise as a stressor to cause beneficial adaptation for many body systems is sometimes under-rated. One would imagine that exercise, either as a community activity or part of a treatment strategy for various patient groups, is a powerful example of the advances of modern society and modern medicine. In most communities today thousands of people of all shapes, sizes and ages can be seen pounding the pavements as they jog or power walk by. They can be heard grunting and straining as they lift weights, pedal stationary bicycles or climb make-believe stairs and skip rope, jump the trampoline or join with others in team activities. Hundreds of research papers and book chapters have been, and are still being, written documenting the benefits to be gained from exercise. When trying to measure advances in this area it is somewhat disconcerting to realize that similar issues were being published and discussed around 400 BC! Herodicus, for example, stressed the importance of therapeutic gymnastics in conservative medicine while at a similar time Hippocrates wrote:

> Eating alone will not keep a man well; he must also take exercise. For food and exercise, while possessing opposite qualities, yet work together to produce health. For it is the nature of exercise to use up material but of food and drink to make good deficiencies. And it is necessary as it appears to discern the power of various exercises, both natural and artificial, to know which of them tends to increase flesh and which to lessen it. And not only this, but also to proportion exercise to bulk of food, to the constitution of the patient, to the age of the individual, to the season of the year, to the changes in the winds, to the situation of the region in which the patient resides, and to the constitution of the year.

Of course some of these later listed variables would have been less important if Hippocrates' patients had access to air-conditioned rehabilitation centres, Nike shoes and goretex clothing! By about AD 200 Galen (of cardinal signs of inflammation fame) was being somewhat evaluative when he wrote: 'To me it does not seem that all movement is exercise, but only when it is vigorous. But since vigour is relative, the same movement might be exercise for one and not for another' ... 'The criterion of vigorousness is change of respiration; those movements which do not alter the respiration are not called exercise. But if anyone is compelled by any movement to breathe more or less faster, that movement becomes exercise for him' (Green, 1951). Thus, approximately 2,500 years ago exercise was not only seen as having both a preventive and therapeutic role, but the concept of specific exercise prescription and evaluation had been identified – maybe Galen, in fact, was the originator of the anaerobic threshold debate! A contemporary definition of exercise is: '... physical activity that is planned, structured, repetitive and purposeful in the sense that improvement or maintenance of one or more components of physical fitness is an objective' (Casperson *et al.*, 1985).

The ability of a person to adapt to repeated bouts of physical exercise over a period of weeks such that exercise capacity is improved can be termed physical training (Booth and Thomason, 1991). Changes in cells, organs or body systems that persist for appreciable periods as a consequence of physical training are known as exercise adaptation (Booth and Thomason, 1991). One of the benefits of exercise adaptation is that there is less disruption of homoeostasis after physical training than before. Less disruption of homoeostasis allows the person to perform physical activity for a longer period, at the same absolute power, before fatigue (Booth and Thomason, 1991). If exercise is to be used successfully as a treatment strategy to cause beneficial adaptation in musculoskeletal, neurological, cardiorespiratory and related systems, then it must be prescribed in a dose that is adequate to stress these systems and their associated tissues. Such disruption of homoeostasis is necessary to cause beneficial adaptation.

Exercise prescription – adequate disruption of homoeostasis

Homoeostasis is the means whereby integrated physiological processes operate in an attempt to maintain a stable internal environment. When the environment changes, homoeostasis is not maintained and, over time, a different homoeostasis may be achieved as the body adapts to the changed environment. Adaptation can be defined as a semipermanent change(s) occurring in the structural and/or functional properties of cells, tissues and organ systems. Short-term adaptations are those for which a person has existing control systems, e.g. increased heat production resulting from shivering in response to cold and increased respiration in response to increased arterial carbon dioxide concentration. Such adaptations are almost immediate and generally only last a short time. (Rowell, 1986). On the other hand, long-term adaptations involve structural alterations within limits set by the genetic code. Immunological adaptation via immunization or acclimation to altitude are examples of long-term adaptations. The stimulus for these adaptations is altered use or altered stress placed upon the tissues or the organ causing long-term disruption to the homoeostatic relationship. The altered stress can either be an increase or a decrease and the adaptation that results will be specific to the stress applied.

With the foregoing in mind a simpler definition of exercise pertinent to those with chronic musculoskeletal disorders could be that exercise is the disruption of homoeostasis caused by physical activity. This definition identifies a concept vital to the efficacious use of exercise as a therapeutic intervention by physiotherapists – namely disruption of homoeostasis. The importance of disturbed homoeostasis and body system disruption is well illustrated by various studies (Saltin *et al.*, 1968; Saltin and Rowell, 1980; Blomqvist and Stone, 1983) which have examined adaptation to underuse and inactivity (bed rest) and increased use (exercise).

Underuse and inactivity (bed rest) cause a decrease in maximal oxygen consumption ($\dot{V}_{O_2\,max}$, with the decrement being related to the duration of the underuse although adaptation occurs at a faster rate during the first part of an inactivity period. For example 21 days of complete bed rest caused a reduction in $\dot{V}_{O_2\,max}$ from 3.3 to 2.4 litres per minute (Saltin *et al.*, 1968). In the same study the prolonged inactivity caused a 26% decrease in cardiac output and stroke volume at $\dot{V}_{O_2\,max}$. The systemic arteriovenous oxygen difference remained the same. In some studies plasma volume also falls but probably not enough to be the whole explanation for the decreased stroke volume (Rowell, 1986). Muscle capillary density also decreases after inactivity; however, so does muscle fibre size, hence more capillaries become available for each muscle fibre and average diffusion distances are decreased (Saltin and Rowell, 1980). This probably means oxygen diffusion ability remains about the same. Physical activity (or training, rehabilitation or conditioning) increases $\dot{V}_{O_2\,max}$. The size of the increase depends partly on the $\dot{V}_{O_2\,max}$ before exercise training, and partly on the age of the person. The higher the $\dot{V}_{O_2\,max}$ and age before the training, the smaller will be the change after training. The greater the muscle mass involved in the training the greater will be the adaptation, provided that exercise dose is sufficient (Clausen, 1977).

Because $\dot{V}_{O_2\,max}$ = heart rate$_{max}$ $\times$ stroke volume$_{max}$ $\times$ arteriovenous difference$_{max}$, the increase in $\dot{V}_{O_2\,max}$ seen after physical training could be explained by increases in any or all of the three factors in the equation. Maximal heart rate does not increase and it has been established in young people that increases in maximal cardiac output (heart rate $\times$ stroke volume) are achieved entirely by an increase in maximal stroke volume (Rowell, 1986). Muscle capillary density rises at the same rate as cardiac output with even greater relative increases (approximately 40%) in muscle oxidative enzyme activity (Saltin and Rowell, 1980).

Submaximal responses to exercise are also altered after physical training with the major changes being:

1. decreased vasomotor outflow to visceral organs at any given submaximal $\dot{V}_{O_2\,max}$;
2. decreased heart rate in proportion to the decreased vasomotor outflow;
3. reduction in sympathetic nervous activity at any given submaximal $\dot{V}_{O_2\,max}$, in direct proportion to the decrease in heart rate (Rowell, 1986).

In essence this means that physical training does not alter the relationship between sympathetic nervous system activity, heart rate and regional vascular resistance; however, because $\dot{V}_{O_2\,max}$ increases, the range of $\dot{V}_{O_2\,max}$ over which these responses occurs is expanded.

So, how should a physiotherapist prescribe exercise to minimize the effects of inactivity and disuse? Exercise is uniquely anti-homoeostatic because it involves integrated activity of a variety of body systems. Depending upon the amount of muscle mass that is active, varying amounts of activation of these body systems will occur. The major body systems affected by inactivity and

Table 9.2 Favourable adaptations to exercise

Cardiovascular/cardiorespiratory (dynamic exercise) (Schiable and Scheuer, 1985)

- Increased stroke volume
- Decreased heart rate for any given amount of work
- Eccentric hypertrophy of the left ventricle of the heart
- Increased maximal oxygen consumption
- Increased arteriovenous oxygen difference in working muscle
- Increased activity of oxidative enzymes
- Increase in number of mitochondria

Musculoskeletal/neurological

- Increased bone mass (Snow-Harter and Marcus, 1991)
- Hypertrophy of muscle fibres
- Increased strength tendon/bone junction
- Increased strength ligament/bone junction
- Increased rate of collagen synthesis and organization after connective tissue damage
- Change in motor unit activation (McDougall *et al.*, 1980; Sale, 1988)

Behavioural

- Possible improvement in self-image and self-esteem
- Possible decrease in depression
- Possible increased ability to sleep at night (Sonstroem, 1984; Dunn and Dishman, 1991)

disuse are the cardiovascular, cardiopulmonary, neurological and musculoskeletal. The aim of any exercise programme should be to cause favourable adaptation (Table 9.2). In order to cause adaptation in one or more body systems one has to upset the homoeostasis of that system by selecting an appropriate dose of treatment. The major components of an exercise dose are the type of exercise to be performed, and the frequency, duration and intensity of the exercise.

Type of exercise to be performed

Large-muscle-mass dynamic exercise has the greatest effect on cardiovascular and neuromusculoskeletal systems. Bicycling, walking, running and swimming all provide this type of exercise. The specific choice for any patient will depend on patient preference, desirable amount of impact or loading of musculoskeletal elements and access to safe and pleasant environments. Provided that other elements of the dose are appropriate and depending upon the initial ability level of the patient, large-muscle-mass dynamic exercise can result in gains of approximately 30% in maximal exercise time, $\dot{V}O_{2\,max}$ and activity of muscle oxidative enzymes (Saltin and Rowell, 1980). The major advantage of increasing $\dot{V}O_{2\,max}$ is that submaximal activities become relatively easier. Walking up one flight of stairs in a typical sedentary person could necessitate working at 70% $\dot{V}O_{2\,max}$. After a training or rehabilitation programme, this person's $\dot{V}O_{2\,max}$ could increase by 20–30% and, because the oxygen cost of walking up the stairs remains the same, the person is now working at a lesser percentage of $\dot{V}O_{2\,max}$ and hence the stair climbing is easier.

Frequency, duration and intensity of exercise

In general large-muscle-mass dynamic exercise at 50–60% $\dot{V}O_{2\,max}$ three times per week for 20–30 min each session will cause beneficial adaptations (Table 9.2). There is a large body of literature documenting such adaptations in many types of population groups including the elderly and those with chronic disorders [for reviews see Cross (1980) and Green and Crouse (1993)]. If one is dealing with a disordered or damaged system, then the exercise stimulus applied should be sufficient to disrupt homoeostasis but should not be so great that it will cause the system to fail. Let us take an example of a muscle we are all familiar with – the heart. When myocardial fibres are stretched during diastole, force of contraction or work produced increases. If, however, the fibres are already lengthened such as with congestive cardiac failure, more length is required to produce less contraction and, at levels less than normal, the system fails.

How does the physiotherapist efficiently and effectively use exercise to prevent sequelae of inactivity and disuse for those with chronic disorders of the musculoskeletal system?

1. Examination must provide suitable data that can quantify the baseline situation. Physical testing may need to provide information about a variety of submaximal and maximum or symptom-limited levels. This testing may involve small components or may involve testing of gross activities activating a number of muscles and a greater proportion of more body systems.
   (a) $\dot{V}O_{2\,max}$ is a useful indicator of physical function, being dependent upon the cardiovascular system's ability to deliver blood to working muscles and the cellular ability to use the oxygen delivered for energy production (Hartung *et al.*, 1993).
   (b) $\dot{V}O_{2\,max}$ or $\dot{V}O_{2\,peak}$ can be directly measured in a laboratory using instruments that can quantify power (ergometers) such as treadmills, stationary cycles and arm crankers. The term $\dot{V}O_{2\,max}$ is generally reserved for the value obtained when exercise activates the maximum amount of active muscle mass, for example, treadmill walking or running. Unless subjects are elite arm-exercising or cycling athletes, the maximal values obtained during arm crank or cycle ergometry are generally lower than during treadmill exercise and are referred to as $\dot{V}O_{2\,peak}$. In the case of disabled individuals, such as after spinal cord injury, then the value obtained during ergometry that activates the maximal amount of muscle under voluntary control should be known as $\dot{V}O_{2\,max}$.
   (c) $\dot{V}O_{2\,max}$ or $\dot{V}O_{2\,peak}$ can be estimated from a variety of submaximal tests, for example, heart rate response to standard submaximal exercise on an appropriate ergometer. Prediction of $\dot{V}O_{2\,max}$ is possible because it is assumed there is a linear relationship between heart rate and $\dot{V}O_2$ or workload (Astrand, 1960; Hartung *et al.*, 1993).
   (d) $\dot{V}O_{2\,max}$ can also be predicted from 'field' tests which could be used in a clinical or community setting. For example, distance run or walked in a specified time (Cooper, 1968) or heart rate response to submaximal stepping workloads (Margaria *et al.*, 1965). The latter method involves lifting body mass against gravity, hence heavier people will do more work for any given step height.
   (e) Tests to measure or predict $\dot{V}O_{2\,max/peak}$ will also provide information about the heart rate response to any given power, and, in addition, depending on the sophistication of the measuring instruments, can identify submaximal and maximal venous lactate response to any given power and respiratory parameters such as ventilatory equivalents for oxygen and carbon dioxide (McArdle *et al.*, 1986). This information can be used to identify when homeostasis begins to be upset and hence which intensity of exercise would be sufficient to cause adaptation.

2. The physiotherapist and patient should be clear about the goals or the adaptations to be achieved and how results will be measured. The major adaptations to exercise are summarized in Table 9.2. The results should be measured in the same way as the original testing procedures.

3. The exercise programme must consist of an appropriate type of exercise, adequate intensity, frequency and duration to cause the targeted adaptations.

4. Results must be frequently evaluated and prescription parameters altered in order that the stimulus remains sufficient, particularly when some gains have been achieved. If the dose is not altered, it becomes less of a disruptor to homoeostasis and therefore has less potential to cause adaptation.

The following case vignette will illustrate some of these points. Eleanor was a 30-year-old woman who had had low back pain for 8 years after a fall down a flight of stairs at work. She had not worked since the accident and had become quite sedentary. A friend of hers with a similar problem had recently commenced an exercise programme and was achieving good results. Eleanor came to the physiotherapist saying that she also wished to begin an exercise programme to increase her physical fitness. She had a letter from her general practitioner stating she would be able to do a maximal exercise test. Eleanor was not a smoker and except for her low back pain her general health was good. She was taking four to six panadol per day for the back pain and two valium to help relax her muscles.

After a familiarization session in the exercise testing laboratory and after giving informed consent, Eleanor returned to do a cycle ergometer test. She was anxious about using the mouthpiece and headgear to measure oxygen consumption and did not want any blood taken for venous lactate estimation therefore it was decided to only measure heart rate. Bipolar electrocardiographic electrodes were placed on Eleanor's chest and the test was performed. The results are depicted in Figure 9.1.

On the basis of this test it was decided with Eleanor that she should exercise on a stationary cycle at 20 W for 30 s, then rest for 30 s, and repeat this exercise prescription 40 times per session four times per week. The physiotherapist accompanied Eleanor to the local gymnasium and went through the first exercise session with her. Eleanor mon-

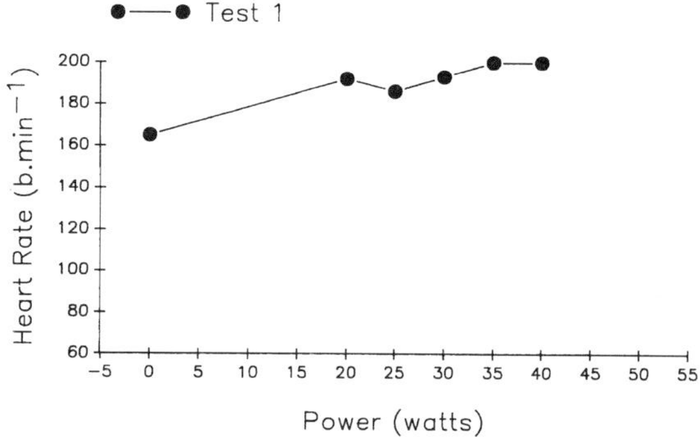

Figure 9.1 Results of Eleanor's first cycle ergometer test

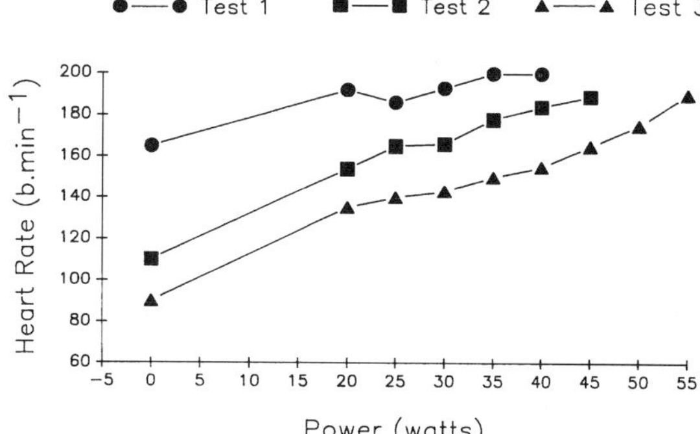

Figure 9.2 Results of Eleanor's first, second and third cycle ergometer tests

itored her heart rate each fifth minute to ensure adequate stress to her cardiovascular homoeostasis. She also kept an activity diary listing the amount of time she exercised, her exercise heart rate and her comments about each session. After a week Eleanor was asked to ring the physiotherapist to talk about her progress. Three weeks later Eleanor returned to the laboratory for another cycle ergometer test (Test 2) and, on the basis of the results, her exercise intensity was increased to 25 W. Twelve weeks later Eleanor returned for a further test (Test 3). Figure 9.2 depicts the results of the cycle ergometer tests in the exercise laboratory. The results of the third test were used to increase exercise intensity again. Eleanor came back to the laboratory each 6–8 weeks thereafter, and exercise intensity was adjusted each time.

These graphs show the decreased heart rate for the same power output at each test and the increased duration and power achieved with each successive test. These changes reflect favourable adaptation to the exercise. Three months after she commenced her programme, Eleanor had started swimming and aquarobics twice per week in addition to cycling three times per week at the gym. Her valium usage was infrequent and she had discontinued panadol. Eleanor still had some back pain, although she felt better able to cope with this. Eleanor had begun working three half days per week at the local library and was finding this quite manageable and enjoyable. She was thinking about enrolling in a librarian assistants course at a local technical college.

The exercise programme had caused demonstrable adaptation in her cardiovascular system, namely a lower heart rate in response to any given submaximal load. Presumably these adaptations were due to an increase in her stroke volume and an increase in the oxidative capacity of her leg muscles.

This case vignette demonstrates that outcome measures should be valid – in this case heart rate response to exercise – and that exercise dose needs constant evaluation and adjustment as performance improves. This ensures a sufficient homoeostatic disruption to continue to cause beneficial adaptation. The same principles can be applied to most, if not all, patients with chronic musculoskeletal disorders. Adequate rehabilitation of these patients involves attention both to the signs and symptoms related to the disorder itself, and prevention or reversal of sequelae of the inactivity and disuse secondary to the musculoskeletal disorder.

Changing role for physiotherapy in arthritis management

J. Stenmark

The most common types of arthritis are osteoarthritis (OA), rheumatoid arthritis (RA) and gout. The most common arthritides that physiotherapists see and treat in practice are OA, RA, ankylosing spondylitis (AS), juvenile chronic arthritis (JCA), systemic lupus erythematosus (SLE) and scleroderma.

Physiotherapy is recognized as one of the fundamental components of comprehensive care for individuals with arthritis, and physiotherapists are key members of the arthritis patient care team. Treatment programmes that include physical modalities, rest, exercise and posture training have been advocated since the early days of physiotherapy (Swain, 1930). By 1960, a relatively standardized approach to treatment of those with arthritis included, in some combination, modalities such as heat, hydrotherapy, traction, massage, exercise and mobility retraining. Recommended types of exercise included passive, active-resisted and range-of-motion. Isometric exercises usually constituted the strengthening component of the treatment programme. Home exercise programmes rarely took into consideration disease fluctuations and did not include measures to encourage adherence to exercise (Haralson, 1990).

In Western societies, where arthritis and musculoskeletal disorders affect more than 10% of the population (Australian Bureau of Statistics, 1989), it is impossible that even the majority of the people who may require treatment will be able to consult a physiotherapist. More emphasis therefore needs to be placed on patient education and health promotion, group exercise programmes and self-help skills. As the population ages (Australian Bureau of Statistics, 1989), the impact of arthritis on society in terms of lost productivity and health care costs will escalate, in addition to the increased numbers of people with disability.

The goals of physiotherapy management in arthritis remain largely unchanged, but the role of the physiotherapist and the strategies used to achieve these goals has undergone considerable change in the last decade. The educational role of the physiotherapist in arthritis management has emerged to gain equal importance to the 'hands-on' role. This educational role centres on exercise prescription and involves the physiotherapist planning management of the 'whole person' aiming to provide the patient with some skills to exert control over their health, thereby maximizing health status. Whether the physiotherapist works in a traditional clinical setting (private practice or hospital), conducts exercise or hydrotherapy classes in a community centre, or is involved in health promotion and education, he or she should be encouraging patients to exercise by giving appropriate exercise guidelines and enhancing compliance.

Traditional medical management of arthritis emphasizes medication and rest (Zvaflier *et al.*, 1988) to control inflammation and gain resolution of the acute condition. Physiotherapy treatment goals during acute episodes are similar for all types of arthritis, namely alleviation of pain, prevention of deformity, and the restoration of function. At other stages of the disease process, programmes will vary depending upon whether the arthritis is inflammatory or non-inflammatory (degenerative). Physiotherapists must be aware that arthritis is not just about treating physical signs and symptoms. The associated problems and disability can change peoples lives, sometimes permanently. For the person with arthritis the major life changes include the challenge of coping with persistent pain, and not being able to carry out activities they need or might like to do. Such changes inevitably lead to alterations in how people with arthritis see themselves. These alterations include changes in their self-esteem, in mood, and in how family and friends react to and feel about them, often resulting in major consequences at work, home and in leisure activities. These real life consequences of chronic arthritis need to be given adequate attention in the traditional medical treatment. Medical treatment is vital in rheumatoid and other types of arthritis, particularly in the area of pharmacological intervention. In RA, medications may slow the progression of the disease (see Chapter 2). In OA, medications are used predominantly for pain control. Surgical intervention such as joint replacement may offer more permanent relief of pain and restoration of function. Physiotherapists in the clinical setting are often eager to treat and 'cure' the problem at hand (e.g. painful neck) and often pay little attention to evaluating the needs and status of the person as a whole. This involves taking into account social, work-related and disease parameters, and the current level of ability. Because of this limited perspective more encompassing strategies such as increasing physical capacity are often overlooked.

When specific joints and regions require treatment, the traditional clinical physiotherapy approach is important and applicable. Modalities such as joint mobilization, manipulation, heat, cold, transcutaneous electrical stimulation, interferential, ultrasound, massage and posture re-education are commonly used (Haralson, 1990).

Emphasis on joint range of movement and strengthening will also retain importance in the treatment of the patient with arthritis, particularly in the acute and subacute stages. However, a balanced, integrated programme of exercise to promote maximal physical function should be encouraged in order to achieve all the goals of management.

Consequences of the disease process

The common features of all types of arthritis are pain and discomfort in affected joints and impaired and/or restricted mobility. In Australia, activity impairment has been estimated to occur in 37% of people with arthritis (IMG Consultants, 1982). A disabled person can be defined as a person who has any restriction or lack of ability (resulting from an impairment) to perform an activity in the manner or within the range considered normal for a human being (World Health Organization, 1980). In Australia the most frequently reported group of disabling conditions are diseases of the musculoskeletal system and connective tissue, including the arthritides. A handicap can be defined as a disadvantage for an individual resulting from an impairment or disability that prevents fulfilment of a normal role for that individual (World Health Organization, 1980). Diseases of the musculoskeletal system and connective tissue including the arthritides were also the most commonly reported primary disabling conditions causing handicap in Australia (Australian Bureau of Statistics, 1988). Arthritis can thus impact upon and limit many aspects of a person's life. It has an adverse effect on the socioeconomic status of individuals as the condition progresses (Meenan *et al.*, 1981). A higher than normal divorce rate has also been reported among with arthritis (Yelin *et al.*, 1987) and a significant number attribute poor self-esteem to their arthritis (Kaplan and Kozin, 1981).

Consequences of inactivity or decreased activity

An early and common change people make after the onset of arthritis is cessation of leisure-time activities (Yelin, *et al.*, 1980). Since leisure activities are often associated with exercise, not only social isolation but also inactivity result. In addition, there is a tendency in Western society to 'slow down' and decrease activity as one ages. As there is increasing incidence of arthritis with increasing age, the likelihood of decreased activity is high in those with arthritis.

Inactivity or disuse has consequences for many body systems, organs and tissues. For example, the beneficial effects of movement on all joint tissues, particularly articular cartilage have been demonstrated (Dieppe, 1984). With inactivity, cartilage becomes fibrosed and atrophied, and loses its elasticity, becoming prone to damage. Thus movement and exercise are essential for the maintenance of healthy articular cartilage, for joint lubrication and to maintain the extensibility of the collagenous connective tissues within and around joints (Salter, 1989). Maintenance of full range of motion decreases the tendency towards adaptive shortening of connective tissue and muscles around joints and minimizes the tendency to stiffen with age (Twomey and Taylor, 1987). Ligaments can also become atrophied with disuse. Regular exercise makes for thicker stronger ligaments (Frank *et al.*, 1984). Disc nutrition is dependent on movement, and regular and large-range spinal movements are important to ensure adequate disc nutrition (Adams and Hutton, 1986).

Bones need the stress of weight-bearing activity to maintain and increase mass and hence prevent osteoporosis (Pocock *et al.*, 1986; Chow *et al.*, 1986; Sambrook and Eisman, 1987). Inactivity and prolonged immobilization increase calcium loss from bone when mechanical stress or gravitational force on the skeleton is removed. This occurs in bed rest (Krolner and Toft, 1983), space flight (Vogel and Whittle, 1976), immobilization of limbs (Andersson and Nilsson, 1979) and paralysis (Whedon, 1984) causing rapid and extensive bone loss. In contrast, athletes who exercise more intensively and consistently than the average person, usually have above average bone mass (Huddlestone *et al.*, 1980; Lane *et al.*, 1985). The effects of exercise on bone are site-specific and result in greater bone density in those body areas subjected to higher stress levels (Bailey *et al.*, 1986; Huddlestone *et al.*, 1980). Cross-country runners have greater bone density in their legs and backs, for example, whereas tennis players show greater bone mass in their dominant arm (Huddlestone, 1980).

The changing role of the physiotherapist in arthritis management

Acute and subacute stages

The physiotherapist needs to have current knowledge about the different pathologies associated with different types of arthritis, and the different stages that will occur in these conditions. When selecting and applying modalities or giving advice about rest and modification of activity in an acute episode, the physiotherapist must be mindful of the specific changes occurring in the tissues. The physiotherapist should, even in the acute stage, aim to involve the patient in minimizing the effects of disuse and inactivity as far as possible. This could mean prescription of a gentle exercise programme for unaffected regions or, if appropriate, a cycling, walking or arm-exercise programme. The intensity, frequency and duration of such exercise should be sufficient to maintain current activity level; however the dose needs to be modified in the light of the disease activity. Consultation with both the medical practitioner and the patient is particularly important at this stage. Information must also be provided to the patient (in a manner to encourage retention) about the changes that are occurring in the disease, why the chosen strategies have been chosen and what the expectation of outcome should be. Psychological support for the patient and family is also an important component.

Subacute or chronic stage

Once an acute exacerbation has passed, the physiotherapist, with other health professionals and with active participation by the patient, should provide a programme that will promote the health of the patient. This programme will include strategies to maximize the physical abilities of the patient, to maximize the patient's autonomy and psychological well being and allow maximal possible participation in work, leisure and social activities. In each instance specific programme goals should be identified and agreed to by health professionals and the patient. Baseline measures should be made to enable evaluation of progress. These measures should be reliable and valid. For a comprehensive discussion about measurement, and some of the tools appropriate for clinical measurement, the reader is referred to a recent publication by Domholdt (1993). The treatment strategies chosen should be of a dose adequate to cause beneficial adaptation. Such adaptation might be increased muscle strength or increased maximal oxygen consumption ($\dot{V}_{O_2\,max}$).

The key features of the changing role of the physiotherapist in the management of those with arthritis are the increased importance of generalized exercise, education, self-efficacy skills and understanding of factors influencing compliance.

The use of exercise as treatment for those with arthritis by physiotherapists

Minor (1991) in her review of the research surrounding exercise in arthritis states that the two major questions to be addressed by studies of conditioning exercise are:

1. Can persons with arthritis exercise regularly and vigorously enough to improve general health status and physical fitness?
2. Does participation in aerobic exercise result in increased disease activity?

Several prospective trials and field tests of conditioning exercise have investigated the effectiveness and safety of physical activity to improve fitness and decrease disability (Ekblom *et al.*, 1975; Nordemar, 1981; Nordemar, *et al.*, 1981; Harkcom *et al.*, 1985; Minor *et al.*, 1989). These studies indicated that many persons with arthritis can safely participate in appropriate exercise programmes to improve psychosocial status, functional status, and physical fitness. Some of these studies (Minor *et al.*, 1988; Nordemar *et al.*, 1981) also reported good subject retention and maintenance of exercise behaviours. Regular exercise of moderate intensity, for example 50–60% $\dot{V}_{O_2\,max}$ can also raise the pain threshold, improve energy levels, lessen depression and improve physical self-concept and belief in self-efficacy (Minor *et al.*, 1989; Perlman *et al.*, 1990; Holman *et al.*, 1989).

A notion that is often perpetuated in the community and by physiotherapists is that osteoarthritis (OA) is a 'wear and tear' disease, causing people to think that exercise will make joints 'wear out' faster and thereby make their arthritis worse. OA is now considered a multifactorial group of disorders. Rather than habitual exercise being a causative OA agent, disuse is a major factor. Regular routine exercise does not increase one's chances of developing OA, in fact exercise is essential to maintain normal joint function (Dieppe, 1984; Eichner, 1989; White *et al.*, 1993). This concept also applies to OA of the spine because intensive physical rehabilitation has been found to restore function and decrease pain (Deyo *et al.*, 1986). There is no evidence for prescribing more rest, medications, supports or for being inactive for people with OA (Deyo *et al.*, 1986).

Ankylosing spondylitis (AS) is a progressive disease, often affecting young patients during their most productive years. Regardless of the course of the disease, the psychosocial and rehabilitative needs of the patient deserve careful consideration (Calabro and Mody, 1965). The main objective of active treatment is to delay and possibly stop the progression of the disease. Education of the patient in self-management should be a prime objective of early management of AS (Dieppe *et al.*, 1985). More than with any other type of arthritis, specific exercises have been established as an essential component of management, with spinal extension exercises being the key component of any AS exercise programme. Regular training and spinal extension exercises twice daily have been recommended as a minimum (Dieppe *et al.*, 1985) The literature surrounding exercise and AS seems to indicate that, at the very least, exercise may exert a stabilizing effect, preserving mobility and preventing further deterioration in function (Dudley, 1968; Carette *et al.*, 1983; Rasmussen and Hansen, 1989). Treatment for AS is ameliorative rather than curative, involving active participation of the patient. The responsibility for involvement in exercise lies with the patient and necessitates a degree of self-management which may be facilitated by attending a self-help group that emphasizes exercise (Barlow *et al.*, 1992, 1993).

Weight-bearing exercise alone does not prevent osteoporosis in the postmenopausal woman. Exercise has been encouraged in combination with adequate calcium and sex-hormone levels (Prince *et al.*, 1991; Sambrook, 1993). Preventive physiotherapy for the middle aged and elderly should stress the necessity for adequate levels of physical activity. There is little doubt that the incidence of osteoporotic bone fractures in elderly persons could be reduced substantially if exercise levels were adequate during youth and maintained into retirement. This reduced risk of fracture may relate as much to the maintenance of muscle strength and neuromuscular coordination as to the associated maintenance of bone mass (Twomey, 1993). Active older people do have significantly better coordination, balance and muscular strength than their sedentary peers, which reduces the risk of falling (Rikli and Busch, 1986; Arthritis Foundation, 1992). The positive effects of exercise on bone density in women is dependent upon the presence of normal or adequate oestrogen levels. Super athletes who become amenorrhoeic have significantly lower spinal bone density than their peers (Baker and Demers, 1988; Drinkwater, 1990). Weight-bearing exercise is of particular benefit in bone remodelling though there may be some benefit to bone density from the pull of muscle on bone (Dixon, 1989). Hydrotherapy is a good medium in which to rehabilitate after specific injuries such as hip and spinal fractures, as it allows graduated introduction of active weight-bearing activities. Weight-bearing exercises with the full effects of gravity are, however, a stronger stressor to prevent bone loss.

Arthritis patients have not previously been encouraged to use exercise to increase their aerobic capacity. This is particularly true for patients with RA because of the concern that exercise may cause a disease exacerbation. The results of published studies provide evidence that this concern is unfounded. It is possible to increase fitness in patients with RA and other inflammatory diseases without causing exacerbation of symptoms (Minor, 1991).

Guidelines for physiotherapists in the use of exercise for those with arthritis

General guidelines are recommended although they will need modification depending on the type of arthritis that the person has and their current ability level. It is most important that the physiotherapist and the patient understand the goal(s) of the exercise programme. For example exercise could be used to strengthen or increase endurance of localized muscle groups, or could be used to increase flexibility of particular body regions. This section will focus on the use of exercise to increase 'fitness' or 'aerobic capacity' or 'functional reserve', i.e. exercise involving large muscle mass designed to cause favourable adaptations in cardiovascular, cardiopulmonary and neuromuscular systems. To cause such adaptations, large-muscle-mass activities are the most appropriate and include walking, water exercise (including hydrotherapy and aquarobics), light jogging and cycling. To have a favourable stress on bone, it is preferable to achieve a combination of weight-bearing and non-weight-bearing activity each week. High

impact exercises such as running and contact sports are not recommended for inflammatory arthritis, moderate to severe osteoarthritis, established osteoporosis or AS. The type of exercise should be chosen after consideration of the preferences of the patient, the ease of access to the desired activity and any specific considerations relating to existing disabilities. Baseline measures of ability should be conducted in order to prescribe exercise doses most precisely, and to monitor improvements. Many methods are available for these baseline measures. These range from fully equipped cardiovascular laboratories to practical tests using a stopwatch and a measured distance. The heart rate response to a known amount of exercise is the guiding principle for tests. The reader is referred to McArdle *et al.* (1986) for more detailed information.

It is important to find the correct balance between rest and exercise for inflammatory arthritis, so that symptoms are not exacerbated. To achieve this balance, the following should be kept in mind.

1. When joints are inflamed, rest is needed, the amount and type will depend on how inflamed the joint is.
2. If joints ache only on certain movements, rest from those movements, is needed.
3. Joints that are stiff, yet have little pain, need more exercise.
4. Joints that feel weak and unstable require more support and exercise (Arthritis Foundation, 1992).

It may be useful to provide exercise guidelines to patients with arthritis. These may need modification for the individual patient. An example is provided below.

Guidelines for people with arthritis who wish to exercise

1. Begin the programme slowly.
2. Increase the amount of exercise gradually – both in terms of effort and amount (this should be based on discussions with your physiotherapist).
3. Move your joints slowly and smoothly – do not jerk them.
4. Be aware of pain and swelling and carefully assess the effect that exercise has on individual joints and whole limbs.

5. If pain occurs after exercise and lasts more than 2 h, it means that your exercise programme may need to be revised by:
   (a) doing less
   (b) avoiding too many repetitions
   (c) performing them with less effort (discuss this with your physiotherapist).
6. Muscles and joints are exercised more effectively when they are warmed up. It may be a good idea to exercise after a bath or shower. Always start your exercise gently with a warm up period.
7. Give muscles time to relax in between movements and activities.
8. If you are on medication, exercise is best when the medication is having its maximum effect.
9. Do not hold your breath while exercising – keep your breathing regular.
10. Do not push through pain (Arthritis Foundation, 1992).

Hydrotherapy as a medium for exercise

Hydrotherapy utilizes the physical properties of warm water to enhance exercise. The uplifting effect of buoyancy makes some movements easier and gives a feeling of weightlessness. Turbulence is used to make movements easier or harder while maintaining some support for the joints (Williams, 1994). Physiotherapists have a role in delivering hydrotherapy services to the person with arthritis. The use of warm water as an exercise medium provides a number of benefits for the person with arthritis. These include decrease in pain and relaxation of muscles, increased circulation and reduction in stiffness. The buoyancy of the water assists movements allowing a greater range and quality of movement. Walking may be possible in the water for people otherwise unable to stand. Water allows greater mobility for those who are severely restricted. Water offers a controlled resistance to movement and thus helps to strengthen grossly weak muscles (Sayce and Fraser, 1991).

A number of psychological benefits have been claimed and these include:

1. satisfaction from participating in a self-help activity;
2. social interaction outside the home which reduces isolation;
3. the ability to achieve a greater amount of mobility makes the person feel good about themselves and encourages a positive attitude (Arthritis Foundation, 1992).

Hydrotherapy is also useful in the rehabilitation phase after hip and knee surgery and osteoporotic fractures. There is also often a higher compliance with hydrotherapy compared with other recommended exercise programmes (Minor *et al.*, 1989).

Education and self-efficacy as treatment

Patient education can be defined as any combination of learning experiences designed to facilitate voluntary behaviour changes conducive to health (Green *et al.*, 1980) and is considered as health education applied to persons with a diagnosed condition. In clinical practice there is opportunity to educate our patients through our treatments, behaviour and advice. It has been shown, however, that increasing a person's knowledge about a disease and proper management is NOT enough to actually change behaviour (Bartlett, 1984; Cumming *et al.*, 1988). A feeling of being in control and able to change behaviour is critical to maximizing health status. Health status in arthritis can be measured by a number of factors including pain levels, visits to the physician, ability level and psychological status (Lorig *et al.*, 1987). The thrust of patient education is teaching people to become active self-managers and to gain confidence in their ability to control their health condition, their pain and ultimately their sense of well-being.

Enhancing a feeling of being able to cope in the arthritis patient is desirable, because the unpredictability of the course of arthritis is a common problem (Daltroy and Liang, 1988). Self-efficacy concerns the patient's judgement of his or her coping capabilities in designated areas of function. Converging findings show that the effects of therapeutic interventions on health behaviour are partly mediated by changes in perceived self-efficacy (O'Leary, 1985). Improved self-efficacy is associated with improvements in health status, therefore most arthritis patient education programmes aim to enhance self-efficacy for specific behaviours such as exercise regimens, relaxation practice and medication compliance. Self-efficacy theory was developed by Bandura (1977) within the framework of social learning theory. He postulated that people's perceptions of their capabilities affect how they behave, their level of motivation, their thought patterns and their emotional reactions in taxing situations. Self-efficacy theory provides a basis for one common mechanism through which people exercise influence over their own motivation and behaviour. Self-efficacy is behaviour-specific so that someone may have a high self-efficacy for a particular task but not for another. Perceived self-efficacy can affect health behaviour in a number of ways. Judgements of self-efficacy determine behaviour choice, i.e. which activities will be attempted or avoided. Assessing patients' perceptions of their self-efficacy to manage pain and enhancing these perceptions with further instruction in pain-management skills when they are low may have great clinical utility (O'Leary, 1985).

It has been demonstrated that self-efficacy can be changed, and that changes in self-efficacy are associated with changes in behaviour and cognitive status such as pain and stress levels (Lorig *et al.*, 1987). Enhancing self-efficacy is perhaps the most important aspect of patient education in arthritis. Lorig (1991) has documented four specific self-efficacy enhancing mechanisms, namely: skills mastery, modelling, re-interpreting physiological symptoms and signs, and persuasion.

Skills mastery

Skills mastery means one must master one part of the skill or some small skill, before moving on to the next task. This is the most important mechanism in enhancing self-efficacy and forms the basis for many patient education programmes. Skills mastery is achieved by dividing skills into small manageable tasks and ensuring successful completion of each task. Short-term goals are set for different behaviours. The key word is mastery. One can only enhance self-efficacy if each task is mastered successfully. Setting short-term goals relates very well to the prescription of exercise and can assist in compliance. It is important that the goal is personal, positive, specific and realistic. For example, when setting goals about exercise, it is important not to be over-ambitious about what one may achieve in the coming week. It is better to set a goal to do a small amount of exercise successfully, achieve that task and gradually increase the amount, rather than be overambitious and only achieve half of the stated goal. This approach can be a very powerful tool for therapists to use not only in education programmes, but in the clinical setting to foster compliance with home programmes. When working out exercise prescription based on baseline measures the physiotherapist should aim to set an exercise amount that will have a favourable outcome, yet which is achievable.

Modelling

Modelling uses the principle that the person who is coping well with their problems and disabilities acts as a 'model' for the person who is coping less well. This allows the person with arthritis to see another person with similar or worse problems who is successfully coping with their disease. It is one of the reasons why support groups are so popular and successful. This strategy has implications for the use of group exercise or group education sessions.

Re-interpreting physiological signs and symptoms

When a patient experiences symptoms such as pain and fatigue, they will be interpreted according to the patient's knowledge and beliefs about their disease. Health professionals need to discover what their patient with arthritis believes about particular symptoms and signs and why they have those beliefs, and then work on changing those beliefs as necessary. For example, people with rheumatoid arthritis commonly experience fatigue as a symptom of their disease, thus the need to balance activity and rest. It is only in recent years that it has been established that many with rheumatoid arthritis are at times subclinically depressed and that fatigue is a common symptom of depression. In this situation rest will only heighten feelings of depression and exacerbate fatigue. It is therefore important to teach those with RA to recognize fatigue and try to determine the underlying causes.

Persuasion

This is the least successful method. It can take many forms, most commonly fear arousal which is more popular than effective, for example,

> 'If you don't exercise, your . . . . joints won't work.'
> 'if you keep smoking, you'll die.'

The use of fear is ineffective in changing behaviour. If people think that the consequences are inevitable, then they think that there is no point in changing the behaviour. Urging people to do a little more (exercise), however, if your assessments suggest they are capable of this, can be an effective use of exercise behaviours and persuasion.

Compliance

A problem facing all health professionals is the failure of patients to adhere to the regimens prescribed by health-care workers. An important determinant of compliance may be patients' perceptions of their ability to carry out the prescribed procedures and thus affect their own health (O'Leary, 1985). Treatments need to be applied in ways that instil and strengthen a patient's belief both in treatment effectiveness and their own abilities to effect positive changes in their health.

It is well accepted that compliance with exercise is one of the most difficult behaviours to influence (Dishman, 1982). When prescribing exercise regimens physiotherapists should provide patients with the tools and guidelines that will foster compliance. Questioning the patient about non-compliance can often discover issues that can be simply overcome by the physiotherapist and patient. It is important that people are successful and have positive experiences with exercise from the beginning in order to continue in an exercise programme (Minor, 1991). A number of strategies have been proposed to enhance the exercise experience. For example exercise should be incorporated into daily activities and become a habit, and short-term goals should be recorded and achievement rewarded. Some people exercise better with a friend or other people and this needs to be organized. People with arthritis should be encouraged to exercise when they are least stiff, or tired, or when they have least pain and when medications are maximally active. Social motivators to exercise are effective so the development of an exercise programme related to a leisure activity is a useful strategy.

The exact amount of patient compliance with physiotherapy is unknown. Compliance with exercise regimens ranges from 30 to 51% (Dishman, 1982; Feinberg, 1988) and rates of compliance drop as time passes (Deyo, 1982; Sluijs and Knibbe, 1991). These findings would make it seem worth while to bring patients back for checks at future intervals to examine programmes and problems with compliance.

In physiotherapy, one can distinguish short-term supervised compliance and long-term non-supervised compliance (Sluijs and Knibbe, 1991). Short-term compliance can be defined as compliance with a specific regimen during the treatment period. This can be called supervised compliance because contact with the health-care provider has direct influence and control over the process (Sluijs and Knibbe, 1991). Long-term compliance occurs after the treatment period. When treatment is stopped, the influence of the health-care provider is minimal. In this phase, compliance behaviour must be self-regulatory in order to be maintained (Kok, 1988). The physiotherapist should determine whether short-term or long-term compliance (or both) is the goal and subsequently derive a plan about the goal and strategy concerning the patient's compliance. If short-term compliance is the purpose of treatment, all regular contacts can be utilized to apply reinforcement for desired behaviours. Discovering specific appropriate cues for each patient is also helpful when taking into account the desired behaviour. Stimulating long-term compliance by self-regulation of the patient does require extra skill and effort from the therapist (Sluijs and Knibbe, 1991). It is helpful to have good knowledge of the patient's ideas and perceptions about the illness and disability in order to adjust the prescribed regimen to existing coping patterns. Teaching the patient how to appraise performances and outcomes in such a way that feelings of competence and self-efficacy are intensified is also desirable.

Summary

In total management of the patient with arthritis it is crucial to examine the disease process, the age of the patient and their activity levels. Goals of management should reflect the active approach possible with RA and other inflammatory disorders. The physiotherapist should measure physical capacity and functional levels in these patients and teach them that moderate exercise (following appropriate guidelines) will in fact relieve pain and inflammation, maintain and increase health and function, prevent deformities and provide much psychological support. A wellness focus should be one of the main aims of management. In spite of the challenges imposed, the focus should be on health and fitness rather than arthritis and disability.

This positive approach should include teaching people to become active self-managers of their arthritis. Treatment language should not focus on terms such as flexibility and range-of-movement but rather on language such as 'you will have more function, be less tired and feel better'. One advantage of performing regular exercise is that it gives a person a sense of control over life. When treating a patient with arthritis, education regarding self-management principles and careful exercise prescription is of paramount importance. Conditioning exercise is an appropriate addition to comprehensive arthritis management. The physiotherapist should contribute to the health of the community through their role in exercise prescription and education.

For patients with arthritis:

1. Moderate aerobic exercise undertaken with correct guidelines will not cause disease exacerbation (Nordemar *et al.*, 1981; Minor, 1991).
2. Inactivity is a major factor in the development of disability (with or without arthritis) (Minor, 1991).
3. Inactivity may be a major factor in OA development (Minor, 1991).
4. Older people who exercise regularly have fewer falls (Rikli and Busch, 1986) due to better balance and co-ordination.

Clinical treatment of acute and chronic arthritis has, and will continue to have, an undeniably important role in the total management of the arthritis patient. Physiotherapy will remain one of the most critical components of arthritis patient care, the more so if it is designed to ensure a healthy lifestyle, increased function and decreased pain. Unquestionably, physical management will continue to evolve as researchers examine both traditional and newer approaches to treatment for patients with arthritis.

References

Adams, M.A. and Hutton, W.C. (1986). The effect of posture on diffusion into lumbar vertebral discs. *J. Anat.* **147**, 121–34.

Andersson, S.M. and Nilsson, B.E. (1979). Changes in bone mineral content following ligamentous knee injuries. *Med. Sci. Sports Exerc.* **11**, 351–3.

Arthritis Foundation (1992). *Osteoporosis: Prevention and Self-management Course*, Leader's Manual, Victoria, Kew, Australia.

Astrand, I. (1960). Aerobic work capacity in men and women with special reference to age. *Acta Physiol. Scand.*, **49** (Suppl 169), 1–92.

Australian Bureau of Statistics (1988) Disability and Handicap Survey Cat. No. 4120.0.

Australian Bureau of Statistics (1989). National Health Survey Cat. No. 4370.1.

Bailey, D.A., Martin, A.D., Houston, C.S. and Howie, L.J. (1986). Physical activity, nutrition, bone density and osteoporosis. *Austra. J. Sci. Med. Sports*, **18**, 3–7.

Baker, E. and Demers, L. (1988). Menstrual status in female athletes: correlation with reproductive hormones and bone density. *Obstet. Gynecol.*, **72**, 683–7.

Bandura, A. (1977). *Social Learning Theory* Englewood Cliffs, New Jersey: Prentice-Hall.

Barlow, J.H., Macey, S.J. and Struthers, G. (1992). Psychosocial factors and self-help in ankylosing spondylitis patients. *Clin. Rheumatol.* **11**, 220–5.

Barlow, J.H., Macey, S.J. and Struthers, G. (1993). Health Locus of control, self-help and treatment adherence in relation to ankylosing spondylitis. *Patient Educ. Counsell.* **20**, 153–66.

Bartlett, E. (1984). Behavioural diagnosis: A practical approach to patient education. *Patient Counsell. Hlth Educ.* **4**, 29–35.

Bergner, M., Bobbitt, R.A., Kressel, A. *et al.* (1976). The sickness impact profile: conceptual formulation and methodology for the development of a health status measure. *Int. J. Hlth Serv.* **6**, 393–415.

Bergquist-Ullman, M. and Larsson, U. (1977). Acute low back pain in industry. *Acta Orthop. Scand.* (Suppl.), **170**, 1–117.

Biering-Sorensen, F. (1983). A prospective study of LBP in a general population. II. Location, character, aggravating and relieving factors. *Scand. J. Rehabil. Med.* **15**, 81–8.

Bigos, S.J. and Battié, M.C. (1987). Acute care to prevent back disability – ten years of progress. *Clin. Orthop. Relat. Res.* **221**, 121–30.

Blomqvist, C.G. and Stone, H.L. (1983). Cardiovascular adjustments to gravitational stress. In *Handbook of Physiology. The Cardiovascular System. Peripheral Circulation and Organ Blood Flow* (J.T. Shepherd and F.M. Aboud, eds), Sect. 2, Vol. 111, Part 2, pp. 1025–63, Bethesda, Maryland: American Physiological Society.

Booth, F.W. and Thomason, D.B. (1991). Molecular and cellular adaptation of muscle in response to exercise: perspectives of various models. *Physiol. Rev.* **71**, 541–85.

Brady, S., Mayer, T. and Gatchel, R.J. (1994). Physical progress and residual impairment quantification after functional restoration. *Spine*, **19**, 395–400.

Cady, L.D., Bischoff, D.P., O'Connell, E.R. *et al.* (1979). Strength and fitness and subsequent back injuries in fire fighters. *J. Occup. Med.*, **21**, 269–72.

Calabro, J.J. and Mody, M.E. (1965). Management of ankylosing spondylitis. *Am. J. Occup. Ther.* **19**, 225–8.

Carette, S., Graham, D., Little, H. *et al.* (1983). The natural disease course of ankylosing spondylitis. *Arthritis Rheum.* **26**, 186–90.

Casperson, C.J., Powell, K.E. and Christenson, G.M. (1985). Physical activity, exercise and physical fitness: definitions and distinctions for health related research *Public Health Rep.*, **100**, 126–31.

Chöler, U., Larsson, R., Nachemson, A. and Peterson, L.E. (1985). *Pain in the Back*, Stockholm: Spri Rapport.

Chow, R.K., Harrison, J.E., Brown, C.F. and Hajek, V. (1986). Physical fitness effect on bone mass in post menopausal women. *Arch. Phys. Med. Rehabil.*, **67**, 231–4.

Clausen, J.P. (1977). Effect of physical training on cardiovascular adjustments to exercise in man. *Physiol. Rev.*, **57**, 779–815.

Cooper, K.H. (1968). A means of assessing maximal oxygen intake: correlation between field and treadmill testing. *J. Am. Med. Assoc.*, **203**, 201–4.

Cross, D.L. (1980). The influence of physical fitness training as a rehabilitation tool. *Int. J. Rehabil. Res.*, **3**, 163–75.

Cutler, R.B., Fishbain, D.A., Rosomoff, H.L. *et al.* (1994). Does nonsurgical pain centre treatment of chronic pain return patients to work? *Spine*, **19**, 643–52.

Cumming, R., Barton, G., Fahey, P. *et al.* (1988). The Western Sydney Health Study – results of a shopping centre survey. *Med. J. Austr.*, **148**, 277–80.

Daltroy, L. and Liang, M. (1988). Patient education in rheumatic diseases: a research agenda. *Arthritis Care Res.* **1**, 161–9.

De Rosa, C.P. and Porterfield, J.A. (1992). A physical therapy model for the treatment of low back pain. *Phys. Ther.* **72**, 261–9.

Deyo, R.A. (1982). Compliance with therapeutic regimens in arthritis: issues, current status and a future agenda. *Semin. Arthritis Rheuma.*, **12**, 233–44.

Deyo, R.A. (1987). Reducing work absenteeism and diagnostic costs for backache. In *Clinical Concepts in Regional Musculo-skeletal Illness* (N.M. Hadler, ed.), pp. 25–50, London: Grune and Statton.

Deyo, R.H., Diehl, A.K. and Rosenthal, M. (1986). How many days of bed rest for acute low back pain? *N. Engl. J. Med.*, **315**, 1064–70.

Dieck, G., Kelsey, J., Goel, V. *et al.* (1985). An epidemiological study of the relationship between postural asymmetry in the teen years and subsequent back and neck pain. *Spine*, **10**, 872–7.

Dieppe, P. (1984). Osteoarthritis: are we asking the right questions? *Br. J. Rheumatol.*, **23**, 161–5.

Dieppe, P.A., Doherty, M., Macfarlane, D. and Maddison, P. (1985). *Rheumatol. Med.*, pp. 72–81. London: Churchill Livingstone.

Dillane, J.B., Fry, J. and Kalton, G. (1966). Acute back syndrome: a study from general practice. *Br. Med. J.* **2**, 82–4.

Dishman, R.K. (1982). Compliance adherence in health related exercise. *Hlth Psychol.* **3**, 237–67.

Dixon, A. (1989). Osteoporosis, the future *Arthritis Update*, p. 7.

Doliber, C.M. (1984). Role of the physical therapist at pain treatment centres. *Phys. Ther.*, **64**, 905–9.

Domholdt, E. (1993). *Physical Therapy Research Principles and Applications*. Philadelphia: W.B. Saunders.

Drinkwater, B.L. (1990). Physical exercise and bone health. *J. Am. Med. Wom. Assoc.*, **45**, 91–6.

Dudley, H.F. (1968). Ankylosing spondylitis. *Lancet*, **ii**, 1230–344.

Dunn, A.L. and Dishman, R.K. (1991). Exercise and the neurobiology of depression. *Exerc. Sport Sci. Rev.*, **19**, 41–98.

During, H., Goudfrooij, H., Keeson, W. *et al.* (1985). Towards standards for posture. *Spine*, **10**, 83–7.

Edwards, B. (1988). Back pain patients who thought they would never get back to work. *Physiother. Today*, **1**, 1–4.

Edwards, B.C., Zusman, M., Hardcastle, P. *et al.* (1992). A physical approach to the rehabilitation of patients disabled by chronic low back pain. *Med. J. Aust.*, **156**, 167–72.

Eichner, E.E. (1989). Does running cause osteoarthritis? *Physician Sports Med.*, **17**, 147–54.

Ekblom, B., Lovgren, O., Alderin, M., Friedstrom, M. and Satterstrom, G. (1975). The effect of short-term physical training on patients with rheumatoid arthritis. *Scand. J. Rheumatol.*, **7**, 33–42.

Feinberg, J. (1988). The effect of patient–practitioner interaction on compliance: a review of the literature and application in rheumatoid arthritis. *Patient Educ. Counsell.*, **11**, 171–87.

Frank, C., Akeson, W.H., Woo, S.L.Y. *et al.* (1984). Physiology and therapeutic value of passive joint motion. *Clin. Orthop. Relat. Res.*, **185**, 113–25.

Frymoyer, J.W. and Cats-Baril, W. (1987). Predictors of low back pain disability. *Clin. Orthop. Relat. Res.*, **22**, 89–98.

Frymoyer, J.W., Pope, M.H., Clements, J. *et al.* (1983). Risk factors in low-back pain. *J. Bone Joint Surg.*, **65A**, 213–18.

Ganora, A. (1984). Chronic back pain: diagnosis, treatment and rehabilitation. *Patient Manag.*, 55–79.

Gottlieb, H., Strite L.C., Koller R. *et al.* (1977). Comprehensive rehabilitation of patients having chronic low back pain. *Arch. Phys. Med. Rehabil.*, **58**, 101–8.

Green, J.S. and Crouse, S.F. (1993). Endurance training, cardiovascular function and the aged. *Sports Med.*, **16**, 331–41.

Green, L., Krueter, M. and Deeds, S. (1980). *Health Education Planning: A Diagnostic Approach*. Palo Alto, California: Mayfield Publishing Co.

Green, R.M. (1951). A translation of *Galen's Hygiene* (De sanitate tuenda) In Berryman, J.W. (1989). The tradition of the "six things non natural". Exercise and Medicine from Hippocrates through Ante-Bellum America. In *Exercise and Sport Sciences Reviews*, (K. Pandolf, ed.), pp. 515–59. Baltimore: Williams and Wilkins.

Haralson, K. (1990). Physical Therapy and arthritis – origins and evolution. *Arthritis Care Res.*, **3**, 173–7.

Harkcom, T.M., Lampman, R.M., Banwell, B.F. and Castor, C.W. (1985). Therapeutic value of graded aerobic exercise training in rheumatoid arthritis. *Arthritis Rheum.*, **28**, 32–9.

Hartung, G.H., Krock, L.P., Crandall, C.G. *et al.* (1993). Prediction of maximal oxygen uptake from submaximal exercise testing in aerobically fit and nonfit men. *Aviat. Space and Environ. Med.*, **64**, 735–40.

Hippocrates: Regimen (trans. by W.H.S. Jones) (1967). In Berryman, J.W. (1989). The tradition of the "six things non natural". Exercise and Medicine from Hippocrates through Ante-Bellum America. In *Exercise and Sport Sciences Reviews* (K. Pandolf, ed.) pp. 515–59. Baltimore: Williams and Wilkins.

Holman, H., Mazonson, P. and Lorig, K. (1989). Health education for self-management has significantly early and sustained benefits in chronic arthritis. *Trans. Assoc. Am. Physicians*, **102**, 204–8.

Howell, D.W. (1984). Musculoskeletal profile and incidence of musculoskeletal injuries in light weight women rowers. *Am. J. Sports Med.*, **12**, 278–82.

Huddlestone, A.L., Rockwell, D. and Kulund, D. (1980). Bone mass in lifetime tennis athletes. *J. Am. Med. Assoc.*, **244**, 1107–9.

IMG Consultants (1982). *The Community Impact of Arthritis on the Australian Community*, Charles E. Frosst (Aust) Pty. Ltd.

Jull, G. and Janda, V. (1987). Muscles and motor control in low back pain – assessment and management. In *Physical Therapy of the Low Back* (L. Twomey and J. Taylor, eds.), pp. 253–78, New York: Churchill Livingstone.

Jette, A.M. (1980). The functional status index: reliability of a chronic disease evaluation environment. *Arch. Phys. Med. Rehabil.*, **61**, 395–401.

Kaplan, S. and Kozin, F. (1981). A controlled study of group counselling in rheumatoid arthritis. *J. Rheumatol.*, **8**, 91–9.

Katz, S., Ford, A.B., Moskowitz, R.W. *et al.* (1963). Studies of illness in the aged: the index of ADL: a standardised measure of biological and psychosocial function. *J. Am. Med. Assoc.*, **185**, 914–19.

Keefe, F.J. and Block, A. (1982). Development of an observation method for assessing pain behaviour in chronic low back pain patients. *Behav. Ther.*, **13**, 363–75.

Kelsey, J.L. (1982). *Epidemiology of Musculoskeletal Disorders*. New York: Oxford University Press.

Kendall, P.H. and Jenkins, J.M. (1968). Exercises for backache: a double blind controlled trial. *Physiotherapy*, **54**, 154–7.

Kishino, N.D., Mayer, T., Gatchel, R. *et al.* (1985). Quantification of lumbar function. Part 4: Isometric and isokinetic lifting simulation in normal subjects and low back dysfunction patients. *Spine*, **10**, 921–7.

Klausen, K., Anderson, L. and Bell, I. (1981). Adaptive changes in work capacity, skeletal muscle capillarisation and enzyme levels during training and detraining. *Acta Physiol. Scand.*, **113**, 9–16.

Kok, G. (1988). Health motivation, health education from a social psychological point of view. In *Topics in Health Psychology* (S. Mass *et al.*, eds), New York: Wiley Press.

Krolner, B. and Toft, B. (1983). Vertebral bone loss: an unheeded side-effect of therapeutic bed rest. *Clin. Sci.*, **64**, 537–40.

Kucera, M. (1986). Back pain and skeletal conditions during intensive training in children and adolescents. In *Children and Exercise, XII*, (J. Rutenfranz, R. Mocellin and F. Klimt, eds), pp. 329–36, Illinois: Human Kinetics Publishers.

Lane, N.E., Bloch, D.A., Jones, H.H. *et al.*, (1985). Long distance running, bone density and osteoarthritis. *J. Am. Med. Assoc.*, **255**, 1147–51.

Lidstrom, A. and Zachrisson, M. (1970). Physical therapy on low back pain and sciatica. *Scand. J. Rehabil. Med.*, **2**, 37.

Lindström, I., Öhlund, C., Eek, C. *et al.*, (1992). The effect of graded activity on patients with subacute low back pain: a randomised prospective clinical study with an operant-conditioning behavioural approach. *Phys. Ther.*, **72**, 279–90.

Lorig, K. (1991). *Commonsense Patient Education*. Melbourne, Australia: Fraser Publications.

Lorig, K., Konkol, L. and Gonzalez, V. (1987). Arthritis patient education: a review of the literature. *Patient Educ. Counsell.*, **10**, 207–52.

MacDougall, J.D., Elder, G., Sale, D. *et al.*, (1980). Effects of strength training and immobilisation on lumbar muscle fibres. *Eur. J. App. Physiol.*, **43**, 25–34.

Máčková, J., Máček, M., Vávra, J. *et al.*, (1986). Relationships among some muscle functions, aerobic power and age during childhood and adolescence in Czechoslovakian children. In *Children and Exercise XII* (J. Rutenfranz, R. Mocellin and F. Klimt, eds), pp. 321–7, Illinois: Human Kinetics Publishers.

Maitland, G.D. (1986): *Vertebral Manipulation* (5th edn). London: Butterworths.

Margaria, R., Aghemo, P. and Rovelli, E. (1965). Indirect determination of maximal O_2 consumption in man. *J. Appl. Physiol.*, **20**, 1070–3.

Mayer, T.G. and Smith, S. (1985). Quantification of lumbar function. Part 2: sagittal plane trunk strength in chronic low back pain patients. *Spine*, **10**, 765–72.

Mayer, T.G., Smith, S., Kondraske, G. *et al.*, (1985). Quantification of lumbar function. Part 3: Preliminary data on isokinetic torso rotation testing with myoelectric spectral analysis in normal and low back pain patients. *Spine*, **10**, 912–20.

Mayer, T., Tabor, J., Bovasso, E., and Gatchel, R.J. (1994). Physical progress and residual impairment quantification after functional restoration. Part 1: lumbar mobility. *Spine*, **19**, 389–94.

McArdle, W., Katch, F.I. and Katch, V.L. (1986). *Exercise Physiology*. Philadelphia: Lea and Febiger.

McNeill, T., Warwick, D., Anderson, G. and Schultz, A. (1980). Trunk strengths in attempted flexion, extension and lateral bending in healthy subjects and patients with low back disorders. *Spine*, **5**, 529–37.

Meenan, R.F., Yelin, E.H. and Nevitt, M. (1981). The impact of chronic disease: a sociomedical profile of rheumatoid arthritis. *Arthritis Rheum.*, **24**, 544–9.

Mellin, G., Härkäpää, K., Vanharanta, H. *et al.*, (1993). Outcome of a multimodal treatment including intensive physical training of patients with chronic low back pain. *Spine*, **18**, 825–9.

Minor, M. (1991). Physical activity and management of arthritis. *Ann. Behav. Med.*, **13**, 117–24.

Minor, M.A., Hewett, J.E., Webel, R.R. *et al.*, (1988). Exercise tolerance and disease related measures in patients with rheumatoid and osteoarthritis. *Int. J. Rheumatol.*, **15**, 905–11.

Minor, M.A., Hewett, J.E., Webel, R.R. *et al.*, (1989). Efficacy of physical conditioning exercise in patients with rheumatoid arthritis and osteoarthritis. *Arthritis Rheum.*, **32**, 1396–405.

Nachemson, A.L. (1982). The natural course of low back pain. In *American Academy of Orthopaedic Surgeons Symposium on Idiopathic Low Back Pain* (A.A. White III, and S. Gordon, eds), pp. 46–51, St. Louis: C.V. Mosby.

Nordemar, R. (1981). Physical training in rheumatoid arthritis: a controlled long term study, II – functional capacity and general attitudes. *Scand. J. Rheumatol.*, **10**, 25–30.

Nordemar, R., Ekblom, B., Zachrisson, L. and Lundqvist, K. (1981). Physical training in rheumatoid arthritis: a controlled long-term study I. *Scand. J. Rheumatol.*, **10**, 17–23.

Nouwen, A., Van Akkerveeken, P. and Versloot, J. (1987).

Patterns of muscular activity during movement in patients with chronic low back pain. *Spine*, **12**, 777–82.

O'Leary, A. (1985). Self-efficacy and health. *Behav. Res. Ther.*, **23**, 437–51.

Patrick, D.L., Peach, H. and Gregg, I. (1982). Disablement and care: a comparison of patient views and general practitioner knowledge. *J. R. Coll. Gen. Pract.*, **32**, 429–34.

Perlman, S.G., Connell, K.J., Clark, A. *et al.*, (1990). Dance-based aerobic exercise for rheumatoid arthritis. *Arthritis Care Res.*, **3**, 29–35.

Pocock, N.A., Eisman, J.A., Yeates, M.G. *et al.*, (1986). Physical fitness is a major determinant of femoral neck and lumbar spine bone mineral density. *J. Clin. Invest.*, **78**, 618–21.

Prince, R.L., Smith, M., Dick, I.M. *et al.*, (1991). Prevention for post menopausal osteoporosis. A comparative study of exercise, calcium supplementation and HRT. *N. Engl. J. Med.*, **325**, 1189–95.

Ransford, A.O., Cairns, D. and Mooney, V. (1976). The pain drawing as an aid to the psychological examination of patients with low back pain. *Spine*, **1**, 127–34.

Rasmussen, J.O. and Hansen, T.M. (1989). Physical training for patients with ankylosing spondylitis. *Arthritis Care Res.*, **2**, 25–7.

Rikli, R. and Busch, S. (1986). Motor performance of women as a function of age and physical activity level. *J. Gerontol.*, **41**, 645–9.

Roland, M. and Morris, R. (1983). A study of the natural history of back pain. Part 1 development of a reliable and sensitive measure of disability in low-back pain. *Spine*, **8**, 141–4.

Rosensteil, A.K. and Keefe, F.J. (1983). The use of coping strategies in chronic low back pain. Relationships to patient characteristics and current adjustments. *Pain*, **17**, 33–44.

Rowell, L.B. (1986). *Human Circulation Regulation during Physical Stress*. New York: Oxford University Press.

Sale, D.G. (1988). Neural adaptation to resistance training. *Med. Sci. Sports Exerc.*, **20**, S135–S145.

Salter, R.B. (1989). The biologic concept of continuous passive motion of synovial joints. *Clin. Orthop. Relat. Res.*, **242**, 12–25.

Saltin, B. and Rowell, L. (1980). Functional adaptations to physical activity and inactivity. *Fed. Proc.*, **39**, 1506–16.

Saltin, B., Blomqvist, G., Mitchell, J.H. *et al.*, (1968). Response to exercise after bed rest and after training. *Circulation*, **38**, Suppl. VII, VII–1–VII–78.

Sambrook, P. (1993). Keynote Address to the Regional Osteoporosis Co-ordinators Workshop held May 7, at Arthritis Foundation NSW.

Sambrook, P. and Eisman, J. (1987). Osteoporosis, The Australian Perspective. *Mod. Med. Austr.*, **30**, 14–27.

Sargeant, A.J., Davies, C.T. and Edwards, R.H. (1977). Functional and structural changes after disuse of human muscle. *Clin. Sci. Mol. Med.*, **52**, 337–42.

Sayce, V. and Fraser, I. (1991). *Exercise Beats Arthritis*, pp. 78–80. Victoria, Australia: Fraser Publications.

Schiable, T. and Scheuer, J. (1985). Cardiac adaptations to chronic exercise. *Prog. Cardiovasc. Dis.*, **27**, 297–324.

Sluijs, E.M. and Knibbe, J.J. (1991). Patient compliance with exercise: different theoretical approaches to short-term and long-term compliance. *Patient Educ. Counsell.*, **17**, 191–204.

Snook, S.H., Campanelli, R.A. and Hart, J.W. (1978). A study of three approaches to low back injury. *J. Occup. Med.*, **20**, 478–81.

Snow-Harter, C. and Marcus, R. (1991). Exercise, bone mineral density and osteoporosis. *Exerc. Sport Sci. Rev.*, **19**, 351–88.

Sonstroem, R.J. (1984). Exercise and self esteem. *Exerc. Sport Sci. Rev.*, **12**, 123–55.

Spratt, K.F., Lehmann, T.R., Weinstein, J.N. and Sayre, H.A. (1990). A new approach to the low-back physical examination – behavioural assessment of mechanical signs. *Spine*, **15**, 96–102.

Swain, L.T. (1930). Arthritis. *Physiother. Rev.*, **10**, 308–10.

Troup, J., Martin, J. and Lloyd, D. (1981). Back pain in industry: a prospective survey. *Spine*, **6**, 61–9.

Twomey, L. (1993). Physical activity and ageing bones. *Patient Manag.*, **17**, 31–4.

Twomey, L.T. and Taylor, J.R. (1987). *Physical Therapy of the Low Back*. New York: Churchill Livingstone.

Valkenburg, H. and Haanen, H. (1982). The epidemiology of low back pain. In *American Academy of Orthopaedic Surgeons Symposium on Low Back Pain* (A. White and S. Gordon, eds), pp. 9–22, St Louis, C. V. Mosby.

Vogel, J.M. and Whittle, M.L. (1976). Bone mineral changes: the second manned skylab mission. *Aviat. Space Environ. Med.*, **47**, 396–400.

Waddell, G. (1987). A new clinical model for the treatment of low back pain. *Spine*, **12**, 632–44.

Waddell, G., Somerville, D., Henderson, I. and Newton, M. (1992). Objective clinical evaluation of physical impairment in chronic low back pain. *Spine*, **17**, 617–28.

Weber, H. (1978). Lumbar disc herniation. Part 1. *J. Oslo City Hosp.*, **28**, 89.

Whedon, G.D. (1984). Disuse osteoporosis: physiological aspects. *Calcifi. Tissue Int.*, **36**, (Suppl.), 146–50.

White, J.A., Wright, V. and Hudson, A.M. (1993). Relationship between habitual physical activity and osteoarthritis in ageing women. *Public Health*, **107**, 459–70.

World Health Organization (1980). *International Classification of Impairments, Disabilities and Handicaps*, Geneva.

Williams, L. (1994). Hydrotherapy. *Arthritis Today*, 4:1 (March–May), pp. 2–3, Perth: Arthritis Foundation of WA.

Yelin, E., Lubeck, D. and Holman, H. (1987). The impact of rheumatoid arthritis and osteoarthritis: the activities of patients with rheumatoid arthritis and osteoarthritis compared to controls. *J. Rheumatol.*, **14**, 71–716.

Yelin, E., Meenan, R., Nevitt, M. and Epstein, W. (1980). Work, disability in rheumatoid arthritis: effects of disease, social and work factors. *Ann. Intern. Med.*, 551–6.

Zvaflier, N.J., Bennett, C.B. and Hess, E.V. (1988). *Rheumatoid Arthritis in Primer on the Rheumatic Diseases*. (H.R. Schumacher, ed.) (9th edn), pp. 48–51, Atlanta, Georgia: Arthritis Foundation.

Index